# Exam Review and Study Guide for Perinatal/Pediatric Respiratory Care

**Robert Harwood, MSA, RRT**

Assistant Professor
Department of Cardiopulmonary Care Sciences
College of Health and Human Sciences
Georgia State University
Atlanta, Georgia

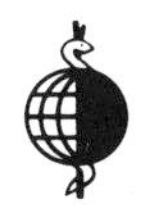

**F. A. DAVIS COMPANY • Philadelphia**

F. A. Davis Company
1915 Arch Street
Philadelphia, PA 19103



Printed in the United States of America

Last digit indicates print number: 10 9 8 7 6 5 4 3 2 1

*Publisher, Health Professions:* Jean-François Vilain
*Senior Editor:* Lynn Borders Caldwell
*Developmental Editor:* Marianne Fithian
*Production Editor:* Stephen D. Johnson
*Cover Designer:* Alicia R. Baronsky

*I dedicate this book to my wife, Kris, and daughters Jessica and Lauren for their constant love and support.*

# Preface

This exam review and study guide has been written with three goals in mind. The first goal is to provide a general review of perinatal/pediatric respiratory care for students and practitioners preparing for the perinatal/pediatric specialty examination offered by the National Board for Respiratory Care (NBRC). Many respiratory care departments require therapists to pass this examination in order to practice in these specialized areas. The second goal of this book is to serve as a reference guide for students taking a neonate/pediatric course. The third goal is to provide a reference book for respiratory care practitioners who are being cross-trained from adult care to perinatal/pediatric care.

Managed care has required respiratory care practitioners to become multiskilled in order to meet the demands of the respiratory care department. This exam review and study guide will provide entry-level knowledge for therapists to meet this challenge and give those who are educating practitioners an organized and concise plan to help meet the department goals.

In general the exam review and study guide will:

- Assist the student and practitioner to identify strengths and weaknesses in knowledge of perinatal/pediatric respiratory care
- Acquaint the student and practitioner with the format of the questions on the examination
- Help the student and practitioner set priorities for study time
- Provide the student with the reference lists from which further study can be pursued
- Provide the practitioner with a general review of the practice of perinatal/pediatric respiratory care
- Assist those practitioners being cross-trained or returning to the profession with basic knowledge in perinatal/pediatric respiratory care.

This exam review and study guide will not:

- Replicate the examination or any questions on the examination
- Offer a student a guarantee of passing the examination.

This exam review and study guide is divided into 16 chapters. Chapter 1 contains the NBRC Detailed Content Outline and information about test preparation and test-taking skills. A 120-question pretest with answers precedes Chapter 1. Before moving on to the other chapters, take the pretest as a way of determining your strengths and weaknesses.

Each chapter is written in outline form using the NBRC Detailed Content Outline along with references to well-known textbooks, refereed journals, and websites. Chapter 2, Developmental Care of the Newborn, is the only chapter not specifically identified on the NBRC Detailed Content Outline. It is such an important aspect of care for newborns and infants that it must be placed at the beginning of the book. Although not a part of the examination now, I believe it will become a part of future examinations.

Following each chapter there are review questions. These questions are written in essay, true and false, fill in the blank, fill in the table, and matching formats. At the end of the study guide there is a 120-question post-test with answers and rationales for each answer. Take this examination after completing the book. These questions and rationales are developed from the information in the exam review and study guide and will offer the student a greater challenge than the pretest.

**Robert Harwood**

# Acknowledgments

I would like to express my sincere appreciation to all those who helped in developing this exam review and study guide: Lynn Borders Caldwell for bringing this idea to F. A. Davis and providing guidance, support, and many dinners along the way; Marianne Fithian at F. A. Davis for her guidance and suggestions and for seeing this project through to completion; and the following people who reviewed the manuscript proposal:

Walter C. Chop, MS, RRT
Program Director
Respiratory Therapy Department
Southern Maine Technical College
South Portland, Maine

Furman Cummings, MEd, RRT, CPFT
Coordinator
Respiratory Care Department
Florida A & M University/Tallahassee
Tallahassee, Florida

Tarilyn S. Dobey, MEd, RRT
Clinical Instructor
Respiratory Therapy Department
University of Missouri-Columbia
Columbia, Missouri

Thanks also to the following reviewers who reviewed the proposal and spent many hours critiquing each chapter and giving helpful suggestions:

James Joseph Bierl, MS, RRT
Associate Professor
Respiratory Care Department
Erie Community College
Buffalo, New York

Melanie Ciesielski, BS, RRT
Educator
Respiratory Care Program
Forsyth Technical Community College
Winston-Salem, North Carolina

R. Bruce Steinbach, BA, RRT
Chairman, Respiratory Care Department
Pitt Community College
Greenville, North Carolina

Margaret A. Swanson, MS, RRT
Professor of Health Occupations
Respiratory Care Program
Illinois Central College
Peoria, Illinois

To the outstanding faculty in the Cardiopulmonary Care Sciences Department at Georgia State University for their support and understanding over the last year. Last but not least to the respiratory care practitioners in the Atlanta area for their educational support and friendship.

**Robert Harwood**

# Contributors

Kris Harwood, RNC, IBCLC
Board Certified Lactation Consultant
NCC Certified in High Risk Neonates
Formerly, Dekalb Medical Center Neonatal Intensive Care Unit
Visiting Nurse Health Systems
Lactation Consultant and Case Manager
Atlanta, Georgia

Jenene Woods, MBA, OTR/L
Developmental Therapist
NIDCAP® Reliable
Dekalb Medical Center, Neonatal Intensive Care Unit
Decatur, Georgia

# Contents

# Pretest

1. The Dubowitz method for clinical assessment uses a standard scoring system that evaluates:

   a. The need for resuscitation

   b. Morbidity and mortality of the infant

   c. Motor response

   d. Gestational age

2. The normal respiratory rate of a normal full-term infant is:

   a. 15 to 20 breaths per minute

   b. 20 to 25 breaths per minute

   c. 30 to 60 breaths per minute

   d. 60 to 90 breaths per minute

3. It is noticed that while assessing vital signs on a newborn, the baby's chest sinks in while the abdomen rises. This type of breathing is called:

   a. Paradoxical

   b. Retractive

   c. Diaphragmatic

   d. Grunting

4. An umbilical artery catheter has been inserted for blood gas monitoring. A chest radiograph has been taken to confirm proper placement. Which of the following is the correct low position placement for this catheter?

   a. Above the diaphragm

   b. Below the diaphragm

   c. Between the ductus venosus and diaphragm

   d. Between the diaphragm and ductus arteriosus

5. A 35-week-gestational-age newborn has been brought from labor and delivery to the nursery because of respiratory distress. The respiratory rate is 75 breaths per minute; mild nasal flaring, substernal retractions, and mild acrocyanosis are noted. At this time, it would be appropriate to recommend which of the following:

   I. Measure saturation with pulse oximetry.

   II. Put in an oxygen environment.

   III. Intubate and apply CPAP.

   IV. Put the newborn in a warm environment.

a. I and II only

b. II and IV only

c. I, II, and IV only

d. I, II, III, and IV

6. The Apgar score taken at 5 min will determine:

a. Gestational age

b. The effectiveness of resuscitation attempts

c. Morbidity and mortality

d. Laboratory evaluations

7. Which of the following may affect the accuracy of a capillary blood gas?

I. Using the finger instead of the heel of the foot to obtain blood

II. Inadequate peripheral perfusion at the puncture site

III. Not warming the site for an adequate time

a. I only

b. II only

c. II and III only

d. I, II, and III

8. A 2500-gm newborn has been ordered for an oxygen hood at 35% oxygen. An appropriate flowrate for the oxygen hood would be:

a. 2 to 3 L/min

b. 4 to 5 L/min

c. 5 to 10 L/min

d. >15 L/min

9. When using an oxygen hood to provide supplemental oxygen to a newborn, it is important to:

I. Provide humidification to prevent mucosal drying.

II. Monitor the $FIO_2$ as close to the newborn as possible.

III. Ensure heated humidification.

a. I only

b. II only

c. II and III only

d. I, II, and III

10. Which of the following are effects of cooling in the newborn?

I. Apnea

II. Increased oxygen consumption

III. Hypoglycemia

IV. Jaundice

a. I and II only

b. II and III only

c. I, II, and III only

d. I, II, III, and IV

11. The Apgar scoring system does NOT assess which of the following signs?

a. Chest excursion

b. Respiratory effort

c. Heart rate

d. Reflex irritability

12. Which of the following are an infant's physiological reactions to excessive noise levels in the NICU?

I. Hypoxia

II. Increased blood pressure (BP)

III. Apnea

IV. Bradycardia

a. I and II only

b. III and IV only

c. I, III, and IV only

d. I, II, III, and IV

13. Acrocyanosis in a full-term newborn would be seen:

a. Around the lips

b. In the hands and feet

c. In the mucous membranes of the nose

d. Around the neck and ears

14. In the NICU, nonverbal signs of an infant's stress would include:

I. Yawning

II. Squirming

III. Hiccuping

IV. Hand on the face

a. II and III only

b. II, III, and IV only

c. I, II, and III only

d. I, II, III, and IV

15. To prevent heat loss by convection, it would be important to:

I. Warm therapeutic gases.

II. Avoid drafts.

III. Cover cold objects the infant touches.

a. I only

b. II only

c. II and III only

d. I, II, and III

16. Jaundice in the newborn is a result of:

a. High levels of hemoglobin

b. Prematurity

c. High serum bilirubin levels

d. Low $PaO_2$ levels

17. A 6-month-old infant has been admitted for an upper respiratory tract infection. It has been ordered that the infant receive oxygen at 40%. Which of the following would be the best device by which to achieve this $FIO_2$?

a. Head hood

b. Venturi mask

c. Oxygen tent

d. Partial rebreathing mask

18. Which of the following represent normal umbilical artery blood gases in the fetus?

| | pH | $PCO_2$ (mm Hg) | $PO_2$ (mm Hg) |
|---|---|---|---|
| a. | 7.32 | 38 | 27 |
| b. | 7.24 | 49 | 16 |
| c. | 7.35 | 35 | 40 |
| d. | 7.21 | 20 | 50 |

19. Which of the following is/are true when administering a small-volume nebulizer (SVN) treatment by hand bagging through an endotracheal tube?

I. Use the same $FIO_2$ to power the SVN as the ventilator.

II. Bagging rate should be the same as the ventilator rate.

III. Inspiratory bagging pressure should be the same as the ventilator inspiratory pressure.

a. I only

b. II only

c. I and III only

d. I, II, and III

20. What is OSHA's standard for acceptable sound level in the NICU?

a. 120 db

b. 100 db

c. 80 db

d. 60 db

21. What is the proper placement of a thermistor probe for the controller of a humidifier device to ensure the proper inspired temperature for a patient in an isolette receiving mechanical ventilation?

a. At the wye adaptor within the isolette

b. Proximal to the humidifier on the exhalation side outside the isolette

c. On the expiratory side of the patient's circuit inside the isolette

d. On the inspiratory side of the patient's circuit outside the isolette

22. Which of the following causes a right-to-left shunt to occur in the fetus?

   I. Foramen ovale

   II. Ductus venosus

   III. Ductus arteriosus

   a. I only

   b. II only

   c. I and III only

   d. I, II, and III

23. A patient receiving an $FIO_2$ of 0.30 via head hood has a transcutaneous $PO_2$ ($P_{TC}O_2$) electrode attached to the upper right chest area. The respiratory care practitioner notices that the $PO_2$ is steadily climbing from a previous stable value of 56 mm Hg. There have been no adjustments in the $FIO_2$ or changes in the infant's status. Which of the following is suggested to do at this time?

   a. Decrease the $FIO_2$ to 0.25.

   b. Recalibrate the low-point $P_{TC}O_2$ value.

   c. Obtain an arterial blood gas to correlate the $PO_2$.

   d. Ensure that the electrode is firmly attached to the skin.

24. A 4-hour-old newborn has a chest radiograph return. On inspection, the heart size appears large. After measurement, the transthoracic ratio is found to be 50%. This would indicate:

   a. A normal size heart

   b. A small chest

   c. An enlarged heart

   d. A congenital heart problem

25. A 40-week-gestational-age newborn is presented, and a 1-min Apgar score has been completed with the following results:

   Body appearance: pink, blue extremities
   Pulse: 148 beats/min
   Grimace: cough, sneeze
   Activity: some flexion of extremities
   Respirations: good crying with regular respirations

   Based on these assessments you should:

   a. Provide routine care and transfer the infant to the well-born nursery.

   b. Begin blow-by oxygen at 5 to 8 L/min.

   c. Begin PPV with 100% oxygen until extremities turn pink.

   d. Continue tactile stimulation, blow-by oxygen at 5 L/min, and transfer to NICU.

26. The normal heart rate of a newborn infant is:

   a. 80 to 100 beats/min

   b. 100 to 120 beats/min

   c. 120 to 170 beats/min

   d. 150 to 190 beats/min

27. Bradycardia in the newborn infant is a heart rate:

    a. Less than 140 beats/min

    b. Less than 120 beats/min

    c. Less than 100 beats/min

    d. Less than 160 beats/min

28. When changing the site of a $P_{TC}O_2/P_{TC}CO_2$ electrode, it is noticed that there is blistering of the site located beneath the electrode. The respiratory care practitioner should:

    a. Change the site more often.

    b. Reduce the temperature to 37°C.

    c. Apply ointment to the skin prior to placing the electrode on the infant.

    d. Discontinue the transcutaneous monitoring.

29. What size endotracheal tube would be required for a newborn infant weighing 1500 gm?

    a. 4.0

    b. 3.0

    c. 2.5

    d. 3.5

30. The appropriate depth of insertion for a 3.5-mm ID endotracheal tube should be at which cm mark?

    a. 7 to 8

    b. 6

    c. 9

    d. 10

31. It has been 45 min since extubating a 5-year-old. The child is receiving a cool aerosol with 28% oxygen. The child is now showing signs of mild retractions and mild stridor on inspiration. The $SpO_2$ is at 93%. Which of the following would you recommend at this time?

    a. Change to a heated aerosol.

    b. Increase the $FIO_2$ to 0.40.

    c. Administer racemic epinephrine with a small-volume nebulizer.

    d. Administer albuterol with an MDI and spacer device.

32. Which of the following is NOT measured by a pulmonary artery catheter?

    a. Cardiac output

    b. Pulmonary artery pressure

    c. Systemic vascular resistance

    d. Central venous pressure

33. For a newborn with PPHN, which of the following set of blood gases would have the greatest effect in helping to reduce pulmonary hypertension?

| **pH** | **$PaCO_2$ (mm Hg)** | **$PaO_2$ (mm Hg)** |
|---|---|---|
| a. 7.29 | 60 | 60 |
| b. 7.55 | 30 | 80 |
| c. 7.40 | 50 | 60 |
| d. 7.19 | 60 | 30 |

34. What size oral endotracheal tube would be appropriate for a 4-year-old child?

a. 4.0 mm ID

b. 4.5 mm ID

c. 5.0 mm ID

d. 5.5 mm ID

35. It is recommended that cuffed endotracheal tubes be used in children at what age?

a. 5 years

b. 7 years

c. 4 years

d. Greater than 8 years

36. What is the correct suction pressure used for an intubated newborn infant?

a. 120 to 130 mm Hg

b. 100 to 120 cm $H_2O$

c. 80 to 120 cm $H_2O$

d. < 100 mm Hg

37. Indications for bag and mask ventilation include:

I. Apnea

II. Acrocyanosis

III. Heart rate less than 100 beats/min

IV. $SpO_2$ < 92%

a. I and III only

b. II and III only

c. I, III, and IV only

d. I, II, III, and IV

38. Which of the following may be the cause of meconium staining in a newborn at birth?

I. Intrauterine hypoxia

II. Reduction in lung fluid

III. Gestational age less than 32 weeks

a. I only

b. II only

c. III only

d. I, II, and III

39. In order to prevent aspiration of meconium by a newborn delivered by vaginal birth, the respiratory therapist should recommend to first:

    a. Suction the mouth and upper airway.

    b. Deliver the newborn and resuscitate with bag and mask.

    c. Suction the stomach with a nasogastric tube.

    d. Intubate and then resuscitate with bag and 100% oxygen.

40. What would you tell the parents of a 3-month-old infant with BPD on mechanical ventilation who have asked you when their child will be ready to be discharged from the hospital?

    I. When the infant's oxygen requirement is stable for 1 week and the infant is able to receive this concentration at home

    II. When the infant's weight gain is stable and the infant is on a specific diet

    III. When the parents have been educated in the care of the infant and knowledge of the equipment

    IV. When the infant is no longer on mechanical ventilation

    a. I and II only

    b. II and III only

    c. I, II, and III only

    d. I, II, III, and IV

41. A ball-valve mechanism developed in the lung of a severely meconium stained newborn will cause which radiologic change?

    a. Enlarged heart

    b. Pleural effusion and pneumopericardium

    c. Hyperinflation

    d. Elevated diaphragm

42. It is suspected that an infant is developing a pneumothorax, so a transillumination is performed. The transillumination is unable to detect the potential pneumothorax. What should be recommended next to determine the pathology?

    a. Needle biopsy

    b. Chest radiograph

    c. Continual observation for deterioration

    d. Insertion of a chest tube

43. A premature newborn is receiving mechanical ventilation when the newborn suddenly develops tachypnea and tachycardia, the BP drops from 45/35 to 30/20, and the infant desaturates to 82%. A transillumination shows a large pneumothorax in the right chest. It has been decided to insert a chest tube. Placement of the chest tube should be:

    a. Between the clavicle and 1st rib, midclavicular line

    b. Between the 2nd and 3rd intercostal rib, anterior aspect, midclavicular line

    c. In the 7th or 8th intercostal space, lateral aspect

    d. In the 8th or 9th intercostal space, lateral aspect

44. The following set of blood gases has been obtained from a newborn in respiratory distress receiving 100% oxygen on mechanical ventilation:

| | **Preductal** | **Postductal** |
|---|---|---|
| pH | 7.29 | 7.23 |
| $PaCO_2$ (mm Hg) | 51 torr | 59 torr |
| $PaO_2$ (mm Hg) | 65 torr | 30 torr |

These values would be indicative of:

a. Hypovolemia

b. Premature lungs

c. Ductal shunting

d. Cyanotic heart disease

45. Hyaline membrane formation is a result of:

a. Oxygen toxicity sloughing epithelial cells and forming a membrane on the surface of the alveoli

b. The pulmonary capillaries leaking fluid that contains fibrin-protein, which forms a membrane

c. Type II alveolar pneumocytes overproducing thick mucus, which forms a membrane

d. Degenerated macrophages lining the alveoli, which form membrane

46. A patient has a 4.0-mm oral endotracheal tube in place. What French suction catheter size would be used to suction this tube?

a. 8

b. 6

c. 7

d. 5

47. A 16-year-old has a peripheral arterial line placed in the right radial artery. Active bleed-back of arterial blood within an arterial line toward the transducer may be the result of:

a. Blood clot at the end of the arterial catheter

b. Dysfunctional fast-flush device

c. Not enough pressure in the pressurized bag

d. Three-way stopcock positioned off the patient

48. A right-to-left shunt may reverse to a left-to-right shunt at the ductus arteriosus as a result of:

I. Fluid administration raising the systemic blood pressure with a partially patent ductus arteriosus

II. Oxygenation causing a decrease in pulmonary vasculature resistance with a closed ductus arteriosus

III. Decrease in systemic blood pressure and increase in pulmonary vascular pressure with a closed ductus arteriosus

a. I only

b. II only

c. III only

d. II and III only

49. Bronchopulmonary dysplasia (BPD) develops in infants because of:

    I. The association with congenital heart disease

    II. Treatment with high oxygen concentrations

    III. Treatment with high ventilatory pressures

    IV. The infant being postmature

    a. I and II only

    b. II and III only

    c. III and IV only

    d. I, II, and III only

50. Which of the following is associated with an infant who has developed a pneumomediastinum?

    a. Cardiac tamponade

    b. Subcutaneous emphysema in the neck

    c. Shifting of the mediastinum to the affected area of air entrapment

    d. Loss of the thymus shadow on chest radiograph

51. The classic radiologic pattern of an infant with RDS is described as:

    a. Hyperlucent lung fields

    b. Bilateral white-out with increased pulmonary vascular markings

    c. Reticulogranular infiltrates or "ground-glass appearance"

    d. Spongelike appearance

52. Which of the following is correct when diagnosing an infant with BPD?

    a. The infant is on mechanical ventilation for more than 30 days with $SpO_2$ values in acceptable range.

    b. The infant is on PIP > 25 cm $H_2O$ and $FIO_2 > 0.50$ for greater than 1 month of age with $SpO_2$ values within acceptable range.

    c. The infant remains on oxygen > 28 days with $SpO_2$ values in an acceptable range following treatment of respiratory distress.

    d. The infant remains on oxygen at an $FIO_2$ of 0.40 or more for at least 2 months with $SpO_2$ values in acceptable range.

53. Which of the following hemodynamic changes is/are present in the pulmonary system of a newborn with persistent pulmonary hypertension?

    I. Systemic hypertension

    II. Increased pulmonary vascular resistance

    III. Increased pulmonary artery pressure

    IV. Underdeveloped left ventricle

    a. I only

    b. II and III only

    c. I and IV only

    d. I, II, and III only

54. Resolution of RDS (if no lung injury from mechanical ventilation) due to macrophages removing the hyaline membrane can occur within:

a. 10 h after onset

b. 24 to 36 h after onset

c. 48 to 72 h after onset

d. 5 to 7 days after onset

55. Which of the following ventilator adjustments would increase mean airway pressure for a patient on volume-targeted ventilation?

I. Increase tidal volume.

II. Decrease inspiratory flow rate.

III. Increase PEEP.

IV. Increase $FIO_2$.

a. I and III only

b. II, III, and IV only

c. I, II, and III only

d. I, II, III, and IV

56. The hyperoxia test performed on a newborn shows a $PaO_2$ of 150 torr. The diagnosis based on this test is:

I. Congenital heart disease

II. Persistent fetal circulation

III. Lung disease

a. I only

b. II only

c. III only

d. I and II only

57. A laboratory examination that is done to differentiate gram-positive bacteria from gram-negative bacteria is:

a. Gram stain

b. Cytologic

c. Acid-fast stain

d. Methylene blue stain

58. A 28-week premature infant has just been administered the appropriate amount of Exosurf. How long following this administration should suctioning be avoided?

a. 10 min

b. 30 min

c. 60 min

d. 2 h

59. The site that is used to determine a preductal $PaO_2$ would NOT include:

I. Right radial

II. Right brachial

III. Umbilical artery

a. I only

b. II only

c. III only

d. I and II only

60. Which of the following drugs would reduce pulmonary vascular resistance in a newborn with PPHN?

a. Sodium bicarbonate

b. Tolazoline

c. Prostaglandin $E_1$ inhibitor

d. Indomethacin

61. In general the age of a child who may not be able to use an MDI for treatment would be:

a. Less than 5 years

b. 6 to 7 years

c. 8 to 10 years

d. < 10 years

62. Respiratory care procedures requiring direct contact with bodily fluids require the use of which of the following?

I. Gown

II. Gloves

III. Eye protection

a. I only

b. II only

c. I and III only

d. I, II, and III

63. The most common complication following placement of a tracheostomy in a child in the first 24 h is:

a. Infection of the tracheostomy site

b. Bleeding from the tracheostomy site

c. Blocked airway

d. Scarring of the trachea

64. A 1400-gm newborn has been on mechanical ventilation for 2 days. Over the past day, the infant has had three chest tubes inserted into the right lung. The ventilator settings are increasing. A chest radiograph has returned with the following findings: "increased air trapping with large cyst formation throughout the right lung." Based on this radiographic finding, what would be the correct diagnosis for this infant?

a. Choanal atresia

b. Pulmonary interstitial emphysema

c. Meconium aspiration

d. Transient tachypnea

65. When administering nitric oxide, it would be important to monitor the level of NO, $NO_2$, and:

    a. Adult hemoglobin

    b. Cardiac output

    c. Methemoglobin

    d. Urine output

66. An 8-month-old infant is receiving ribavirin from a SPAG unit in line with a Servo 900C. It is noticed that the PEEP level has increased from 4 to 8 cm $H_2O$ over the last 2 h. Which of the following would be appropriate?

    a. Increase the flowrate from the SPAG unit.

    b. Reduce the driving pressure of the ventilator.

    c. Check the exhalation valve for proper function.

    d. Increase the ventilator inspiratory flowrate.

67. Which of the following is the best treatment for ventricular fibrillation?

    a. Administration of lidocaine

    b. Cardioversion at 100 J/s

    c. Defibrillation

    d. Administration of atropine

68. Upon entering a child's room, you notice that the child is slumped over the patient table. You would first:

    a. Open the airway.

    b. Call for help.

    c. Check for pulse.

    d. Establish unresponsiveness.

69. Prior to going to a patient's room to perform therapy, you read in the chart from the previous respiratory care practitioner that postural drainage and percussion was done with the patient lying on his abdomen, hips supported. Percussion was performed over the middle third of ribs on the right back. The area on which the therapy was performed would be the:

    a. Right lower lobe medial basal

    b. Right lower lobe superior segment

    c. Right lower lobe anterior segment

    d. Right lower lobe later segment

70. A heat moisture exchanger should NOT be used for infants where humidification is required for:

    a. 10 h or less

    b. 48 h or less

    c. 96 h or less

    d. 5 to 7 days

71. The nasal cannula of a newborn infant running at 1 L/min at an $FIO_2$ of 0.21 has been discontinued. Over the next 2 h, it is noticed that there are increased episodes of apnea and bradycardia. Which of the following should be recommended at this time?

a. Replace the nasal cannula at 21% and 1 L/min.

b. Replace the nasal cannula at 40% and 3 L/min.

c. Place the infant on CPAP of 10 cm $H_2O$.

d. Replace the nasal cannula at 2 L/min and at 40%.

72. A 41-week-gestational-age infant is being treated for meconium aspiration and is graded a (+) 1 meconium aspiration. Which of the following treatments would be appropriate for this infant?

a. Intubation and mechanical ventilation

b. Nasal prong CPAP at 4 to 6 cm $H_2O$ and $FIO_2$ of 1.0

c. High-frequency oscillation

d. Head hood with an $FIO_2$ of 0.30 to 0.40

73. Which of the following would exclude an infant from going home on mechanical ventilation?

a. $FIO_2$—0.28

b. PEEP—5 cm $H_2O$

c. PIP—20 cm $H_2O$

d. 4.0-mm ID endotracheal tube in place

74. The cuffless tracheostomy tube of an infant at home receiving mechanical ventilation should be changed:

a. Daily

b. Every second day

c. Weekly

d. Biweekly

75. Which of the following tests is most definitive to determine the presence of PPHN?

a. Hypoxia test

b. Hypercarbia test

c. Hyperoxia hyperventilation test

d. Pre-postductal shunting test

76. Which of the following multifactorial risk factors is/are implicated in the development of BPD?

I. Low gestational age (< 34 weeks)

II. Race (Caucasian)

III. Gender (males)

IV. Immature lungs from low birth weight (< 1500 gm)

a. I and IV only

b. II only

c. II, III, and IV only

d. I, II, III, and IV

77. An infant at home has been weaned from mechanical ventilation and is on heated aerosol receiving an $FIO_2$ of 0.21 going to a 5.0-mm, cuffless tracheostomy tube. The physician's orders state to wean the infant from the tracheostomy tube. Weaning from the tube should begin with which of the following?

    a. Replace the cuffless tracheostomy tube with a fenestrated tracheostomy tube one size larger.

    b. Replace the cuffless tracheostomy tube with a cuffed tracheostomy tube of the same size.

    c. Plug the cuffless tracheostomy tube every 2 h for 30 min and increase the time the tube is plugged.

    d. Replace the 5.0-mm cuffless tracheostomy with a 4.0-mm cuffless tracheostomy tube.

78. Which of the following is the major hemodynamic problem associated with a ventricular septal defect (VSD)?

    a. Right-to-left shunting across the ductus arteriosus

    b. Right-to-left shunting across the foramen ovale

    c. Left-to-right shunting across the ductus arteriosus

    d. Left-to-right shunt, blood directed into the right ventricle

79. Which of the following are common signs and symptoms of respiratory infection in the child?

    I. Fever

    II. Cough

    III. Vomiting

    IV. Dyspnea

    a. I and II only

    b. III and IV only

    c. II, III, and IV only

    d. I, II, III, and IV

80. A 10-year-old male is in the ED for acute exacerbation of asthma. His initial PEF upon admission is 130 L/min (personal best is 320 L/min). Over the next 3 h, he has received 12 puffs of albuterol MDI, oral theophylline, and prednisone, and he is on a 50% air entrainment mask. Following this, another PEF shows 125 L/min. A further examination reveals the patient to be tachypneic and febrile with the use of accessory muscles. At this time it should be suggested to:

    a. Admit to the hospital.

    b. Give two more puffs of albuterol, then discharge to home.

    c. Discharge to home.

    d. Intubate and mechanically ventilate.

81. Coarctation of the aorta occurs in the newborn:

    a. Between the pulmonary trunk and branching of pulmonary arteries

    b. In the arch of the aorta near the ductus arteriosus

    c. In the abdominal aorta

    d. At the area of the aortic valve as it leaves the left ventricle

82. The major hemodynamic effect associated with an atrial septal defect (ASD) is:

a. Right-to-left shunting across the ductus arteriosus

b. Hypoplasia of the pulmonary artery and reduced PAP

c. Stenosis of the aorta and an increase in afterload

d. Left-to-right shunting through the opening in the atrial septum

83. When an asthmatic patient is being discharged with MDI steroids, it would be important to tell the patient, in order to reduce the risk of oropharyngeal candidiasis, to:

I. Rinse the mouth following use of the MDI.

II. Actuate the MDI 2 to 3 in away from the open mouth.

III. Use a spacer device with the MDI.

IV. Following the MDI actuation, inhale in short, intermittent breaths.

a. I and II only

b. II and III only

c. I and III only

d. I, II, and IV only

84. Which of the following are major defects associated with tetralogy of Fallot?

I. Ventricular septal defect

II. Pulmonic infundibular stenosis

III. Aorta overriding the ventricular septum

IV. Right ventricular hypertrophy

a. I and II only

b. II and III only

c. III and IV only

d. I, II, III, and IV

85. A chest radiograph of the heart of an infant with tetralogy of Fallot may show a very distinguishable shape referred to as a(n):

a. "Snowman" appearance

b. "Boot-shaped" appearance

c. "Sail" appearance

d. "E" sign appearance

86. Care and treatment of a patient with bronchiolitis cultured with respiratory syncytial virus (RSV) with no previous history of respiratory disease and with mild symptoms includes:

I. Isolation

II. Mist tent with 30% to 40% oxygen

III. Bronchodilator therapy (with presence of wheezing)

IV. Handwashing

V. Administration of ribavirin

a. I, II, and IV only

b. I, II, IV, and V only

c. I, II, III, and IV only

d. I, II, III, IV, and V

87. It has been determined that a 14-year-old child on mechanical ventilation because of exacerbation of asthma has developed auto-PEEP. Which of the following maneuvers will help reduce auto-PEEP?

I. Increase expiratory time.

II. Decrease flowrate.

III. Administer bronchodilator therapy.

IV. Decrease delivered tidal volume.

a. I and II only

b. II and IV only

c. I, III, and IV only

d. I, II, III, and IV

88. The sweat chloride test is diagnostic for cystic fibrosis (CF) if:

a. NaCl level is 22 mEq/L or less

b. NaCl level is less than 28 mEq/L

c. NaCl level is 30 to 50 mEq/L

d. NaCl level is greater than 60 mEq/L

89. A term infant on oxygen and in severe respiratory distress has a chest radiograph return showing a distinguishable "egg-shaped" heart. This would indicate the infant to have:

a. Transposition of the great vessels

b. Patent ductus arteriosus

c. Ventricular septal defect

d. Tetralogy of Fallot

90. The common cause of upper airway obstruction is:

a. Secretions

b. Laryngospasm

c. Bronchospasm

d. Soft tissue

91. Which of the following would NOT be associated with a child who has epiglottitis?

I. Most common infectious agent is mycoplasma pneumonia.

II. Lateral neck radiograph shows enlarged supraglottic area.

III. Symptoms of distress occur within 7 to 8 h.

IV. High temperature

a. I only

b. II and III only

c. I and IV only

d. I, III, and IV only

92. The most common infectious agent of bronchiolitis in a 1-year-old infant is:

    a. Parainfluenza virus

    b. *Haemophilus influenzae type B*

    c. Respiratory syncytial virus

    d. Adenovirus

93. A 3-year-old has been admitted to the floor with a diagnosis of upper respiratory tract infection. You have been asked to assess the infant and return to the physician with your findings. It would be appropriate to first begin the examination by:

    a. Listening to breath sounds

    b. Assessing the extremities

    c. Obtaining a capillary blood gas

    d. Assessing the eyes, ears, nose, and throat

94. A positive expiratory pressure (PEP) device is used to provide which of the following?

    a. A PEEP effect to increase the $PaO_2$ levels

    b. A prolonged expiratory phase to prevent premature collapse of airways

    c. Greater deposition of aerosol particles when administered with a small volume nebulizer

    d. A cough when a pressure of > 10 cm $H_2O$ is used

95. Which of the following would NOT be a symptom of foreign body aspiration into the larynx?

    a. Aphonia

    b. Hoarseness

    c. Stridor

    d. Pain radiating to the sternum or back

96. In asthma, hyperresponsiveness and inflammation of the airways result from:

    I. Allergens

    II. Viral infections

    III. Pollution

    a. I only

    b. II and III only

    c. I and II only

    d. I, II, and III

97. A 7-year-old known asthmatic is presented to the ER with a 2-day history of wheezing and "cold" symptoms. Initial assessment reveals the following:

    Sensorium: alert
    Speech: halting
    Breath sounds: diminished
    PEF = 60% of predicted
    Heart rate: 148 beats/min
    Respiratory rate: 48 breaths per minute
    $SpO_2$: 85%

As the ED therapist, you would suggest doing which of the following FIRST?

a. Apply oxygen to keep $SpO_2$ >90%.

b. Administer inhaled corticosteroids.

c. Administer IV aminophylline.

d. Obtain ABGs.

98. The following information has been obtained from a patient after performing a respiratory physical assessment:

Inspection: Dyspneic
Palpation: Decreased fremitus on the right side
Percussion: Flatness on the right side
Auscultation: Absent breath sounds over the right lower lung area

The patient has which of the following based on these findings?

a. Pneumothorax

b. Consolidation

c. Atelectasis

d. Pleural effusion

99. Respiratory isolation requires which of the following?

I. Single room

II. Gloves to be worn upon entering the room

III. Mask to be worn upon entering the room

IV. Gown to be worn upon entering the room

a. I and III only

b. I, II, and III only

c. I, III, and IV only

d. I, II, III, and IV

100. A 12-year-old has the following laboratory data returned:

Sodium: 138 mEq/L
Chloride: 4.2 mEq/L
Calcium: 9.7 mg/dL
Potassium: 3.0 mEq/L

Based on this information this patient would have which of the following?

a. Hypernatremia

b. Hypochloremia

c. Hypercalcemia

d. Hypokalemia

101. A patient is receiving 3 L/min of oxygen from a nasal cannula attached to a liquid oxygen system. There is 60 lb of oxygen in the system. What is the duration of flow in days?

a. 3 days

b. 4 days

c. 5 days

d. 6 days

102. For which of the following age groups will a PEF measurement be unreliable?

a. Younger than 5 years of age

b. 6 to 8 years of age

c. 8 to 10 years of age

d. 10 to 12 years of age

103. Which of the following will have the greatest effect in reducing the spread of RSV between hospital personnel?

a. Gowning

b. Gloving

c. Wearing goggles

d. Hand washing

104. Which of the following is the best explanation of how to perform a PEF maneuver when instructing a 10-year-old?

a. "Breathe in normally, then exhale as fast as possible, and for as long as possible."

b. "Breathe in normally, then slowly exhale as long as possible."

c. "Take in a deep breath, then exhale as hard and fast as possible."

d. "Take in a deep breath, then exhale hard and as long as possible."

105. A chest radiograph has been returned on an infant in respiratory distress. The chest radiograph shows air-filled bowels in the thoracic cavity with a mediastinal shift away from the affected side. Based on the chest radiograph, the infant has:

a. Pulmonary interstitial emphysema

b. Diaphragmatic hernia

c. Pneumomediastinum

d. Pneumopericardium

106. Common symptoms and signs of epiglottitis include:

I. Distress

II. Drooling

III. Dyspnea

IV. Dysphagia

V. Diuresis

a. I and II only

b. II and III only

c. I, II, III, and IV only

d. I, II, III, IV, and V

107. Clinically, which of the following would be included in assessing the need for mechanical ventilation for the asthmatic?

I. Pulsus paradoxus

II. Exhaustion

III. $PaCO_2 > 55$ mm Hg and rising

IV. Fixed chest from hyperinflation

V. $PaO_2 < 60$ on $FIO_2 > 0.60$

a. I, II, and III only

b. II, IV, and V only

c. II, III, IV, and V only

d. I, II, III, IV, and V

108. Adjusting the flowrate from 4 to 8 L/min will do which of the following to the flow curve delivered by a pressure-limited, time-cycled ventilator?

a. Make it more sigmoidal shaped

b. Make it more linear shaped

c. Make it more square shaped

d. Make it sine wave shaped

109. A 2500-gm infant has been intubated, and CPAP of 4 cm $H_2O$, $FIO_2$ of 0.60 has been initiated as a result of the following ABGs:

pH: 7.31
$PaO_2$: 40 mm Hg
$PaCO_2$: 37 mm Hg

Over the next 2 h, CPAP has been adjusted with the following blood gas results:

| CPAP (cm $H_2O$) | 5 | 6 | 7 | 8 |
|---|---|---|---|---|
| pH | 7.33 | 7.36 | 7.28 | 7.24 |
| $PaCO_2$ (mm Hg) | 38 | 39 | 58 | 63 |
| $PaO_2$ (mm Hg) | 42 | 50 | 51 | 51 |

Given these values, which CPAP value would you recommend?

a. 5

b. 6

c. 7

d. 8

110. To affect the $PaCO_2$ of a patient receiving HFO, which of the following controls could be adjusted?

I. Amplitude

II. Rate

III. MAP

IV. PEEP

a. I only

b. III only

c. II and IV only

d. I and II only

111. A newborn is being ventilated with the following settings:

PIP: 17 cm $H_2O$
Flowrate: 10 L/min
Itime: 0.5 s
Etime: 1.5 s

Rate: 30 breaths per minute
$FIO_2$: 0.60

The physician has ordered 6 cm $H_2O$ PEEP. An ABG following this change shows the $PaO_2$ increased from 34 to 58 mm Hg and the $PaCO_2$ has increased from 49 to 60 mm Hg. Given this situation, what adjustment should be made to the ventilator settings?

a. Increase the $FIO_2$.

b. Reduce the flowrate.

c. Increase PIP.

d. Discontinue PEEP.

112. The following end-tidal $CO_2$ waveform has appeared on a child following intubation. The child is being ventilated with a resuscitation bag. Based on the end-tidal $CO_2$ waveform, which of the following is recommended?

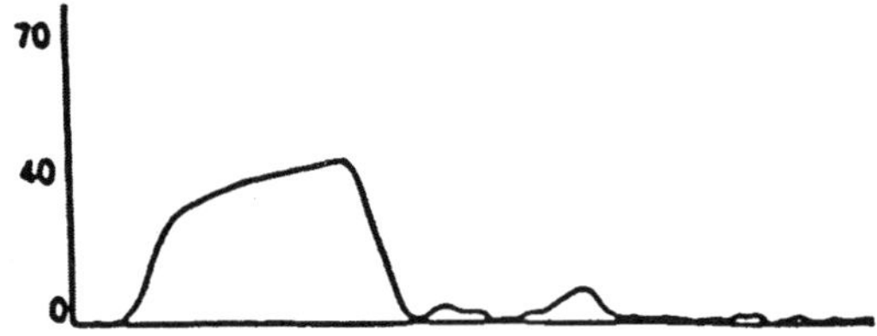


a. Increase the bagging rate.

b. Increase the $FIO_2$.

c. Reintubate the patient.

d. Increase the compression of the bag.

113. What is the mean arterial pressure when the systolic blood pressure is 96 mm Hg and the diastolic pressure is 54 mm Hg?

a. 60 mm Hg

b. 68 mm Hg

c. 75 mm Hg

d. 81 mm Hg

114. An infant on a pressure-limited, time-cycled ventilator has the volume-pressure loop shown in the accompanying figure. Which of the following ventilator changes is suggested at this time?

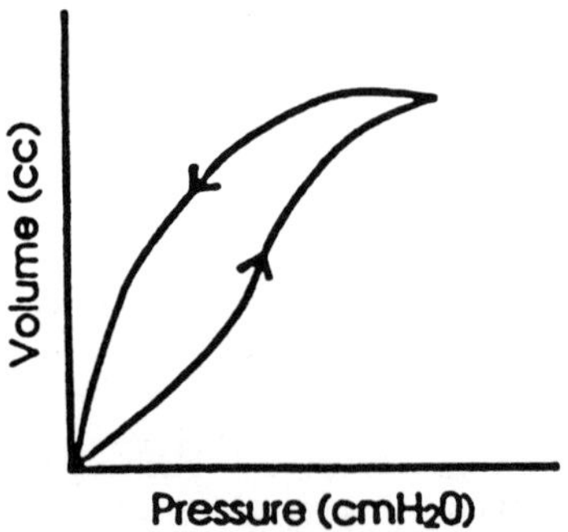

a. Decrease the PIP.

b. Decrease the tidal volume.

c. Increase PEEP.

d. Administer a bronchodilator.

115. A child intubated with a 6.0-mm ID cuffed endotracheal tube is on volume-targeted ventilation. A flow-volume loop is obtained and appears as in the accompanying figure.

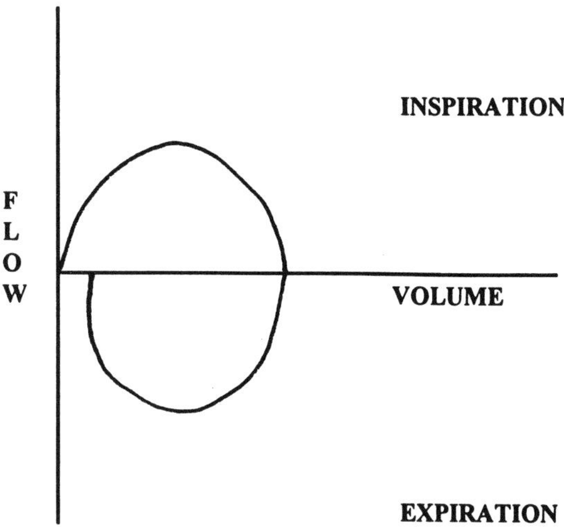


This flow-volume loop would indicate:

a. Excessive delivered tidal volume

b. Inadequate flowrate

c. Leakage around the endotracheal tube

d. Obstruction in the endotracheal tube

116. Excessive bubbling in the water-sealed chamber of a chest drainage system from a patient on mechanical ventilation would indicate:

a. A normally functioning water-sealed compartment

b. Excessive suction pressure

c. Leakage in the patient or the drainage system

d. Obstruction in the drainage tubing from the patient's chest tube

117. A pharmacological agent that is used to control the bleeding caused by removal of lung tissue for biopsy during flexible bronchoscopy is:

a. Lidocaine

b. Epinephrine

c. Fentanyl

d. Glycopyrrolate

118. A child has the following hemodynamic data obtained following insertion of a pulmonary artery catheter:

CVP: 5 mm Hg
PAP: 38/10 (19) mm Hg

PCWP: 7 mm Hg
CO: 6.0 L/min

What is the pulmonary vascular resistance?

a. 160 dyn/s/$cm^{-5}$

b. 200 dyn/s/$cm^{-5}$

c. 250 dyn/s/$cm^{-5}$

d. 275 dyn/s/$cm^{-5}$

119. A child has been diagnosed with bacterial infection and atelectasis in the right lower lung field. On chest radiograph, a right pleural effusion is seen. A thoracentesis is performed, and a cloudy, turbid fluid is withdrawn. This would indicate which type of pleural effusion fluid?

a. Hemothorax

b. Transudate

c. Hydrothorax

d. Exudate

120. Decannulation from venovenous extracorporeal membrane oxygenation (ECMO) is indicated when:

a. Chest radiograph shows improvement and oxygen saturation is stable.

b. Ventilator settings are PIP < 20 cm $H_2O$, rate < 10 breaths per minute, PEEP < 5 cm $H_2O$, and $FIO_2$ < 0.50.

c. The patient's oxygen index is 40 to 50.

d. The patient is permanently off ECMO.

## ANSWER KEY TO PRETEST

| | | | |
|---|---|---|---|
| 1. d | 31. c | 61. a | 91. a |
| 2. c | 32. c | 62. d | 92. c |
| 3. a | 33. b | 63. b | 93. b |
| 4. b | 34. c | 64. b | 94. b |
| 5. c | 35. d | 65. c | 95. d |
| 6. b | 36. d | 66. c | 96. d |
| 7. c | 37. a | 67. c | 97. a |
| 8. c | 38. a | 68. d | 98. d |
| 9. d | 39. a | 69. b | 99. a |
| 10. c | 40. c | 70. d | 100. d |
| 11. a | 41. c | 71. a | 101. c |
| 12. d | 42. b | 72. d | 102. a |
| 13. b | 43. b | 73. d | 103. d |
| 14. c | 44. c | 74. c | 104. c |
| 15. d | 45. b | 75. c | 105. b |
| 16. c | 46. a | 76. d | 106. c |
| 17. c | 47. c | 77. d | 107. d |
| 18. b | 48. a | 78. d | 108. c |
| 19. d | 49. b | 79. d | 109. b |
| 20. c | 50. b | 80. a | 110. d |
| 21. d | 51. c | 81. b | 111. c |
| 22. c | 52. c | 82. d | 112. c |
| 23. d | 53. b | 83. c | 113. b |
| 24. a | 54. d | 84. d | 114. a |
| 25. a | 55. c | 85. b | 115. c |
| 26. c | 56. c | 86. c | 116. c |
| 27. c | 57. a | 87. c | 117. b |
| 28. a | 58. d | 88. d | 118. a |
| 29. b | 59. c | 89. a | 119. d |
| 30. c | 60. b | 90. d | 120. d |

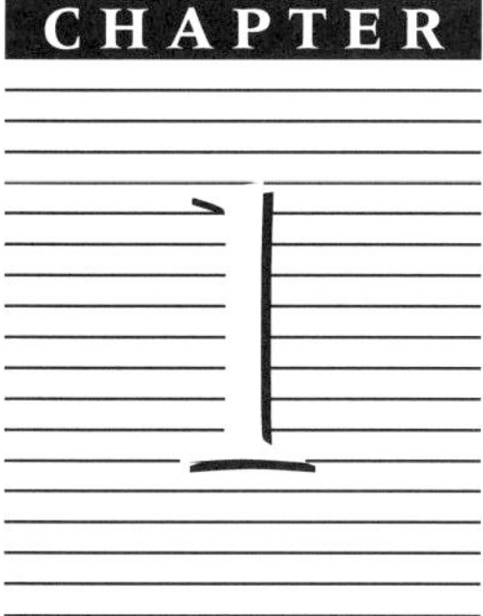

# Preparing for the Examination

## WHAT IS THE PERINATAL/ PEDIATRIC SPECIALTY EXAMINATION (PPSE)?

The roles of respiratory care practitioners expanded throughout the late 1970s and 1980s, with many practitioners specializing in perinatal/pediatric care. Because of this, the American Association for Respiratory Care (AARC) asked the National Board for Respiratory Care (NBRC) to implement a specialty examination for both certified respiratory therapy technicians (CRTTs) and registered respiratory therapists (RRTs). Over the next few years a viability study confirmed the need for such an examination. National research showed the need for greater numbers of respiratory care practitioners in perinatal/pediatric care. The first job analysis survey sent out to a wide professional population was directed at respiratory care practitioners in hospitals and educational institutions, including neonatologists and pediatricians. Based on these responses the NBRC has developed content specifications and examination questions. A second job analysis survey conducted in 1996 has resulted in a revision of the first examination. The test is administered annually in March with the entry-level examination. The cost of the examination is $180 for a new applicant and $150 for reapplication. The application deadline is November 1. To date, 5616 respiratory care practitioners have been credentialed by the NBRC.

## WHO CAN TAKE THE SPECIALTY EXAMINATION?

The NBRC oversees the certification examination and eligibility of candidates. Candidates must have graduated from an accredited or approved respiratory therapy program. Both CRTT-credentialed and RRT-credentialed practitioners are eligible to sit for the examination. Certified practitioners require 1 year of clinical experience (minimum of 10 hours per week for 1 calendar year) in perinatal/pediatric care under the supervision of a medical director of respiratory care or special care area acceptable to the board. Clinical experience must be completed by the last day of the month in which the test is administered. Registered practitioners are eligible for the examination following successful completion of the registry examination and do not require 1 year's experience. After applying for the test, the candidate is sent a handbook that contains a practice examination with answers, directions for taking the examination, and test-taking tips.

## WHAT IS THE FORMAT OF THE EXAMINATION?

Beginning in March 1998, the examination will have 120 multiple-choice questions, an increase of 20 questions from the first examination. Each question has four options. The increase in questions is the result of a job survey identifying therapists performing more tasks than indicated in the previous job analysis. The time limit for the examination has increased from 2 hours to 3 hours because of the increase in examination questions. The questions are developed from a detailed matrix that contains three content areas: clinical data, equipment, and therapeutic procedures. Each content area has a specific number of questions and three levels of complexity: recall, application, and analysis. The greatest number of questions have to do with applications, followed by analysis. The fewest number are recall questions. Table 1–1 shows the subcategories for each content area, the number of questions at each complexity level, and the total number of questions in each category. The complete, detailed PPSE is at the end of this chapter. The following questions are examples of the three levels of complexity.

### Recall Questions

Recall questions test the recall of isolated information. These questions require memory and include the recall of specific facts, concepts, principles, procedures, or theories.

TABLE 1–1. ***Perinatal/Pediatric Respiratory Care Specialty Examination Matrix***

| Content Area | Recall | Application | Analysis | Number of Items |
|---|---|---|---|---|
| I. Clinical data | 8 | 11 | 15 | 34 |
| A. Review existing data in the patient record | 3 | 5 | 0 | 8 |
| B. Collect and evaluate additional pertinent clinical information | 4 | 4 | 11 | 19 |
| C. Recommend procedures and modifications | 1 | 2 | 4 | 7 |
| II. Equipment | 3 | 9 | 4 | 16 |
| III. Therapeutic procedures | 14 | 34 | 22 | 70 |
| A. Maintain records and explain therapy | 2 | 3 | 0 | 5 |
| B. Conduct therapeutic procedures to maintain a patent airway and remove bronchopulmonary secretions | 1 | 3 | 2 | 6 |
| C. Conduct therapeutic procedures to achieve adequate ventilation and oxygenation | 1 | 4 | 5 | 10 |
| D. Evaluate patient's response to respiratory care | 2 | 7 | 2 | 11 |
| E. Recommend modifying the respiratory care plan based on the patient's response | 2 | 2 | 5 | 9 |
| F. Modify therapeutic procedures based on patient's response | 3 | 7 | 3 | 13 |
| G. Conduct techniques in an emergency setting and assist physician | 2 | 5 | 4 | 11 |
| H. Initiate and conduct pulmonary rehabilitation and home care | 1 | 3 | 1 | 5 |
| Total number | 25 | 54 | 41 | 120 |

(Adapted from *NBRC Horizons,* p 5, 1997.)

Which of the following is used to determine the need for resuscitation immediately following birth?

a. Dubowitz

b. Ballard

c. Apgar

d. Silverman

Answer c is correct.

## Application Questions

This type of question requires more than simple recall but less than problem solving. Application questions test the simple application of limited data.

A 2100-gm infant receiving mechanical ventilation has had numerous episodes of bradycardia and desaturation less than 90%. The respiratory care practitioner should FIRST do which of the following?

a. Suction the endotracheal tube.

b. Obtain an arterial blood gas.

c. Increase the rate on the ventilator.

d. Auscultate the chest.

The correct answer is d.

## Analysis Questions

Analysis questions test the evaluation of data for the solution of a specific problem. The questions often are based on a clinical report that requires the candidate to choose a therapeutic regimen or differential diagnosis. The candidate may have to make a value judgment concerning the effectiveness, appropriateness, or best course of action, given a specific situation.

An 1800-gm infant born 2 weeks earlier is on a pressure-limited, time-cycled ventilator with a PIP at 18 cm $H_2O$, rate of 23 bpm, $FIO_2$ of 0.50, and PEEP 4 cm $H_2O$. Arterial blood gas analysis shows pH 7.34, $PaCO_2$ 47 mm Hg, $PaO_2$ 66 mm Hg, and $SpO_2$ 97%. Based on the blood gas values, which of the following should be recommended?

a. Reduce PEEP.

b. Reduce $FIO_2$.

c. Increase the PIP.

d. Suggest no changes at this time.

Answer b is correct.

## WHAT HAPPENS AFTER THE EXAMINATION?

The testing agency will mail the results to you no later than 10 business days following the test. Test scores are reported as raw scores and scaled scores. The raw score is the number of questions answered correctly. The total scaled score is derived from the raw score, and it is used to determine passing or failing. The minimum passing scaled score is 75. From year to year, tests may change in difficulty as questions are replaced, but the scaled score remains 75. Candidates receiving a failing score may request, within 60 days of the examination results, a rescoring of the answer sheet submitted. A written request and a $15 fee are required. This is sent to the NBRC executive office. Following successful completion of the PPSE, you will receive a certificate recognizing the achievement and competence in the field of perinatal/pediatric respiratory care.

## TO WHOM DO I APPLY FOR THE EXAMINATION?

Applications may be obtained by writing or calling:

National Board for Respiratory Care, Inc.
Executive Office
8319 Nieman Road
Lenexa, KS 66214
(913) 599-4200
E-mail: nbrc-info@nbrc.org
WWW Home Page: http://www.nbrc.org

A study guide for the Perinatal/Pediatric Respiratory Care Specialty Examination will be sent that includes examination policies, examination preparation suggestions, test directions, a 120-question self-evaluation examination with answers, a scoring matrix, an evaluation of your performance on the self-evaluation examination, an application, and other information pertaining to the examination. With the application and fee, the applicant will need to include a 2 × 2 color photograph (passport size photograph) with the applicant's social security number written on the back of the photograph.

When mailing the application, the applicant should use certified mail or certificate of mailing and keep the receipt as proof that the application was sent to the NBRC. If the application is accepted by the admissions committee, the applicant will receive a letter of acceptance approximately 4 weeks after the application deadline. Then, 2 weeks before the examination, the applicant will receive an admission ticket to the test center chosen on the application. If the applicant does not receive this ticket within 6 weeks following the application deadline, he or she should call the NBRC. Tests are administered on Saturday and Sunday (religious preference). On test day, the applicant will need the admission ticket and a valid driver's license (no student ID or employment ID). Check-in is at 8:30 A.M. There is no further admittance to the examination room once the doors are closed.

## WHAT DOES THIS BOOK CONTAIN AND HOW DO I USE THIS BOOK?

This book begins with a chapter dealing with test preparation that includes information about the examination structure, content, number of questions, and examination matrix. Following this, test-taking tips will help the candidate with tools to identify his or her strengths and weaknesses as well as to organize and set priorities for study time. The test-taking tips are followed by a pretest with 120 multiple-choice questions with answers. The pretest questions have been developed in accordance with the PPSE detailed matrix. Following the pretest, there are 16 chapters that have been developed from the matrix as well as material that will enhance the applicant's knowledge in perinatal/pediatric respiratory care. Following each chapter are review questions that follow the content of each chapter. A complete bibliography is included with each chapter, including primary textbooks the reader is likely to own and information from the Internet. The Internet sites are easily located and contain an abundance of information that will assist the reader in preparation for this examination and other educational needs. At the end of this book, there is a post-test with 120 multiple-choice questions with answers and rationale for the answers.

Before taking the pretest, begin with preparation for the examination. In this chapter you will learn how to prepare yourself for the task of test taking. Preparing to take the examination can be overwhelming when you look at the "big picture." By breaking the process into smaller parts, it is easier to manage. The first step to work through is to identify your areas of strengths and weaknesses. A personal study plan will help you through this process. Go through each of the chapters in the book quickly to get an idea of your strengths and weaknesses with that subject matter. Next take the pretest and then correct the pretest. Review the pretest and write down the material that was covered in the questions that were answered incorrectly. Even those questions that you answered correctly but in which you felt unsure of the information should be included in this list. Categorize the content of the question so that it relates to the chapters in the book. Decide in what area of material you have the greatest weakness. For example, if your clinical practice is concerned primarily with neonatal medicine, you might find that pediatric medicine is your weak area. This would be a good starting point for studying based on your assessment of the pretest. Once this has been completed, the second step is to invest time completing the study plan (see Test-Taking Tips).

The final step is to pull all of the information together to take the final practice examination. Take this examination 1 week before the examination date. Go through all of the questions you answered incorrectly by referring to the rationale and going back into the chapter and reviewing this information.

## TEST-TAKING TIPS

### Tip 1: Create a Personal Study Plan

Now that priorities have been set for studying, the next activity is to write target dates for reviewing each area and subject. Based on your needs assessment, choose the material that has the highest priority or was labeled the greatest weakness. For example, an individual may choose to review pediatric assessment and pediatric diseases because these two areas were labeled the weakest. A typical week can be planned by using a calendar to schedule the topics to be covered and the dates when these topics are completed. Keep this separate from your other schedules by placing it in the area where you intend to study. Also include on this schedule the times you eat, sleep, work, and other activities so that you can develop a complete overview of your day-to-day schedule.

You will need to begin studying approximately 6 to 8 weeks before the examination date. Some individuals need more time, some less. Only you can gauge this time period. Give yourself adequate time to review all the subject matter, complete review questions, and pretests and post-tests. Do not begin studying so long before the examination that you will burn out. Intensive, organized study is the most efficient.

### Tip 2: Make Your Study Time Organized and Efficient

1. Do not study for longer than 1 hour without taking a break. Drill work involving rote memory is fatiguing. Take a break when you feel you need one.
2. Study the most difficult material during the time of day when you are most awake.
3. Apply the facts you learn. This is done by relating material learned in clinical situations. Discuss material with other practitioners and apply your knowledge to patient care.
4. Study similar subjects at separate times. Separate your study periods according to information with similar subject matter. For example, separate neonatal diseases and pediatric diseases according to whether invasive or noninvasive monitoring is required.
5. Memorize actively, not passively. The worst way to memorize is to read something over and over again. Use as many senses as possible. Try to visualize in concrete terms to develop a picture in your head. Talk out loud. Use association in learning materials by relating subject matter to clinical experience.
6. Consistent work habits aid in concentration. Study in the same place every day where there are minimal distractions. Keep only material you will need to study at the desk. Begin studying with a clear goal in mind and when you are going to complete it. Make an outline of what you are going to study, review questions you are going to complete, and preview questions you are going to review. After completing these goals, cross them off your list. This will give you the satisfaction of completing the goal and give you the confidence to continue.
7. There will be times when you cannot concentrate on the subject matter. Go on to another subject, sample tests, or review questions. Also, to get your mind off studying, close your eyes and relax for a few minutes and think of other things. You may find you are studying too much material or reading too quickly to get through the material. Slow down your reading and study smaller amounts of material. You may need to review and rewrite your goals to reflect this change.
8. Form a study group of two or three people and meet 1 day per week for no more than 2 hours.

### Tip 3: Be Prepared

The more prepared you are to take the examination, the more comfortable the examination will be. Preparation includes studying the knowledge base of respiratory care, getting a good night's sleep, and bringing the right tools to the examination. Once the studying is complete, the majority of the preparation is complete; however, the most important thing you can do to prepare yourself adequately is to get a good night's sleep. Plan to arrive at the test center 20 to 30 minutes before the examination so you can acclimate yourself to the environment. If you are unsure of your test site, plan a trip before the test day to become familiar with the area. If the drive is longer than 2 hours, you may want to stay overnight near the test site. This will help relieve test anxiety. Also bring two to three sharpened No. 2 pencils with good erasers with you on test day.

**Tip 4: Prepare Your Body as Well as Your Mind**

Eating a well-balanced breakfast can actually affect your performance on the examination. A breakfast high in carbohydrates and low in fat will increase your energy and not produce a sluggish feeling. Avoid caffeine because its ultimate effect will leave you tired and drowsy in the middle of the examination. Finally, wear comfortable clothes in layers to allow you to adjust as necessary to the temperature of the room.

**Tip 5: Pace Yourself**

You should bring a watch in case the examination site does not have a clock. Place the watch in front of you so you can keep track of your time. The test is to be completed within 3 hours. Within this time frame, 120 questions are to be completed. One technique for pacing the examination is to divide the test booklet into three equivalent sections by bending the corner of the page in the top right-hand corner. The goal should be to complete each of the three sections within 50 minutes to 1 hour. Remember, you will complete the first set of 40 questions faster than the second and third set. As you start to get tired, you will need more time with each question. After every page of questions, look at the clock and gauge your time.

**Tip 6: Be Test Smart**

1. Do not leave any answers blank. If you are unsure of the answer, take a guess and then make a notation next to the question in the test booklet. Return to it at the end of the examination.
2. Do not mark answers in the test booklet and transfer these answers to the score sheet when you have completed the examination. In so doing, you may place an answer in the wrong numbered question on the score sheet. Also, there may not be enough time to complete the transfer of answers from the test booklet to the score sheet.
3. Do not dwell on questions for a long period of time. Inevitably there will be questions for which you will not have a clue. Do not be disturbed by these questions; guess and move on.
4. Feel free to mark in the test booklet, circle or underline key phrases, and perform calculations next to the question. Do calculations mechanically, reciting the steps to yourself as you go. Remember, you cannot use a calculator during the examination.
5. When questions involve comparing values within the stem of the question, remove these values from the question and write them down next to the question in the test booklet. It will be easier to compare values when they are removed from nonessential information.
6. Read the question stem and options completely. Ask yourself, "What is this question about?" You can answer this by looking at the most important information and separating it from peripheral information. On completion, answer only what is there. Do not add anything or put certain qualifications on the statement.
7. Reread all questions containing negative wording such as "not" or "least."
8. Be cautious about changing your answer. Your first "guess" is more likely to be correct than are subsequent "guesses," so have a sound reason for changing your answer.
9. Do not be concerned with people leaving before you. Do not leave the test prematurely. You should plan to have time at the end of the examination to review questions and to check over your score sheet to ensure that all answers are correctly filled in. You may remember facts that will help answer questions you had guessed at earlier.

**Tip 7: When You Use the Same Letter for More Than Three Answers in a Row, Double-Check the Questions to Verify Each Answer**

Test writers usually break up strings of four or more of the same letter or answer. The multiple-choice format is usually set so that three of the same letters in a row are the maximum run of correct answers. If there are four or more of the same letters in a row, and if time allows, it may be beneficial to recheck the answers at the end of the examination.

### Tip 8: Mark Your Answers Clearly on the Score Sheet

Stray marks may invalidate answers. If the answer is too light, it may not be scanned appropriately by the scoring machine. If the answer is too big, it may be interpreted incorrectly as one of the adjacent letters. Before marking the score sheet, be sure the letter you are marking is the one you want.

## BIBLIOGRAPHY

Anderson, D., et al. (1997). *The Occupational Therapy Examination Review Guide.* Philadelphia: F. A. Davis.

Hoffman, G. (May/June 1997). Perinatal/pediatric specialty examination revised. *NBRC Horizons.*

National Board for Respiratory Care. (1997). *Study Guide, Perinatal/Pediatric Respiratory Care Specialty Examination.* Lenexa, Kansas: National Board for Respiratory Care, Inc.

National Board for Respiratory Care. (1985). *Item Writers Guide.* Lenexa, Kansas: National Board for Respiratory Care, Inc.

Quattlebaum, L. (1995). *Test-Taking Strategies* [WWW document]. URL http://c.edu/depts/ucc/testtake.html

*Test Taking Skills* [WWW document]. (1997). URL http://abel.richland.cc.il.us/~kpde;;/testtake.html

Wrenn, C. G., and Larsen, R. P. (1992). *Studying Effectively.* Stanford: Stanford University Press.

Zalaquett, C. (1997). *Test Taking Strategies* [WWW document]. URL http://www.shsu.edu/~counsel/test_taking.html

## NBRC Perinatal/Pediatric Respiratory Care Specialty Examination Detailed Content Outline

| | TOTAL | RECALL | APPLICATION | ANALYSIS |
|---|---|---|---|---|
| **I. SELECT, REVIEW, OBTAIN AND INTERPRET DATA** **SETTING:** In any perinatal/pediatric patient care setting, the Specialist reviews existing clinical data, collects additional clinical data and recommends obtaining additional pertinent data. The Specialist interprets all data to determine the appropriateness of the prescribed respiratory care, and participates in developing the respiratory care plan. | 34 | 8 | 11 | 15 |
| **A. Review Existing Data in the Patient Record** | 8 | 3 | 5 | 0 |
| 1. Maternal history: | | | | |
| a. prenatal [e.g., para, gravida] | | | | X[1] |
| b. medical [e.g., eclampsia, preeclampsia, diabetes, renal failure] | | | | X |
| c. family [e.g., congenital and genetic disorders] | | | | X |
| d. social [e.g., substance abuse] | | | | X |
| 2. Antenatal and intrapartum (labor and delivery) history: | | | | |
| a. maternal bleeding | | | | X |
| b. intrauterine stress testing | | | | X |
| c. amniocentesis results [e.g., L/S ratio] | | | | X |
| d. placental problems [e.g., placenta previa, placental abruption] | | | | X |
| e. premature and/or prolonged ruptured membranes | | | | X |
| f. results of fetal monitoring | | | | X |
| g. anesthesia and analgesia | | | | X |
| h. medications [e.g., corticosteroid, tocolytic, magnesium sulfate] | | | | X |
| i. presentation and type of delivery | | | | X |
| j. presence and character of meconium | | | | X |
| 3. Admission and current respiratory care orders | | | | X |
| 4. Patient history, physical examination, current vital signs, progress notes | | | | X |
| 5. Neonatal assessment [e.g., gestational age, birth weight, physical findings, Apgar scores, breathing pattern] | | | | X |
| 6. Hematologic and/or chemistry studies | | | | X |
| 7. Serologic studies [e.g., Rh, ABO, HIV] | | | | X |
| 8. Pulmonary function values and blood gas results | | | | X |
| 9. Results of respiratory monitoring: | | | | |
| a. noninvasive monitoring data [e.g., pulse oximetry, capnography, transcutaneous] | | | | X |
| b. ventilatory data [e.g., PIP, $P\overline{aw}$, minute ventilation, I:E ratio, PEEP] | | | | X |
| c. pulmonary mechanics [e.g., MIP, PEF, compliance and resistance] | | | | X |
| d. radiographs [e.g., chest, upper airway and abdominal] | | | | X |
| e. noninvasive hemodynamic monitoring [e.g., ECG, blood pressure] | | | | X |
| f. invasive hemodynamic monitoring [e.g., shunt studies ($\dot{Q}s/\dot{Q}t$), $S\bar{v}O_2$, pressure measurements, cardiac output] | | | | X |
| g. neurologic monitoring [e.g., intracranial pressure, EEG, $CO_2$ response] | | | | X |
| 10. Sweat test results | | | | X |
| 11. Culture/sensitivity and Gram stain results [e.g., urine, blood, sputum, CSF] | | | | X |
| 12. Amount and character of pleural drainage | | | | X |
| **B. Collect and Evaluate Additional Pertinent Clinical Information** | 19 | 4 | 4 | 11 |
| 1. Assess patient's overall status by *inspection* to determine: | | | | |
| a. general appearance: | | | | |
| 1) muscle wasting | | | | |
| 2) peripheral edema | | | | |
| 3) flushing and diaphoresis | | | | |
| 4) pattern of cyanosis | | | | |
| 5) dysmorphia | | | | |
| 6) activity level | | | | |
| 7) abdominal configuration | | | | |
| b. respiratory status: | | | | |
| 1) respiratory rate and pattern | | | | |
| 2) chest configuration and movement | | | | X |

| | TOTAL | RECALL | APPLICATION | ANALYSIS |
|---|---|---|---|---|
| 3) accessory muscle activity | | | | X |
| 4) diaphragmatic movement | | | | X |
| 5) intercostal and sternal retractions | | | | X |
| 6) nasal flaring and expiratory grunting | | | | X |
| 7) cough effort | | | | X |
| 8) amount and character of sputum | | | | |
| c. cardiac status: | | | | |
| 1) venous distention | | | | X |
| 2) digital clubbing | | | | X |
| 3) capillary refill | | | | |
| 4) precordial activity | | | | X |
| 2. Assess patient's overall status by *palpation* to determine: | | | | |
| a. pulse rate, rhythm and force | | | | |
| b. asymmetrical chest movements | | | | X |
| c. tactile fremitus, palpable rhonchi, crepitation, tenderness | | | | X |
| 3. Assess patient's overall status by *percussion* to determine: | | | | |
| a. diaphragmatic excursion | | | | X |
| b. areas of altered resonance | | | | X |
| 4. Assess patient's overall status by *auscultation* to determine: | | | | |
| a. respiratory function: | | | | |
| 1) breath sounds [e.g., normal, adventitious, pleural rub] | | | | X |
| 2) upper airway sounds [e.g., stridor] | | | | X |
| b. cardiac function [e.g., heart sounds, blood pressure, murmurs] | | | | X |
| 5. Interview patient and/or family to determine: | | | | |
| a. level of consciousness and orientation to time, place and person | | | | X |
| b. emotional state and ability to cooperate | | | | X |
| c. presence of dyspnea and orthopnea | | | | X |
| d. sputum production, exercise tolerance, activities of daily living | | | | X |
| e. physical environment, social support systems, nutritional status | | | | X |
| 6. Visually inspect radiographs to determine: | | | | |
| a. position of endotracheal or tracheostomy tube | | | | |
| b. position of chest tube or nasogastric tube | | | | |

| | TOTAL | RECALL | APPLICATION | ANALYSIS |
|---|---|---|---|---|
| c. presence and position of foreign bodies | | | | |
| d. position of, or changes in, hemidiaphragms | | | | |
| e. estimation of lung volumes | | | | |
| 7. Visually inspect radiographs to determine presence of, or changes in: | | | | |
| a. air bronchogram | | | | X |
| b. pneumothorax or subcutaneous emphysema | | | | X |
| c. consolidation and atelectasis | | | | X |
| d. pulmonary interstitial emphysema | | | | X |
| e. pneumopericardium and pneumomediastinum | | | | X |
| f. hyperinflation | | | | |
| g. pleural fluid | | | | X |
| h. pulmonary edema/opacification | | | | X |
| i. pulmonary artery catheter, pacemaker, CVP, umbilical artery catheter | | | | X |
| j. mediastinal shift | | | | |
| k. swollen epiglottis and subglottic narrowing | | | | |
| 8. Visually inspect radiographs to determine findings consistent with: | | | | |
| a. bronchopulmonary dysplasia | | | | X |
| b. diaphragmatic hernia | | | | X |
| c. Respiratory Distress Syndrome | | | | X |
| d. cardiac anomalies | | | | X |
| e. abdominal abnormalities | | | | X |
| 9. Perform and/or interpret results of general procedures: | | | | |
| a. vital signs and blood pressure | | | | X |
| b. gestational age assessment | | | | X |
| c. Apgar scoring | | | | |
| d. intake and output | | | | X |
| e. glucose level | | | | X |
| 10. Perform and/or interpret results of respiratory monitoring/evaluation: | | | | |
| a. noninvasive monitoring data [e.g., pulse oximetry ($SpO_2$), capnography, transcutaneous ($TcPO_2$, $TcPCO_2$)] | | | | |
| b. ventilatory data [e.g., PIP, $P\overline{aw}$, minute ventilation, I:E ratio, PEEP] | | | | |
| c. pulmonary mechanics [e.g., MIP, PEF, compliance, resistance, airway] | | | | |
| d. spirometry | | | | |
| e. bronchoscopy | | | | |
| f. transillumination | | | | X |

| | TOTAL | RECALL | APPLICATION | ANALYSIS |
|---|---|---|---|---|
| g. oxygenation [e.g., $PaO_2/P_AO_2$, $P(A\text{-}a)O_2$, oxygen index] | | | | |
| h. blood gas analysis and co-oximetry | | | | |
| i. thoracentesis | | | | X |
| j. tracheal tube cuff pressure | | | | X |
| k. polysomnograms and pneumograms | | | | |
| 11. Perform and/or interpret cardiac monitoring: | | | | |
| a. ECG | | | | |
| b. shunt studies ($\dot{Q}s/\dot{Q}t$) | | | | |
| c. inserting arterial, umbilical and central monitoring catheters | | | | |
| d. invasive pressure measurements [e.g., CVP, PAP, PCWP, arterial pressure] | | | | |
| e. cardiac output | | | | |
| f. blood pressure by Doppler | | | | |
| g. mixed venous sampling | | | | |
| h. pre- and postductal oxygenation studies | | | | |
| **C. Recommend Procedures and Modifications** | 7 | 1 | 2 | 4 |
| 1. Recommend procedures to obtain additional data: | | | | |
| a. noninvasive monitoring data [e.g., pulse oximetry, capnography, transcutaneous] | | | | |
| b. ventilatory data [e.g., PIP, $\overline{Paw}$, minute ventilation, I:E ratio, PEEP] | | | | |
| c. pulmonary mechanics [e.g., MIP, PEF, compliance, resistance, airway graphics] | | | | |
| d. pulmonary function studies [e.g., bronchoprovocation, spirometry] | | | | |

| | TOTAL | RECALL | APPLICATION | ANALYSIS |
|---|---|---|---|---|
| e. transillumination | | | | |
| f. oxygenation data [e.g., $PaO_2/P_AO_2$, $P(A\text{-}a)O_2$, oxygen index] | | | | |
| g. blood gas analysis and co-oximetry | | | | |
| h. cardiac monitoring: | | | | |
| 1) ECG | | | | X |
| 2) inserting arterial, umbilical and central monitoring catheters | | | | X |
| 3) echocardiography | | | | X |
| 4) invasive pressure measurements [e.g., CVP, PAP, PCWP, arterial pressure] | | | | X |
| 5) cardiac output | | | | X |
| i. mixed venous sampling | | | | |
| j. hematologic and/or chemistry studies | | | | X |
| k. evaluation for infection: | | | | |
| 1) culture/sensitivity and Gram stain [e.g., urine, blood, sputum, CSF] | | | | |
| 2) nasal swab/washing for RSV | | | | X |
| l. chest and upper airway radiographs | | | | |
| 2. Determine appropriateness of the respiratory care plan and recommend modifications where indicated: | | | | |
| a. analyze available data to determine pathophysiological state | | | | |
| b. review planned therapy to establish therapeutic goals | | | | |
| c. determine appropriateness of prescribed therapy and goals for identified pathophysiological state | | | | |

| | TOTAL | RECALL | APPLICATION | ANALYSIS |
|---|---|---|---|---|
| **II. SELECT, ASSEMBLE, CHECK, IDENTIFY AND CORRECT MALFUNCTIONS OF EQUIPMENT**<br>**SETTING:** In any perinatal/pediatric patient care setting, the Specialist selects, assembles and checks all equipment used to provide respiratory care, as well as identifies and corrects malfunctioning equipment. | **16** | **3** | **9** | **4** |
| 1. Select, assemble, check and identify/correct malfunctions of equipment | | | | |
| a. oxygen administration devices: | | | | |
| 1) oxygen hoods | | | | X |
| 2) CPAP mask | | | | X |
| 3) nasal CPAP device | | | | X |
| 4) bilevel positive airway pressure device | | | | |
| 5) low-flow devices [e.g., nasal cannula] | | | | X |
| 6) high-flow devices [e.g., air entrainment mask] | | | | X |
| b. humidifiers: | | | | |
| 1) water-based [e.g., bubble, passover, cascade, wick] | | | | X |
| 2) heat moisture exchangers | | | | X |
| c. aerosol generators: | | | | |
| 1) pneumatic nebulizer | | | | X |
| 2) small particle aerosol generator (SPAG) | | | | X |
| d. resuscitation devices: | | | | |
| 1) flow-inflating resuscitator | | | | X |
| 2) self-inflating resuscitator | | | | X |
| e. ventilators: | | | | |
| 1) pneumatic | | | | X |
| 2) electric/microprocessor | | | | X |
| 3) external negative pressure | | | | X |
| 4) high frequency ventilators [e.g., jet, oscillator, flow interrupter] | | | | |
| f. extracorporeal membrane oxygenation (ECMO) system | | | | X |
| g. artificial airways: | | | | |
| 1) oro- and nasopharyngeal airways | | | | X |
| 2) oral and nasal endotracheal tubes | | | | X |
| 3) tracheostomy tubes and buttons | | | | X |
| 4) tracheal speaking devices | | | | X |
| h. intubation equipment – laryngoscope and blades | | | | X |
| i. suctioning devices: | | | | |
| 1) catheters, bulb, meconium aspirators, specimen collectors | | | | X |
| 2) oropharyngeal suction devices (tonsil tip) | | | X | X |
| j. gas delivery, metering and clinical analyzing devices: | | | | |
| 1) low-flow flowmeters | | | X | X |
| 2) air and oxygen proportioners (blenders) | | | | X |
| 3) capnograph | | | | |
| 4) blood gas analyzer and co-oximeter | | | | |
| 5) transcutaneous monitor | | | | |
| 6) pulse oximeter | | | | X |
| k. patient breathing circuits: | | | | |
| 1) continuous mechanical ventilation | | | | X |
| 2) CPAP | | | | X |
| l. environmental devices: | | | | |
| 1) incubators | | | | X |
| 2) aerosol (mist) tents | | | | X |
| 3) heat shield, radiant warmers | | | | X |
| m. hemodynamic monitoring devices: | | | | |
| 1) cardiac leads | | | | X |
| 2) arterial pressure system | | | | |
| 3) central venous catheters | | | | |
| 4) pulmonary artery catheter | | | | |
| 5) cardiac output | | | | X |
| n. pleural drainage devices | | | | X |
| o. apnea monitors | | | | X |
| p. impedance and inductive pneumographs | | | | X |
| q. incentive breathing devices | | | | X |
| r. therapeutic gas measuring devices [e.g., $CO_2$, $He\text{-}O_2$, $N_2$] | | | | |
| s. volume measuring devices [e.g., pneumotachometer] | | | | X |
| 2. Perform quality control and calibration procedures for the following devices: | | | | |
| a. blood gas analyzers | | | | X |
| b. pulmonary function equipment | | | | X |
| c. gas metering devices | | | | X |
| d. hemodynamic monitoring devices | | | | X |

| | TOTAL | RECALL | APPLICATION | ANALYSIS |
|---|---|---|---|---|
| **III. INITIATE, CONDUCT AND MODIFY PRESCRIBED THERAPEUTIC PROCEDURES** **SETTING:** In any perinatal/pediatric patient care setting, the Specialist maintains records and communicates relevant information to other members of the healthcare team. The Specialist also initiates, conducts and modifies prescribed therapeutic procedures to achieve one or more specific objectives. | **70** | **14** | **34** | **22** |
| **A. Maintain Records and Explain Therapy** | 5 | 2 | 3 | 0 |
| 1. Maintain records, record therapy and results using conventional terminology as required by hospital policy and regulatory agencies: | | | | |
| a. specify therapy administered, including date, time, frequency of the medication, and ventilatory data | | | | X |
| b. note and interpret patient's response to therapy: | | | | |
| 1) subjective response to therapy | | | | X |
| 2) vital signs and blood pressure | | | | X |
| 3) auscultatory findings | | | | X |
| 4) cough and sputum production and characteristics | | | | X |
| 5) adverse reactions | | | | X |
| c. verify computations and identify erroneous data | | | | X |
| 2. Communicate information regarding patient's clinical status to: | | | | |
| a. appropriate members of the healthcare team | | | | X |
| b. those responsible for coordinating patient care [e.g., scheduling, avoiding conflicts, sequencing of therapies] | | | | X |
| 3. Explain therapy and protect patient from infections, namely: | | | | |
| a. explain planned therapy and goals to pediatric patient or family in nontechnical, understandable terms to achieve therapeutic outcome | | | | X |
| b. protect patient from nosocomial infection by adherence to infection control policies and procedures | | | | X |

| | TOTAL | RECALL | APPLICATION | ANALYSIS |
|---|---|---|---|---|
| **B. Conduct Therapeutic Procedures to Maintain a Patent Airway and Remove Bronchopulmonary Secretions** | 6 | 1 | 3 | 2 |
| 1. Maintain a patent airway: | | | | |
| a. position patient properly | | | | X |
| b. insert appropriate oro- and nasopharyngeal airways | | | | X |
| c. select appropriate endotracheal tubes | | | | X |
| d. perform endotracheal intubation | | | | |
| e. maintain: | | | | |
| 1) adequate humidification | | | | X |
| 2) proper cuff inflation and position of endotracheal and tracheostomy tubes | | | | |
| f. change tracheostomy tubes | | | | |
| g. extubate the patient | | | | |
| 2. Remove bronchopulmonary secretions: | | | | |
| a. instruct pediatric patients and parents to encourage proper coughing techniques | | | | X |
| b. perform: | | | | |
| 1) postural drainage, percussion and vibration | | | | X |
| 2) nasotracheal or orotracheal suctioning | | | | X |
| 3) alternative airway clearance techniques [e.g., PEP, Flutter® device, Intrapulmonary Percussive Ventilation (IPV®), external percussive devices, autogenic drainage] | | | | X |
| c. suction endotracheal and tracheostomy tubes | | | | X |
| d. administer prescribed agents [e.g., bronchodilators, saline, mucolytics, antibiotics] | | | | X |
| **C. Conduct Therapeutic Procedures to Achieve Adequate Ventilation and Oxygenation** | 10 | 1 | 4 | 5 |
| 1. Achieve adequate spontaneous and artificial ventilation: | | | | |
| a. instruct pediatric patients in proper breathing technique and encourage deep breathing | | | | X |
| b. administer: | | | | |
| 1) bronchodilators | | | | X |
| 2) corticosteroids | | | | |
| 3) ribavirin (Virazole) | | | | X |
| 4) exogenous surfactant | | | | X |
| 5) mucolytics | | | | X |
| 6) proteolytics | | | | X |
| 7) antibiotics | | | | X |

| | TOTAL | RECALL | APPLICATION | ANALYSIS |
|---|---|---|---|---|
| c. select appropriate mechanical ventilation parameters: | | | | |
| 1) tidal volume, rate, minute ventilation | | | | |
| 2) inspiratory pressure, I:E ratio, flow, flow pattern | | | | |
| d. initiate and adjust continuous mechanical ventilation when: | | | | |
| 1) no settings are specified | | | | |
| 2) settings are specified | | | | |
| e. initiate and adjust: | | | | |
| 1) IMV/SIMV and assist-control | | | | |
| 2) pressure support ventilation | | | | |
| 3) bilevel positive airway pressure | | | | |
| 4) settings for high frequency ventilation | | | | |
| f. modify weaning procedures | | | | |
| 2. Achieve adequate arterial and tissue oxygenation: | | | | |
| a. position patient to minimize hypoxemia | | | | X |
| b. administer oxygen (on or off ventilator) | | | | X |
| c. prevent procedure associated hypoxemia [e.g., oxygenate before and after suctioning and equipment changes] | | | | X |
| d. initiate and adjust: | | | | |
| 1) CPAP | | | | |
| 2) peak inspiratory pressure, inspiratory time, tidal volume, I:E ratio, $P\overline{aw}$, PEEP | | | | |
| **D. Evaluate Patient's Response to Respiratory Care** | 11 | 2 | 7 | 2 |
| 1. Adjust and check alarm systems | | | | X |
| 2. Calculate and interpret: | | | | |
| a. $\dot{Q}s/\dot{Q}t$ | | | | |
| b. cardiac output and index | | | | |
| c. pulmonary and systemic vascular resistance | | | | |
| d. $P(A\text{-}a)O_2$, $PaO_2/P_AO_2$, oxygen index | | | | |
| e. compliance values | | | | |
| 3. Determine vital capacity and perform spirometry | | | | X |
| 4. Inspect and auscultate chest and record findings | | | | X |
| 5. Interpret: | | | | |
| a. results of blood gases | | | | |
| b. results of pre- and postductal oxygenation | | | | |
| c. changes in servo pressure during jet ventilation | | | | |

| | TOTAL | RECALL | APPLICATION | ANALYSIS |
|---|---|---|---|---|
| 6. Measure: | | | | |
| a. peak expiratory flow | | | | X |
| b. central venous pressure, pulmonary artery pressures, wedge pressure, cardiac output | | | | X |
| 7. Measure and record vital signs and blood pressure | | | | X |
| 8. Monitor: | | | | |
| a. mean airway pressure | | | | X |
| b. cardiac rhythm | | | | X |
| 9. Monitor and interpret mixed-venous oxygenation studies | | | | |
| 10. Note: | | | | |
| a. patient's subjective response to therapy | | | | X |
| b. patient's responses to mechanical ventilation | | | | X |
| 11. Obtain blood gas sample from indwelling catheters | | | | X |
| 12. Perform: | | | | |
| a. arterial and capillary punctures | | | | X |
| b. transcutaneous gas monitoring and pulse oximetry | | | | X |
| c. capnography | | | | X |
| 13. Recommend and review upper airway and chest radiographs | | | | |
| **E. Recommend Modifying the Respiratory Care Plan Based on the Patient's Response** | 9 | 2 | 2 | 5 |
| 1. Initiate or adjust: | | | | |
| a. ventilator settings [e.g., PIP, inspiratory time, PEEP, rate, tidal volume, I:E ratio, flow, flow waveform, pressure support, $P\overline{aw}$, $F_IO_2$] | | | | |
| b. high frequency ventilator settings [e.g., amplitude, rate, inspiratory time %, $P\overline{aw}$] | | | | |
| 2. Adjust: | | | | |
| a. $F_IO_2$ and oxygen flow | | | | |
| b. ventilatory mode or type of ventilator | | | | |
| c. inspiratory effort (sensitivity) setting | | | | |
| d. weaning, or changing weaning procedures | | | | |
| e. aerosol drug dosage or concentration | | | | |
| f. duration of therapy | | | | |
| g. patient's position | | | | |
| 3. Discontinue any treatment based on patient's response | | | | |

| | TOTAL | RECALL | APPLICATION | ANALYSIS |
|---|---|---|---|---|
| 4. Insert: | | | | |
| a. arterial and umbilical catheters | | | | X |
| b. chest tube | | | | X |
| 5. Institute bronchopulmonary drainage procedures | | | | X |
| 6. Intubate or extubate | | | | |
| 7. Use or change artificial airways (endotracheal tube or tracheostomy) | | | | |
| 8. Use radiant warmer or incubator | | | | X |
| 9. Use pharmacologic agents: | | | | |
| a. sedatives and neuromuscular blockers | | | | |
| b. oral and parenteral bronchodilators, corticosteroids, cromolyn sodium | | | | |
| c. vasoconstrictors, vasodilators | | | | |
| d. antibiotics | | | | |
| e. narcotic antagonists | | | | |
| f. antiviral agents | | | | |
| g. mucolytics and proteolytics | | | | |
| h. exogenous surfactants | | | | |
| **F. Modify Therapeutic Procedures Based on Patient's Response** | 13 | 3 | 7 | 3 |
| 1. Terminate treatment based on patient's adverse reaction to therapy | | | | |
| 2. Modify therapeutic modalities: | | | | |
| a. incentive breathing devices | | | | X |
| b. aerosol therapy: | | | | |
| 1) change type of equipment | | | | X |
| 2) change dilution of medication | | | | |
| c. temperature of inspired gas | | | | X |
| d. patient breathing patterns | | | | X |
| e. aerosol output | | | | X |
| f. oxygen therapy: | | | | |
| 1) change mode of administration | | | | |
| 2) adjust flow | | | | |
| 3) adjust $F_IO_2$ | | | | |
| g. other gas therapy [e.g., $He$-$O_2$, $CO_2$-$O_2$, $N_2$]: | | | | |
| 1) change mode of administration | | | | |
| 2) adjust flow | | | | |
| 3) adjust gas concentration | | | | |
| h. chest physiotherapy (bronchopulmonary drainage): | | | | |
| 1) change position of patient | | | | X |
| 2) alter duration of treatment | | | | X |
| 3) change equipment used | | | | X |
| 4) alter techniques | | | | X |
| 3. Coordinate sequence of therapies with other care | | | | |
| 4. Manage artificial airways: | | | | |
| a. change: | | | | |
| 1) type of humidification equipment | | | | X |
| 2) endotracheal or tracheostomy tube | | | | |
| 3) endotracheal or tracheostomy tube position | | | | X |
| b. suction patient's airway: | | | | |
| 1) initiate suctioning | | | | X |
| 2) change size and type of catheter | | | | X |
| 3) alter negative pressure | | | | X |
| 4) instill irrigating solutions | | | | X |
| 5) alter frequency of suctioning | | | | X |
| 6) alter duration of suctioning | | | | X |
| 5. Change: | | | | |
| a. continuous mechanical ventilation | | | | |
| b. patient breathing circuitry | | | | X |
| c. weaning procedures | | | | |
| d. type of ventilator | | | | |
| 6. Adjust: | | | | |
| a. ventilator settings [e.g., PIP, inspiratory time, PEEP, rate, tidal volume, I:E ratio, flow, flow waveform, $\overline{Paw}$, $F_IO_2$] | | | | |
| b. ventilator alarm settings | | | | |
| 7. Initiate airway graphic monitoring | | | | X |
| **G. Conduct Techniques in an Emergency Setting and Assist Physician** | 11 | 2 | 5 | 4 |
| 1. Initiate, conduct or modify respiratory therapy techniques in an emergency setting, including transport and delivery room: | | | | |
| a. recognize the need for emergency resuscitation | | | | X |
| b. call for help | | | X | X |
| c. establish patent airway | | | | X |
| d. check breathing | | | | X |
| e. use mouth-to-valve or bag-mask ventilation | | | | X |
| f. check pulse and observe chest excursion | | | | X |
| g. perform: | | | | |
| 1) external cardiac compression | | | | X |
| 2) defibrillation | | | | X |
| 3) endotracheal intubation | | | | X |
| 4) transillumination | | | | X |
| h. initiate/interpret ECG monitoring | | | | |

| | TOTAL | RECALL | APPLICATION | ANALYSIS |
|---|---|---|---|---|
| i. insert: | | | | |
| 1) arterial catheter | | | | X |
| 2) umbilical catheter | | | | X |
| j. insert and/or reposition nasogastric tube | | | | X |
| k. recommend: | | | | |
| 1) volume expanders | | | | |
| 2) defibrillation | | | | |
| 3) chest and upper airway radiographs | | | | |
| l. recommend and/or instill medication through endotracheal tube | | | | |
| m. recommend administering: | | | | |
| 1) cardiac stimulants | | | | |
| 2) sedatives, muscle relaxants, anticonvulsants | | | | |
| 3) bicarbonate | | | | |
| n. administer: | | | | |
| 1) bicarbonate | | | | X |
| 2) exogenous surfactant | | | | X |
| 3) cardiac drugs [e.g., epinephrine, atropine] | | | | X |
| o. obtain arterial or capillary blood gas sample | | | | X |
| p. provide supplemental oxygen | | | | X |
| q. relieve tension pneumothorax | | | | |
| 2. Act as an assistant to physician performing special procedures, including: | | | | |
| a. bronchoscopy | | | | |
| b. thoracentesis | | | | X |
| c. percutaneous needle biopsies of the lung | | | | X |
| d. transtracheal aspiration | | | | X |
| e. tracheostomy | | | | |
| f. chest tube insertion | | | | |
| g. noninvasive diagnostic testing [e.g., echocardiography, EEG] | | | | X |
| h. catheter insertion for invasive monitoring [e.g., central venous pressure, pulmonary and arterial catheter] | | | | |
| i. bronchial lavage | | | | X |
| j. polysomnograms and pneumograms | | | | |
| k. cardioversion | | | | X |
| l. cannulation/decannulation for extracorporeal membrane oxygenation (ECMO) | | | | |
| **H. Initiate and Conduct Pulmonary Rehabilitation and Home Care** | 5 | 1 | 3 | 1 |
| 1. Survey and recommend home environment modifications to assure optimal therapeutic goals, safety and infection control | | | | |
| 2. Evaluate patient's progress | | | | |
| 3. Explain goals and instruct patient and family in planned therapy | | | | X |
| 4. Evaluate patient's and family's understanding of therapeutic goals and procedures | | | | |
| 5. Monitor and maintain home respiratory care equipment | | | | X |
| 6. Select ventilator for home use | | | | |
| 7. Provide instructions for: | | | | |
| a. CPR procedures | | | | X |
| b. self-inflating resuscitation bag | | | | X |
| c. ventilator use in the home | | | | X |
| d. tracheostomy care in the home | | | | X |
| e. using apnea monitors | | | | X |
| f. oxygen, aerosol and bronchopulmonary hygiene procedures | | | | X |
| g. infection control | | | | X |
| **Totals** | **120** | **25** | **54** | **41** |

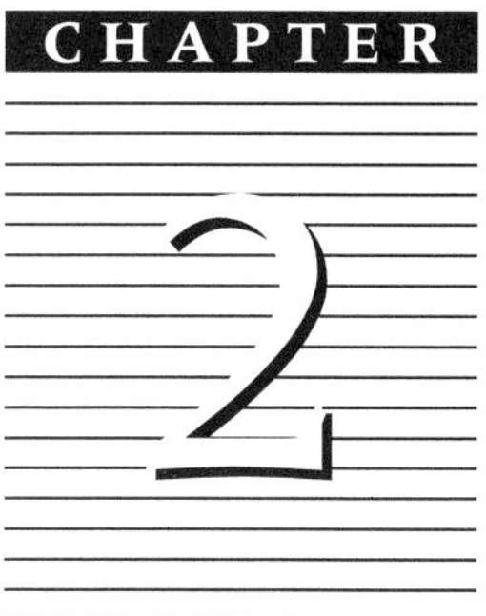

# Developmental Care of the Newborn

## I. History

A. Developmental care is a concept initiated by Dr. Heidelise Als in the early 1970s. As a result of her research and observations, subsequent studies have been conducted that continue to validate her findings. This has influenced the type of care that is delivered in neonatal intensive care units (NICUs) across the country.

B. Traditionally, the intensive care nursery setting has been very high tech and high touch. The developmental care approach embraces a very individualized approach based on the infant's "signals" and behaviors. High-risk infants, especially premature infants, require careful protection from the often harsh environment of the NICU. The health care team needs to be acutely aware of stress and behavior cues from these infants.

## II. Goals and purpose

A. The goal in providing developmentally supportive care is to facilitate not just survival, but also the optimal development of both the physical and the neurological systems. Quality of life for the patient as well as the families involved can be impacted by how these babies are cared for. By providing expert intensive care within a framework of individualized developmental care, outcomes are improved medically as well as neurodevelopmentally.

B. The purpose is to protect the developing brain by mimicking the uterine environment.

1. Interruption of brain development will affect or even arrest further development of specific functions, such as hearing, sucking, swallowing, speech, and vision.
2. Insults to the brain can cause lifelong sequelae, including motoric involvement (i.e., cerebral palsy in varying degrees) and learning disabilities.
3. To protect the fragile infant, the caregiver must be aware of infant signals and cues that signify stress and environmental stimuli, which can negatively impact the brain. Environmental issues include thermoregulation, positioning, handling, light, and noise.

## III. Environmental issues

A. Thermoregulation

1. The goal of thermoregulation is to provide a thermoneutral environment, taking into account ambient air temperature, air flow, relative humidity, and temperature of surrounding objects, which result in reduced oxygen and calorie consumption.
2. Types of heat loss
   a. Radiation heat loss occurs as the result of transfer of heat between two objects that are not in direct contact with each other (from a warm to a cooler object). This is a common source of heat loss in very low birth weight (VLBW) infants.
   b. Conductive heat loss is the transfer of heat from one object to another by direct contact.
   c. Convective heat loss is the transfer of heat from an object to surrounding air. This is the most common source of heat loss in VLBW infants.
   d. Evaporative heat loss occurs when moisture from body surfaces is lost to the environment.
3. Interventions to prevent heat loss
   a. Radiation
      (1) Place infant's bed away from external walls and windows or direct sunlight.
      (2) Use thermal shades on external windows.

(3) Use double-walled incubators or heat shields or cover infant with plastic wrap.
(4) Prewarm incubators, radiant warmers, heat shields.
(5) Use heat lamps only if necessary, monitoring temperature every 15 minutes or less to avoid burns.

b. Conduction
(1) Put warm blankets on scales, x-ray plates, or other surfaces in contact with the infant.
(2) Warm blankets and clothing before use.
(3) Avoid placing infant on any surface that is warmer than the baby (heating pads).

c. Convection
(1) Maintain room temperature to provide a safe thermal environment.
(2) Use enclosed, warmed incubators to transport infants through internal hallways and between external environments.
(3) Open incubator portholes only when necessary and then only for brief periods.
(4) Swaddle infant with warm blankets or stretch transparent plastic across infant between radiant warmer side guards; use caps with adequate insulation.
(5) Monitor incubator temperature to avoid temperatures warmer than infant's body temperature.
(6) Place infants away from air vents, drafts, and other sources of moving air.
(7) Use side guards on radiant warmers to decrease cross currents across infant.

d. Evaporation
(1) Warm oxygen and monitor temperature inside oxygen hood.
(2) Use a warm towel to dry infant, especially head, immediately after birth.
(3) Use caps on the head.
(4) Replace wet blanket with dry, warm ones and place baby in a warm environment.
(5) Delay bath until temperature has stabilized; then give a sponge bath. Bathe in a warm, draft-free area and place on warmed towels and dry immediately. Bathe under heat lamps or radiant warmer.
(6) Provide warm, humidified oxygen.
(7) Increased incubator humidity levels may be necessary for very premature infants.
(8) Position the baby in a flexed manner. If the infant is lying flat, more surface area is exposed, causing more heat loss.

4. Results of temperature instability
   a. Symptoms of hypothermia
   (1) Hypoglycemia
   (2) Metabolic acidosis
   (3) Increased oxygen demand
   (4) Increased metabolic rate
   (5) Decrease in growth
   (6) Clotting disorders
   (7) Shock
   (8) Apnea
   (9) Intraventricular hemorrhage (IVH)
   b. Symptoms of hyperthermia
   (1) Hyperventilation
   (2) Apnea
   (3) Decreased muscle tone
   (4) Decreased heart rate
   (5) Irritability
   (6) Stupor
   (7) Convulsions
   (8) Coma
5. Thermal environments to maintain adequate body temperature in the first 4 days of life (Table 2–1). Ability to control temperature occurs between 36 and 38 weeks. Respiratory distress syndrome limits infant's capacity to maintain appropriate body temperature.
6. Factors of neonatal thermal stress—heat production
   a. Response to cold stress leads to increase in metabolic rate.

TABLE 2–1. ***Environmental Temperature Setting According to Weight of the Infant***

| Weight (gm) | Temperature (degrees centigrade) |
|---|---|
| < 1200 | 34–35.5 |
| 1201–1500 | 33–34.5 |
| 1501–2500 | 32–34 |
| > 2500 | 28–31 |

b. Premies have limited stores of fat and glucose.
c. Heat production causes increased oxygen use, which stresses the cardiac and pulmonary systems.
d. Because of the large surface to mass ratio, metabolic rate increases.
e. Immature skin causes increased evaporative loss.
f. Because of immaturity, there is no shivering response—brown fat is used, which utilizes more oxygen. If the cardiorespiratory system cannot meet demands, hypoxia results, in turn causing anaerobic metabolism and then acidosis. This causes increased glucose metabolism, resulting in hypoglycemia.

7. Factors of neonatal thermal stress—insulation
   a. Limited subcutaneous fat. Brown fat is present at 26 to 30 weeks of gestation.
   b. Limited development of muscle

B. Positioning

1. The goal of positioning is to accomplish the following:
   a. Facilitate development of normal motor patterns, midline orientation, and symmetrical positioning.
   b. Enhance self-quieting skills and behavioral organization.
   c. Provide better lung compliance and lung volumes.
   d. Facilitate the parent-infant relationship because of a more normalized infant appearance.
2. Prone position
   a. To place the infant in prone position, flex the infant's hips and knees with the knees under the hips. Arms are flexed with hands near face. Boundaries (folded blankets) provided at head, sides, and feet. Avoid flat positioning.
   b. Prone position has been found to:
      (1) Lower metabolic rates
      (2) Contribute to better sleep patterns and decreased energy loss
      (3) Decrease aspiration
      (4) Decrease gastroesophageal reflux and increase stomach emptying
      (5) Decrease intracranial pressure
      (6) Increase chest wall stability, increasing oxygenation and pulmonary function
      (7) Prevent infantile scoliosis
      (8) Facilitate flexion and development of early head control
      (9) Produce less gross movement, jerk and twitch movement
      (10) Result in less sleep apnea
3. Supine position
   a. To position the infant in supine position, flex the knees and hips up toward the abdomen. Shoulders should be rounded and flexed forward with hands on chest or abdomen, and head midline, not rotated.
   b. Placing infants in the supine position has been found to:
      (1) Be disruptive and disorganizing for infants
      (2) Increase energy expenditure
      (3) Increase intracranial pressure (ICP)
      (4) Predispose infant to upper airway obstruction
      (5) Promote asymmetrical gait pattern and extensor patterns
      (6) Expose eyes to ceiling lights
4. Side-lying position
   a. To position the infant in side-lying position, the hips and knees are flexed, shoulders are forward and comfortably flexed. Head in line with body or slightly flexed.

b. Side-lying position has been found to:
   (1) Provide better midline development
   (2) Be difficult for maintaining proper neck positioning
   (3) Be preferred over supine position
   (4) Facilitate flexion
   (5) Encourage hand-to-mouth activity (self-quieting behavior)

C. Handling
   1. The goal of handling is to facilitate normal development through sensorimotor experiences appropriate to the infant's developmental level.
   2. Impact of handling
      a. Infant receives sensorimotor information through handling.
      b. With high-risk and premature infants, handling may need to be kept to a minimum to prevent medical complications and assist with energy conservation.

D. Infant communication of stress (Fig. 2–1)
   1. Finger splays—fanning or finger extension
   2. Airplanes—both arms stretched out from sides of body
   3. Salutes—one or both arms come straight out from body often with fingers splayed ("stop sign")
   4. Sitting on air—when supine, both legs shoot straight up in air
   5. Arching—body arches backward
   6. Frantic activity—uncontrollable, unable to settle
   7. Loss of muscle tone—limpness
   8. Gagging, spitting up, bowel straining, hiccoughing
   9. Changes in heart rate
   10. Color changes
   11. Startles
   12. Tremors, twitches
   13. Eye floating—eyes open and "float" into head
   14. Sudden changes in respirations
   15. Irritability

E. Appropriate handling of the infant
   1. Move gently in a nonstressful manner.
   2. Time handling according to infant's response to stimulation.
   3. Caregivers—use hands and body to provide support and containment.
   4. Careful handling during routine caregiving decreases infant stress and reinforces the benefits of therapeutic handling.
   5. Provide time out from stimulation when infant is disorganized or displaying stress signals.

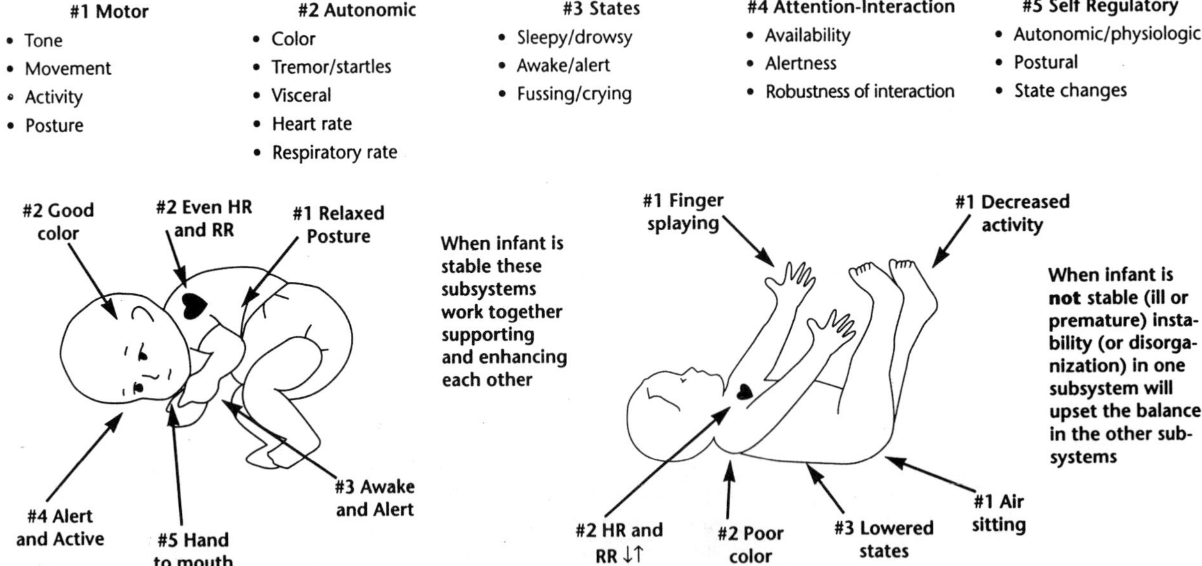


**FIGURE 2–1** Five subsystems of intraorganism functioning in the newborn. (From Als, H: Five subsystems of intraorganism functioning in the newborn. Infant Mental Health Journal 3[4]:229, 1982, with permission.)

## IV. Noxious stimuli

A. The goal is to minimize assault by noxious stimuli, protect the developing systems, and allow for the normal progression of neurological development.

B. Types of noxious stimuli

1. Light
   a. Low lighting decreases retinopathy of prematurity and visual disorders.
   b. Low lighting facilitates better infant behavior and physiological responses.
   c. Low lighting increases infant rest and betters recovery patterns.
2. Noise
   a. Sensory overload can be produced by the following:
      (1) Alarms
      (2) Talking or laughing by the bedside
      (3) Suctioning, mechanical ventilator
      (4) Radios
      (5) Computer printers
      (6) Ringing telephones
      (7) Medical rounds or loud report at bedside
      (8) Closing isolette portholes
      (9) Trash can lids
      (10) Opening and closing drawers
   b. Sound levels in NICU (Table 2–2)
   c. Infant response to loud environment
      (1) Startles
      (2) Apnea or tachypnea
      (3) Bradycardia or tachycardia
      (4) Color changes
      (5) Desaturation
      (6) Hypoxemia
      (7) Alterations in blood pressure leading to increased ICP and possible intracranial hemorrhage
      (8) Hearing loss

## V. Infant states

A. Infant state or level of arousal indicates the level of availability to interact with the environment.

1. The quiet alert state is the optimal time for infant interaction.
2. When brought abruptly out of deep-sleep state, negative responses may occur. These may include the following:
   a. Uncoordinated, jerky movements
   b. Tachypnea or apnea

TABLE 2–2. ***Sound Levels in NICU***

| Location | *Sound Level (dB)* Average | Peak |
|---|---|---|
| SOUND PRODUCED IN PATIENT'S ROOM | | |
| Quiet in patient's room | 58–62 | |
| Talking quietly | 58–64 | |
| Radio playing | 60–64 | |
| Intravenous pump alarming | 61 | 78 |
| Turning the sink faucet on and off | 66 | 76 |
| SOUND PRODUCED INSIDE INCUBATOR | | |
| Using hood top as a writing surface | 59 | 64 |
| Incubator alarm | 67 | 67 |
| Bumping into the metal wastebasket | 62 | 85 |
| Opening a plastic sleeve | 67 | 86 |
| Bubbling in the ventilator circuit | 62 | 87 |
| Tapping hood with fingers | 70 | 95 |
| Closing an incubator cabinet | 70 | 95 |
| Setting a plastic feed bottle on canopy | 84 | 108 |
| Closing a solid plastic porthole | 80 | 111 |

(Adapted from Mishoe, S. C., p 1116, with permission.)

c. Bradycardia
d. Vomiting

B. There are three general states, which include sleep, transitional state, and awake. States labeled A are noisy, unclean, and diffuse (premie states). States labeled B are clean, well-defined states.
1. Sleep states
 a. 1A. Diffuse sleep with momentary regular breathing; eyes closed; no eye movements under closed lids; relaxed facial expression; no spontaneous activity.
 b. 1B. Deep sleep with predominantly regular breathing, eyes closed, no eye movements under closed lids, relaxed facial expression, no spontaneous activity except isolated startles.
 c. 2A. Light sleep with eyes closed; rapid eye movements can be observed under closed lids; low activity level with diffuse or disorganized movements; respirations are irregular, and there are many sucking and mouthing movements, whimpers, facial twitchings, and much grimacing; the impression of a "noisy" state is given.
 d. 2B. Light sleep with eyes closed; rapid eye movements can be observed under closed lids; low activity level with movements and dampened startles; movements are likely to be of lower amplitude and more monitored than in state 1; infant responds to various internal stimuli with dampened startle. Respirations are more irregular; mild sucking and mouthing movements can occur off and on; one or two whimpers may be observed, as well as an isolated sigh or smile.
2. Transitional states
 a. 3A. Drowsy or semidozing; eyes may be open or closed, eyelids fluttering or exaggerated blinking; if eyes open, glassy veiled look; activity level variable, with or without interspersed, mild startles from time to time; diffuse movement; fussing and/or much discharge of vocalization, whimpers, facial grimacing, and so on.
 b. 3B. Drowsy; same as above, but with less discharge of vocalization, whimpers, and facial grimacing.
3. Awake states
 a. State 4: Alert
  (1) 4AL (awake, low keyed). Awake and quiet; minimal motor activity; eyes half-open or open, but with glazed or dull look, giving impression of little involvement and distance; or focused, yet seems to look through, rather than at, object or examiner; or the infant is clearly awake and reactive but has his or her eyes open intermittently.
  (2) 4AH (awake, hyperalert). Awake and quiet; minimal motor activity; eyes wide open; "hyperalert"or giving the impression of panic or fear; may appear to be hooked by the stimulus and may seem to be unable to modulate or break the intensity of the fixation.
  (3) 4B. Alert with bright, shiny look; seems to focus attention on source of stimulation and appears to process information actively and with modulation; motor activity is at a minimum.
 b. State 5: Active
  (1) 5A. Eyes may or may not be open, but infant is clearly awake and aroused, as indicated by his or her motor arousal, tonus, and mildly distressed facial expression, grimacing, or other signs of discomfort; fussing is diffuse.
  (2) 5B. Eyes may or may not be open, but infant is clearly awake and aroused, with considerable, well-defined motor activity. Infant is also clearly fussing but not crying.
 c. State 6: Crying
  (1) 6A. Intense crying, as indicated by intense grimace and cry face, yet cry sound may be very strained, very weak, or even absent.
  (2) 6B. Rhythmic, intense crying that is robust, vigorous, and strong in sound.

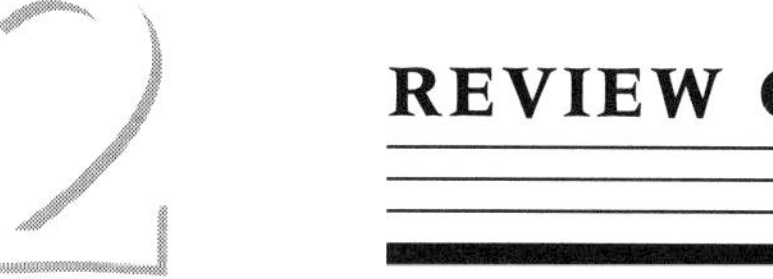

# REVIEW QUESTIONS

1. Define developmental care.

2. Given the following types of heat loss, list two ways to prevent heat loss with each type:

   **Radiant**

   a.

   b.

   **Convective**

   a.

   b.

   **Conductive**

   a.

   b.

   **Evaporative**

   a.

   b.

3. Fill in the temperature that is appropriate for the given weight of an infant.

| Weight (gm) | Temperature (degrees centigrade) |
|---|---|
| < 1200 | |
| 1201–1500 | |
| 1501–2500 | |
| > 2500 | |

4. List four goals of proper positioning of an infant.

   a.

   b.

   c.

   d.

5. Given the following positions, describe how to properly position an infant.

   a. Prone

   b. Supine

   c. Side-lying

6. Of the three positions listed in question 5, which is the best in meeting the goals of positioning? Why?

7. List five ways in which an infant communicates stress (refer to Figure 2–1).

   a.

   b.

   c.

   d.

   e.

8. List two types of noxious stimuli and describe how these stimuli can be avoided in the NICU.

   a.

   b.

9. What is the infant's response to a loud environment? List five responses.

   a.

   b.

   c.

   d.

   e.

10. Give a brief description of the following sleep states, transitional states, and awake states.

    **Sleep State**

    a. 1A

    b. 1B

    c. 2A

    d. 2B

    **Transitional State**

    a. 3A

    b. 3B

    **Awake State 4**

    a. 4AL

    b. 4AH

    c. 4B

    **State 5: Alert**

    a. 5A

    b. 5B

    **State 6: Crying**

    a. 6A

    b. 6B

## BIBLIOGRAPHY

Als, H, et al.(1994). Individualized development care of very low-birth-weight infant. *JAMA* 272(11):853.

Als, H. (1986). A synactive model of neonatal behavioral organization: Framework for the assessment of neurobehavioral development in the premature infant and for support of infants and parents in the neonatal intensive care environment. *Physical and Occupational Therapy in Pediatrics* 6:3.

Catlett, A. T. (1990). Environmental stimulation of the acutely ill premature infant: Physiological effects and nursing implications. *Neonatal Network* 8:19.

Cole, J. G., et al. (1990). Changing the NICU environment: The Boston City Hospital Model. *Neonatal Network* 9:15.

Creger, P. J., and the Staff of Denver Children's Hospital. (1989). *Developmental Interventions for Preterm and High-Risk Infants.* Tucson: Therapy Skill Builders.

Graven, S. N., Bowen, F. W., and Brooten, D. (1992). The high-risk infant environment: Part 1. The role of the neonatal intensive care unit in the outcome of high-risk infants. *Journal of Perinatology* 12:164.

Graven, S. N., Bowen, F. W., and Brooten, D. (1992). The high-risk infant environment: Part 2. The role of caregiving and the social environment. *Journal of Perinatology* 12:267.

Hiniker, P., and Moreno, L. (1993). *Developmentally Supportive Care Theory and Application: A Self-Study Module.* Weymouth, MA: Children's Medical Ventures.

Lotas, M. (1992). Effects of light and sound in the neonatal intensive care unit environment on the low-birth-weight infant. *NAACOG's Clinical Issues* 3:1.

Mishoe, S. (1995). Quiet-hospital zone: Why we should reduce noise levels in the hospital. Editorial. *Respiratory Care* 40(11):1116.

Mishoe, S., et al. (1995). Octave waveband analysis to determine sound frequencies and intensities produced by nebulizers and humidifiers used with hoods. *Respiratory Care* 40(11):1120.

Perez-Woods, R., and Malloy, M. (1992). Positioning and skin care of the low-birth-weight neonate. *NAACOG's Clinical Issues* 3(1):97.

Pickel, M. (1991). Caring for families: What we see is what we get. *Comprehensive Pediatric Nursing* 14:65.

Semmler, C. J., and Butcher, S. D. (1990). *Handle with Care: Articles about the At-Risk Neonate.* Tucson: Therapy Skill Builders.

Vergara, E. (1993). Foundations for practice in the neonatal intensive care unit and early intervention. In the American Occupational Therapy Association: *A Self-Guided Practice Manual,* Vols I and II. Rockville, MD: American Occupational Therapy Association.

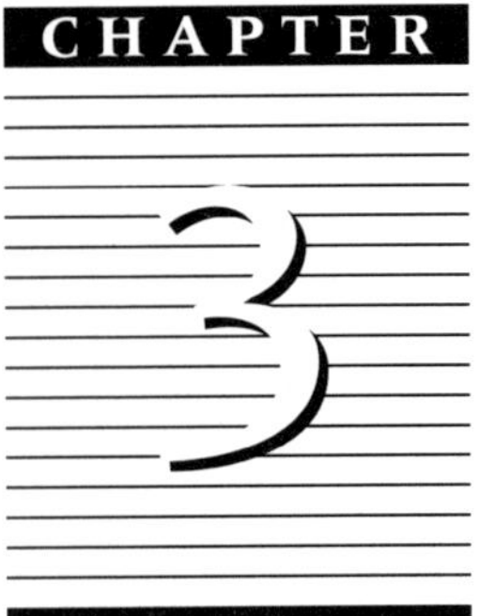

# Fetal Development

**I. General developmental period**

A. Fertilization period (first 21 days)
1. Fertilization of egg by sperm and implantation into uterus.
2. Blood vessels first appear.
3. Heart tubes form that will develop into the heart.
4. Blood cells form from endothelial cells within the yolk sac.
5. Formation of primary germ layer, mesoderm, endoderm, ectoderm, and formation of tissues and differentiation into organs (Table 3–1).

B. Embryonic period (weeks 4 to 7)
1. Embryo forms a C-shaped appearance.
2. Primitive gut forms.
3. Umbilical cord develops.
4. The brain, heart, eyes, ears, nose, and mouth are developing, giving the embryo human characteristics.

C. Fetal period (week 8 to birth)
1. The embryo is now called a fetus.
2. Rapid body growth and organ system maturation occur.

**II. Respiratory system development**

A. Upper airway
1. By the fourth week, branchial arches form and develop into the upper and lower jaws.
2. The branchial arches also form the pharynx, mouth, oropharyngeal airway, and laryngeal cartilages.
3. The tongue develops within weeks 4 to 7.
4. The palate starts to develop in the 5th week and is complete by the 17th week of gestation.
   a. A cleft lip may develop as a result of an incomplete formation of the lip and its extension into the nostril. A cleft palate, which may be unilateral or bilateral, occurs from malformation of the palate.
5. The nasal cavity with nasal concha develops when the oronasal membrane ruptures, allowing the oral and nasal cavity to develop at approximately the 7th week.
6. Nasal sinuses develop during the latter part of fetal development, with further development of the ethmoid, maxillary, frontal, and sphenoidal sinuses continuing into puberty.
7. True and false vocal cords are formed by the 10th week.

B. Lower airway

TABLE 3–1. ***Formation of Organs and Tissues by the Primary Germ Layers***

| Ectoderm | Mesoderm | Endoderm |
|---|---|---|
| Nasal cavity | Connective tissue, bone, cartilage, muscles | Tonsils |
| Nervous system | Blood cells | Thyroid, parathyroid, thymus |
| Sweat glands | Bone marrow | Pharynx |
| Epidermis, hair, nails | Heart, circulatory system | Tongue |
| | Kidneys | Digestive tract |
| | | Respiratory tract |

1. An epithelial groove will give rise to the trachea, bronchi, pulmonary epithelium, and assorted glands.
2. The tracheoesophageal septum divides into the esophagus and laryngotracheal tube.
3. The first lung bud develops from the laryngotracheal tube by 24 to 25 days after fertilization.
4. The laryngotracheal tube, along with the surrounding tissue, develops into the trachea, bronchi, and lungs.
5. Visceral and parietal pleura develop from the lung buds (bronchopulmonary buds).
6. The phrenic nerve innervates the diaphragm within the 4th week, and the diaphragm is completely formed by the 7th week.
7. The lung buds grow and develop further into secondary buds, two on the right and one on the left.
8. This branching continues, with 24 orders of branches present at 16 weeks.

C. Periods of lung maturation
   1. Embryonic period (fertilization to week 5)
      a. Formation of laryngotracheal groove
      b. First appearance of lung bud
      c. Lung bud divides into left and right mainstem bronchus.
   2. The pseudoglandular period (5 to 16 weeks)
      a. During this period, the conducting airways develop and are complete to, and including, the terminal bronchioles.
      b. Mucous glands and goblet cells appear.
      c. Bronchi and bronchioles are lined with cuboidal epithelium.
   3. The canalicular period (17 to 24 weeks)
      a. Enlargement of the conducting airways continues with proliferation of pulmonary blood vessels.
      b. Gas exchange units develop from respiratory bronchioles.
      c. Meconium is present in bowels.
      d. Breathing movements can be detected between 18 to 20 weeks.
      e. Elastic tissue develops beginning at 20 weeks.
      f. Type I and type II alveolar pneumocytes develop, with synthesis and production of surfactant starting by week 24.
   4. The terminal sac period (24 weeks to birth)
      a. Primitive alveoli develop from alveolar ducts.
      b. Further development of the pulmonary capillaries occurs as well as lymphatic proliferation.
      c. The fetus weighs approximately 1000 gm at 26 to 28 weeks.
      d. The fetal lungs represent 2% to 3% of the total body weight. This percentage decreases as the weight of the fetus increases toward the end of gestation.
      e. The air sacs change from a simple cuboidal cellular configuration to a squamous epithelium, allowing greater diffusion of gases.
      f. Reduction in connective tissue, and proliferation of capillaries surrounding the terminal air sacs.
      g. As the lung matures, the number of alveoli increase, and the thickness of the alveolar wall decreases. At approximately 36 weeks, "true" alveoli arise from alveolar ducts.
      h. At birth, the number of alveoli range from 24 to 75 million.
      i. The alveoli continue increasing in number until approximately 8 years of age, when alveoli equal approximately 300 million.
      j. The size of the lung is approximately 1 to 2 $m^2$. With growth, the lung will increase to an adult size of 70 $m^2$ by age 6 to 8 years.

D. Summary of chronological development of the upper and lower airway (Table 3–2)

## III. Pulmonary vasculature

A. Right and left pulmonary arteries begin to develop at approximately 24 to 26 days and are completely formed by 16 weeks' gestation.

B. In the fetus, pulmonary blood flow is low and pulmonary vascular resistance is high. This is caused by an increased constriction of the pulmonary vascular smooth muscle, compression of the pulmonary vasculaturc, and vascular kinking. Because of this, only 5% to 10% of cardiac output enters the lungs.

## IV. Intrauterine breathing movements

A. Occur as early as 12 weeks' gestation.

B. Short, irregular, gasping breathing movements early in gestation are replaced by single, longer breaths similar to gasps.

TABLE 3–2. *Chronological Development of the Upper and Lower Airway*

| Week of Development | Structural Development |
|---|---|
| Embryonic period (up to week 5) | Branchial arches, oral cavity, nasal cavity, pharynx, primitive lung bud, mainstem bronchus |
| Pseudoglandular period (5–16 weeks) | Pulmonary artery/vein, conducting airways, mucous glands, goblet cells, cartilaginous ring |
| Canalicular period (17–24 weeks) | Respiratory bronchioles; alveolar ducts; alveolar sacs; alveolar pneumocytes type I, II; pulmonary vasculature proliferation; surfactant synthesized |
| Terminal sac period (24 weeks–birth) | Increase surfactant secretion, increase lung surface area, increase number of alveoli and capillaries |

C. Further growth matures breathing movements into balanced inspiratory and expiratory phases.

D. Physiological changes in these breathing movements are the result of the following:
   1. Hypoxia, hypocapnia, and alkalosis reduce breathing movements.
   2. Hypercapnia and acidosis increase rate and depth.

E. Peripheral and central chemoreceptors are functional as early as 28 weeks' gestation. Peripheral chemoreceptors and carotid and aortic bodies are responsive to hypoxia. Central chemoreceptors are responsive to hypercarbia.

## V. Fetal lung fluid

A. The lung begins secreting fluid by the 70-day gestation period.

B. This fluid is composed of a combination of sodium, potassium, chloride, bicarbonate, and a small percentage of protein.

C. The presence of lung fluid assists lung growth and the development of the functional residual capacity (FRC).

D. Fetal breathing helps secrete lung fluid and mixes lung fluid with amniotic fluid. This breathing starts at approximately 12 weeks' gestation with short, irregular breaths with gasping. This helps prepare the fetus for extrauterine breathing.

E. Because of this process, amniotic fluid can be analyzed to determine lung maturation.

F. An amniocentesis is a procedure in which amniotic fluid is removed from the uterus.

## VI. Surfactant

A. Surfactant reduces surface tension at the air-liquid interface of the terminal airways and alveoli. This helps maintain alveolar stability and prevents atelectasis.

B. Surfactant is synthesized and secreted by type II alveolar pneumocytes contained within the alveolar walls. Within these cells, storage compartments called lamella inclusion bodies release surfactant into the alveolar airspace.

C. Surfactant is 90% phospholipids and 10% proteins. The phospholipid fraction is primarily dipalmitoyl phosphatidylcholine (PC) or lecithin. Other phospholipids including sphingomyelin make up the smaller portion of surfactant.

D. In the normal newborn's lung, surfactant secretion generally is stimulated by expansion of the lung during inspiration along with hormonal control.
   1. With inflation, surfactant is released into the alveoli, forming a single layer at the alveolar-air interface. As alveoli continue to expand, surface tension increases as the surfactant layer thins along the alveolar walls.
   2. At end-inspiration, surfactant has less effect on reducing surface tension. At this point in the ventilatory cycle, the increased surface tension, along with the natural recoil of the lung, initiates expiration.

E. As air leaves the lung and the alveoli become smaller, the surfactant lining thickens, reducing surface tension and preventing the collapse of alveoli. Without surfactant, surface tension would collapse the alveoli at end-expiration because of the inward force and contraction it has on spheres (Laplace's law of physics).

F. Besides surfactant's ability to reduce surface tension and improve lung compliance, it also helps keep alveoli "dry." Fluid is impeded from entering the alveoli from pulmonary capillary circulation because interstitial pressure is increased from the reduced surface tension.

G. Several routes of surfactant clearance are available that reduce the accumulation within the lung. These routes include, or may be in combination with, ingestion by macrophages, transport to the mucociliary escalator, clearance by lymphatic system, and uptake by type II alveolar pneumocytes to be resynthesized.
H. At birth a large pool of surfactant is released and continues to increase for the first 24 hours. Inadequate surfactant levels may be present in the newborn as a result of the following:
   1. Prematurity
   2. Hypoxia
   3. Malnutrition
   4. Maternal diabetes
   5. Hypothermia
   6. Acidosis

## VII. Amniotic fluid

A. Amniotic fluid is developed from amniotic cells, maternal blood, and fetal urine. The approximately 30 mL in volume at 10 weeks increases to approximately 1500 mL by term.
B. The fetus swallows amniotic fluid, which is absorbed by the gastrointestinal tract. Every 3 hours, amniotic fluid is exchanged by the placenta.
C. Amniotic fluid protects the fetus and acts as a cushion surrounding the fetus. It also allows growth and development, movement, and maintenance of a thermoneutral environment.
D. An excess amount of amniotic fluid is called polyhydramnios. Oligohydramnios is an abnormally small amount of amniotic fluid.

## VIII. Placenta and placental function

A. The placenta is a highly vascular organ that joins the fetus to the mother. It is a unique organ in that not only does it permit the diffusion of oxygen and carbon dioxide but it also provides the functions of the liver, kidney, gastrointestinal tract, and endocrine glands.
B. The placenta is attached to the uterine fundus of the mother by projections called chorionic villi found in the wall of the fundus. Problems and complications can arise if the normal placental attachment does not occur. Some of these problems include the following:
   1. Abruptio placentae—premature separation of the placenta from the uterine wall.
   2. Placenta previa—placenta implanted in the lower uterine segment.
   3. Placenta previa marginalis—placenta covering the cervical os.

## IX. Transfer of oxygen from maternal to fetal blood

A. The umbilical cord connects the placenta to the fetus and provides bidirectional blood flow. Two arteries and one vein are found within the length of the umbilical cord. The arteries have thicker walls than the vein, although the vein is larger in diameter than the arteries. The differences in the vessels take on greater importance when there is a need to obtain a venous or arterial cord sample of blood.
B. Two umbilical arteries bring circulating blood from the fetus to the placenta.
C. As this blood enters the placenta, it is routed to anchoring villi. Maternal blood pressure forces the maternal blood into the placenta through endometrial arteries. This blood surrounds the anchoring villi as the blood pressure decreases. It is here that maternal and fetal blood come in close proximity, separated only by a very thin placental membrane, and diffusion occurs.
D. Fetal blood, which is now oxygenated, will be routed through the placenta, making its way out to the fetus by the umbilical vein. A very important function of the placenta is to exchange oxygen and carbon dioxide between the fetal and maternal blood. Table 3–3 shows the differences between oxygen, carbon dioxide, and pH in the human maternal and fetal blood.
E. Approximately 80% to 90% of the total hemoglobin in the fetus is fetal hemoglobin (HbF). Structurally, HbF is different from adult hemoglobin (HbA) in that HbF lacks a binding site for 2,3-disphosphoglycerate (2,3-DPG). The reactivity of hemoglobin with oxygen depends upon the presence or absence of 2,3-DPG found in the erythrocyte.
F. In the adult, when 2,3-DPG attaches to hemoglobin, it will reduce oxygen's affinity.
G. In the fetus, although the amount of 2,3-DPG is the same as the adult, it is the inability of 2,3-DPG to attach to hemoglobin that gives fetal blood its greater

TABLE 3–3. ***Normal Values of Oxygen, Carbon Dioxide, and pH in Human Maternal and Fetal Blood***

| | *Maternal* | | *Fetal* | |
|---|---|---|---|---|
| | **Artery** | **Vein** | **Artery** | **Vein** |
| $PO_2$ (mm Hg) | 95 | 38 | 22 | 30 |
| $HbO_2$ (% saturation) | 97 | 38 | 50 | 80 |
| $O_2$ Content | 16.4 | 11.8 | 10.9 | 16.2 |
| Hemoglobin (mL/dL$^{-1}$) | 12 | 12 | 16 | 16 |
| $PCO_2$ (mm Hg) | 32 | 40 | 48 | 43 |
| pH | 7.42 | 7.35 | 7.34 | 7.38 |

(Adapted from Scarpelli, p 2.)

capacity for oxygen. As a result, fetal blood is able to transport a large content of oxygen from the placenta to fetal organs in spite of relatively low $PO_2$.

H. This results in a shift of the oxygen dissociation curve to the left of the normal adult curve (Fig. 3–1).

I. At birth, the majority of hemoglobin is of the fetal type, but within the first year of life this changes over to HbA. This is especially important now that the newborn infant must deliver sufficient oxygen to the tissues.

J. To help with oxygen delivery, 2,3-DPG increases twofold at birth, reducing hemoglobin oxygen affinity. This can be seen on the oxygen-dissociation curve as a shift of the fetal curve to the right as it begins to align with the normal adult or maternal curve (Fig. 3–1).

K. After HbF has changed into HbA, the curve will be positioned as a normal adult curve (Fig. 3–1).

## X. Fetal circulation (Fig. 3–2)

A. The umbilical vein leads to the fetal liver, but a small passageway, called the ductus venosus, connects the umbilical vein directly to the inferior vena cava

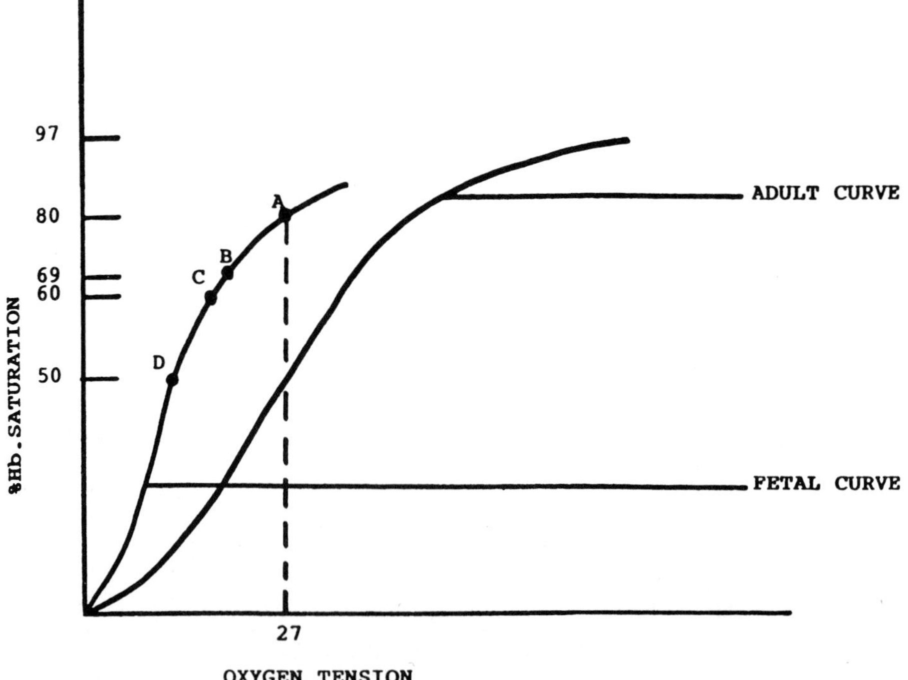


**FIGURE 3–1** Adult and fetal dissociation curve. Point *A* is saturation level in the umbilical vein. Point *B* is saturation in inferior vena cava prior to entering the right atrium. Point *C* is the $SaO_2$ within the right atrium, and point *D* is $SaO_2$ of the blood returning to the placenta and lower extremities. (From Kacmarek, et al, p 145, with permission.)

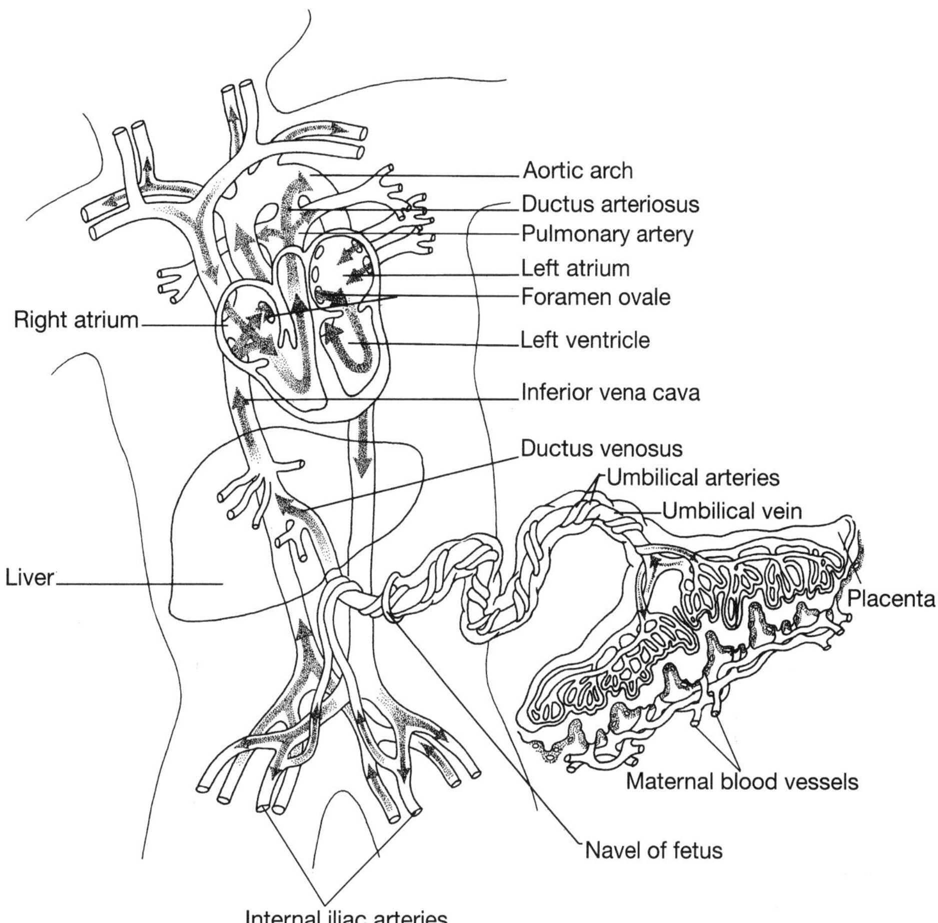


**FIGURE 3–2** Fetal circulation and corresponding anatomy. (From Scanlon, VC, and Sanders, T: Understanding Human Structure and Function. FA Davis, Philadelphia, 1997, p 238, with permission.)

(IVC). Instead of flowing through the system of small veins and capillaries in the liver, much of the umbilical blood (50%) bypasses the liver via the ductus venosus into the IVC.

B. In the IVC, blood shunted through the ductus venosus mixes with deoxygenated blood returning from the tissues of the lower body via the portal circulation and the hepatic circulation. This blood lowers the $SaO_2$ and $PaO_2$ within the IVC. Thus, as the oxygenated blood from the ductus venosus enters the inferior vena cava and mixes, the $SaO_2$ drops from 80% to approximately 67%.

C. The blood enters the right atrium from the IVC, where it mixes with blood returning from the upper body and head. This further reduces the oxygen saturation.

D. The blood flow entering the right atrium is divided into two streams, with the larger stream entering the left atrium by way of the foramen ovale. The foramen ovale is an opening of the interatrial septum between the right and left atria. This opening remains patent because of the increase in blood pressure in the right heart relative to that of the left.

E. The blood enters the left atrium and then mixes with a small amount of deoxygenated blood returning from the lungs by way of the pulmonary veins. This blood enters the left ventricle and is pumped out the aorta. A portion of this blood is directed up to the head and upper extremities. This flow of blood has a higher oxygen content and $SaO_2$ than the flow that is pumped out of the right ventricle.

F. The second stream of blood in the right atrium is pumped to the right ventricle and out the pulmonary artery. About 10% of the blood from the right heart enters the pulmonary arteries and the lung. Very little blood is needed by the lungs at this time because gas exchange occurs within the placenta. The pulmonary arteries are constricted from the low $PaO_2$, pH, lung fluid compressing the vessels, and vascular kinking within the lung.

G. This blood returns to the left atrium by the pulmonary veins and mixes with blood shunted through the foramen ovale.
H. The greater volume of blood leaving the right heart enters the descending aorta by way of the ductus arteriosus. This opening connects the pulmonary arteries and aorta and creates a right-to-left shunt. The saturation of these two blood mixtures results in an oxygen saturation of approximately 50% and a $PaO_2$ of approximately 14 to 17 mm Hg.
I. Blood flow moves through the arch of the aorta, descending aorta, and thoracic aorta. Here, blood is directed to the kidneys, gut, and lower body. A major portion of the blood (about 50% of the cardiac output) enters the placenta for oxygenation.

**XI. Transition from fetal to newborn circulation**

A. By the end of the normal gestational period of 38 to 42 weeks, the lungs of the normal fetus take on the function of gas exchange.
B. Following birth, inflation of the lungs and transition of fetal circulation to newborn circulation occurs.
C. Vaginal birth of the fetus is initiated by contraction of the uterus. The fetus moves through the birth canal and the chest is compressed. As a result, blood flow from the placenta to the fetus decreases, causing fetal blood gas values to change. The $PaO_2$ decreases to approximately 18 mm Hg, and the pH becomes more acidotic (pH 7.28). The small amount of blood flow that is perfusing the lungs is further reduced from vasoconstriction of the pulmonary vasculature in response to acidosis and hypoxia.
D. When the compressed chest passes completely through the vaginal opening of the mother, it recoils, drawing in the first breath to the lungs. With successive breaths, respiratory muscles contract, bringing air into the lungs and overcoming the effects of surface tension.
E. The first breath of the newborn generates an intrapleural pressure between (–)40 cm $H_2O$ and (–)100 cm $H_2O$.
F. Increase in respiratory muscle tone is the result of sympathetic nervous system stimulation and catecholamine stimulation as well as chemoreceptors becoming sensitive to the changes in $PaO_2$ and $PaCO_2$.
G. Air entering the lungs distends alveoli and stimulates the release of surfactant along the alveolar lining so that with expiration, alveoli remain inflated. As alveolar size is established, each successive breath requires less intrapleural pressure.
H. Lung fluid in the alveoli is removed by the pulmonary capillary blood flow and lymphatic blood flow. As air replaces the fluid within alveoli, oxygen diffusing into the pulmonary capillaries increases $PaO_2$ and vasodilates the pulmonary capillaries. This reduces pulmonary vascular resistance, allowing more blood flow and lymphatic flow into the lung, enhancing lung fluid drainage.
I. Within a short time after birth, air completely replaces lung fluid, establishing the FRC that is approximately 25 to 30 mL/kg of body weight.
J. A number of factors contribute to the first and subsequent breaths of the newborn. These include the following:
   1. Neuronal activity from the central and peripheral chemoreceptors
   2. Hypoxia
   3. Hypercapnia
   4. Acidosis
   5. Light, noise
   6. Cooling of the body surface
   7. Tactile stimulation
K. Circulatory adjustments following the first breath
   1. Immediately following birth, the umbilical cord is clamped and cut. The umbilical arteries and vein within the cord constrict.
   2. The ductus venosus will also constrict within a few days and form the ligamentum venosum.
   3. Pulmonary capillary blood flow increases as the $PaO_2$ increases from gas exchange. Vasoactive substances such as bradykinin and prostaglandin (specifically, $PGI_2$ and $PGE_2$), which are released into the lung following inflation, will reduce pulmonary vascular resistance (PVR). Recruitment of small, unperfused alveoli increases the cross-sectional area of the pulmonary circulation, reducing PVR.
   4. Pulmonary venous return increases, and as a result the left atrium pressure increases. This, coupled with the increase in systemic vascular resistance, results in left atrial pressure exceeding right atrial pressure, thereby closing

the foramen ovale. This is a functional closure, which, with changes in right and left heart pressures, can reopen and re-establish a right-to-left shunt.

a. For example, if a newborn develops hypoxia, pulmonary vasoconstriction increases PVR, which in turn reduces pulmonary venous return to the left heart.
b. When left atrial pressure drops below right atrial pressure, the foramen ovale opens, re-establishing a right-to-left shunt. In the normal developing newborn, the foramen ovale closes shortly after birth.

5. Within the 1st hour of life, ductus arteriosus blood flow reduces as it begins to close. This reduces the right-to-left shunt.
6. As systemic vasculature pressure rises, it can force blood through the partially closed ductus, creating a left-to-right shunt and forcing blood into the pulmonary arteries.
7. Over the next few days, the ductus will begin to close but, like the foramen ovale, it can reopen as a result of hypoxemia, resulting in persistent fetal circulation.

3

# REVIEW QUESTIONS

1. List the three general developmental stages of the fetus.

   a.

   b.

   c.

2. What are the three primary germ layers that give rise to all tissues and organs of the fetus?

   a.

   b.

   c.

3. When does the primary lung bud develop?

4. What are the two stages of lung development?

   a.

   b.

5. Fill in the structural development that occurs in each of the periods shown in the accompanying chart.

| Developmental Week | Structural Development |
|---|---|
| Embryonic period (fertilization to week 5) | |
| Pseudoglandular period (Week 5–16) | |
| Canalicular period (Week 17–24) | |
| Terminal sac period (Week 25–birth) | |

6. What contributes to the increase in pulmonary vascular resistance of the developing fetus?

7. What helps establish the FRC in fetal lungs?

8. How does fetal blood transport a large content of oxygen from the placenta to fetal organs in spite of a relatively low $PaO_2$?

9. Trace the normal fetal circulation as blood leaves the placenta by way of the umbilical vein to where it re-enters the placenta by way of the umbilical arteries.

10. Given the fetal anatomic structures listed in the accompanying chart, give the location and function of each one listed.

| Anatomic Structure | Location | Function |
|---|---|---|
| Umbilical vein | | |
| Ductus venosus | | |
| Foramen ovale | | |
| Ductus arteriosus | | |
| Umbilical artery | | |

11. Describe how the first breath of the newborn occurs.

12. Describe the changes in blood flow that occur following the first and subsequent breaths of the newborn.

13. Describe how the ductus arteriosus causes a right-to-left shunt before birth and a left-to-right shunt after birth.

14. Define the following terms.
    a. Polyhydramnios
    b. Oligohydramnios
    c. Placenta previa
    d. Abruptio placentae

## BIBLIOGRAPHY


Avery, G. (1986). *Neonatology, Pathophysiology and Management of the Newborn,* ed 3. Philadelphia: J. B. Lippincott.

Beard, R., and Nathaneilsz, P. (1976). *Fetal Physiology and Medicine: The Basis of Perinatology.* Philadelphia: W. B. Saunders.

Berhardt, T., et al. (1987). Pulmonary mechanics in normal infants and young children during first 5 years of life. *Pediatric Pulmonology* 3:309.

Caminiti, S., and Young, S. (1991). The pulmonary surfactant system. *Hospital Practice* 26:57.

Clark, A. (1988). Human surfactant as prophylactic treatment of respiratory distress syndrome in newborns. *Research Resources Reporter* 12:1.

Fallon, M., Merisalo, R. L., and Kennedy, J. L., Jr. (1983). The frequency of apnea and bradycardia in a population of healthy, normal newborns. *Neuropediatrics* 14:73.

Gabbe, S. (1990). Latest methods of determining fetal lung maturity. *Contemporary Obstetrics/Gynecology* 35:89.

Harper, R. G., and Yoon, J. J. (1987). *Handbook of Neonatology,* ed 2. New York: Year Book Medical Publishers.

Harwood, R. (1990). Intrauterine development and comparative respiratory anatomy. In Kacmarek, R., Mack, C., and Dimas, S. (Eds.). *The Essentials of Respiratory Care,* ed 3. St. Louis: Mosby.

Harwood, R. (1992). Embryology and growth of the respiratory system. In Pierson, D., and Kacmarek, R. (Eds.). *Foundations of Respiratory Care.* New York: Churchill Livingstone.

Harris, P., and Heath, D. (1977). *The Human Pulmonary Circulation,* ed 2. New York: Churchill Livingstone.

Jobe, A. (1986). Surfactant treatment for respiratory distress syndrome. *Respiratory Care* 31:467.

Jacobs, H. (1984). Surfactant kinetics. *Seminars in Perinatology* 8:258.
Korones, S. (1986). *High-Risk Newborn Infants: The Basis for Intensive Nursing Care*. St. Louis: Mosby.
Martin, D. (1988). *Respiratory Anatomy and Physiology*. St. Louis: Mosby.
Moore, K. (1993). *The Developing Human*, ed 4. Philadelphia: W. B. Saunders.
Murray, J. (1986). *The Normal Lung*, ed 2. Philadelphia: W. B. Saunders.
Pawlak, R., and Herfect, L. (1988). *Drug Administration in the NICU: A Handbook for Nurses*. Petaluma, Calif.: Neonatal Network.
Rudolph, A. M., and Heyman, M. A. (1967). The circulation of the fetus in utero. *Circulation Research* 21:163.
Scanlon, V. C., and Sanders, T. (1997). *Understanding Human Structure and Function*. Philadelphia: F. A. Davis.
Scarpelli, E. (1990). *Pulmonary Physiology*, ed 2. Philadelphia: Lea & Febiger.
Stark, A., and Frant, F. (1990). Respiratory distress syndrome. *Pediatric Clinics of North America* 33:533.
Stiles, A. D. (1996). Fetal lung growth. *Neonatal Respiratory Diseases* 6(3):1.
Thibeault, D., and Gregory, G. (1986). *Neonatal Pulmonary Care*. Norwalk, Conn.: Appleton-Century-Crofts.
Tietal, D., and Rudolph, A. (1985). Perinatal oxygen delivery and cardiac function. *Advances in Pediatrics* 32:321.
Walters, D. V., Strang, L. B., and Geubelle, F. (1987). *Physiology of the Fetal and Neonatal Lung*. Victoria, Australia: MTP Press Limited.
Walther, F. J., and Taeusch, H. W. (1991). New approaches to surfactant therapy. *Neonatal Respiratory Diseases* 1(1):1.
Yeomans, R., Bocking, A., and Sigger, J. (1986). Upper airway resistances in fetal sheep: The influence of breathing activity. *Journal of Applied Physiology* 60:160.

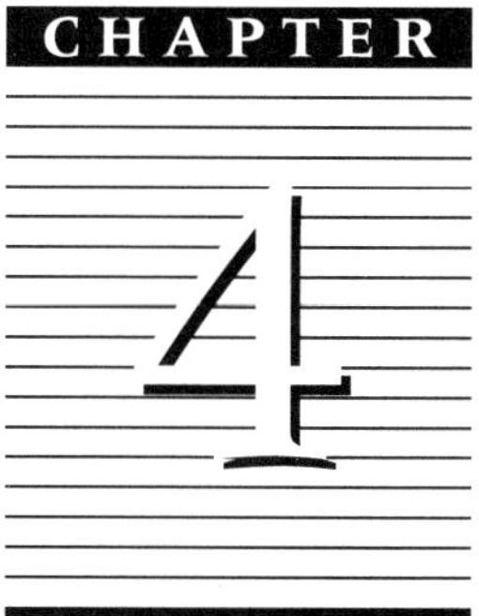

# Perinatal Assessment

## I. Factors related to infants with low birth weight (LBW) and intrauterine growth retardation (IUGR)

A. The primary predictor of infant survival is birth weight. There is an association between cigarette smoking during pregnancy, an increased risk of LBW, and an increased fetal and infant mortality. IUGR, a fetus or infant with a weight in the lowest 10% of the normal population, is also linked to cigarette smoking.
   1. Etiology
      a. Maternal factors causing LBW include smoking, drugs, alcohol, and nutritional deficiencies.
      b. Neonatal and fetal factors causing LBW include infections (rubella, cytomegalovirus [CMV], and chromosomal anomalies).

B. There is a dose relationship between the number of cigarettes smoked during pregnancy and the decline in birth weight. The longer the duration of smoking, the greater the reduction in birth weight. Infants born to smoking mothers are 92 to 300 gm lower in birth weight as compared with infants born to nonsmoking mothers. Also, head circumference and body length are smaller in infants born to smoking mothers.

C. Alcohol also contributes to LBW, as well as to an abnormally developed fetus. The syndrome resulting from the effects of intrauterine exposure to alcohol is called fetal alcohol syndrome (FAS). FAS causes a group of clinical manifestations, including mental retardation, cardiac and genital abnormalities, small head circumference, low-set eyes, and poorly developed extremities. As little as 6 oz of alcohol per week is associated with a reduction in birth weight and other fetal anomalies.

D. Along with cigarettes and alcohol, cocaine also contributes to perinatal mortality. Once cocaine is in the mother's bloodstream, it causes vasoconstriction and reduces blood supply to the fetus. As cocaine passes into the placenta, it causes vasoconstriction, reducing blood flow within the placenta, thus altering and impairing oxygen transport, which results in a lowered partial pressure of arterial oxygen ($PaO_2$). Consequently, cocaine-abusing women have a greater chance of bearing a fetus with LBW, smaller head circumference, smaller body length, lower Apgar score, as well as a greater incidence of spontaneous abortion and fetal death.

## II. Monitoring fetal development

A. Over the past 30 years, because of better medical care, there has been a dramatic decrease in maternal mortality.

B. There has been less of a decrease in perinatal mortality. The fetus is still at risk, even with sophisticated monitoring techniques.

C. Maternal factors leading to a high-risk infant include the following:
   1. No prenatal care
   2. Maternal age less than 16 years or greater than 40
   3. Fetal weight less than 4 lb
   4. Low socioeconomic class
   5. Medical history of the mother
   6. Previous pregnancy problems
   7. Present pregnancy problems
   8. Diabetic mother

D. The fetus is evaluated to determine the actual fetal size and maturity. Improvements in diagnostic technique aid the physician in determining size, position, any anomalies, fetal heart rate, and fetal breathing movements and in analyzing metabolic functions.

E. Amniocentesis is performed to determine a prenatal diagnosis of congenital defects and lung maturity.

F. Testing for congenital abnormalities can be done at approximately 14 to 16 weeks.

G. Examinations of the mother to determine fetal well-being include the following:

1. Ultrasound examination to determine or assess the following:
    a. Gestational age
    b. Length of the fetus
    c. Biparietal diameter (skull)
    d. Placenta location
    e. Multiple gestation
    f. Fetal movement and breathing activity
    g. Volume of amniotic fluid
        (1) An excess amount of amniotic fluid (more than 1500 mL) is known as polyhydramnios.
        (2) A reduced volume of amniotic fluid (less than 500 mL) is known as oligohydramnios.
2. Fetal heart rate (FHR) monitoring
    a. To monitor the heart rate of a distressed fetus, an intrauterine catheter is used, or a FHR monitoring device is placed over the abdomen.
    b. The normal FHR is 120 to 160 beats/min. Tachycardia is a FHR of 180 beats/min or greater. This may be the result of fetal immaturity, fetal hypoxia, or fetal cardiac dysrhythmia. Bradycardia is a FHR of less than 100 beats/min. This may be the result of fetal hypoxia.
    c. FHR patterns are classified according to actual heart rate, variability (irregularity), and alterations.
    d. Baseline FHR is the number of beats per minute maintained over a 10-min interval.
    e. FHR variability or irregularity consists of fluctuations in the recorded FHR.
    f. Accelerations are increases in FHR that accompany other events such as fetal motion and fetal stimulation.
    g. Decelerations are decreases of FHR in response to uterine contraction (Table 4–1).
    h. Decelerations are classified as early, late, or variable (Table 4–2).

## III. Labor and delivery history

A. Risk factors are divided into two groups: antepartum factors, those occurring before birth; and intrapartum factors, those occurring during birth (Tables 4–3 and 4–4).

B. Assessing lung maturation.

1. Because lecithin and sphingomyelin are present in surfactant, measurement of these phospholipids helps determine lung maturity. This test is called the L/S ratio.
2. Throughout gestational development, the concentration of surfactant changes. Surfactant synthesizes beginning at approximately 24 to 26 weeks' gestation and is secreted into the lungs beginning between 25 and 30 weeks. Surfactant contained in lung fluid migrates out of the lungs with the assistance of fetal breathing movements and mixes with amniotic fluid. As a result of this process, an amniocentesis, if needed, is performed to determine the concentration of surfactant.

TABLE 4–1. ***Causes of Reduced Fetal Heart Rate with Early, Late, and Variable Decelerations***

| Early | Late | Variable |
|---|---|---|
| ↓ Cerebral blood flow | ↓ Oxygen transfer | ↑ Peripheral vascular resistance |
| ↓ | ↓ | ↓ |
| Activates vagus nerve | Fetal hypoxia, myocardial depression, vagal stimulation | Fetal hypertension |
| ↓ | ↓ | ↓ |
| Bradycardia | Bradycardia | Stimulation of aortic/carotid receptors |
| | | ↓ |
| | | ↓ Fetal heart rate |

TABLE 4–2. ***Comparison of Early, Late, and Variable Decelerations of Fetal Heart Rate***

| Onset/Cause | Fetal Heart Rate | Comments |
|---|---|---|
| Early decelerations—Early response to uterine contraction. Caused from head compression. | 140–100 beats/min | The fetal heart rate recovers to baseline at the completion of the contraction. |
| Late decelerations—After uterus begins to contract, there are decelerations of fetal heart rate. Caused from uteroplacental insufficiency. | 160–120 beats/min (severe <60 beats/min) | After complete cessation of uterine contractions, the fetal heart rate does not return to baseline. This is an ominous sign of fetal distress. |
| Variable decelerations—These can occur at variable times. Caused from umbilical cord compression reducing blood flow to the fetus. | 140–120 beats/min (severe <90 beats/min) | Change in the position of the fetus or mother alleviating the compression on the umbilical cord. |

3. Sphingomyelin concentrations are comparable to lecithin concentrations up to approximately 34 weeks. At this time, lecithin concentration increases. From this gestational period on, lecithin concentration exceeds sphingomyelin. An L/S ratio of greater than 2:1 indicates that maturation of the lungs has progressed, and thus the incidence of respiratory distress syndrome (RDS) decreases.
4. In normal pregnancies, L/S ratios compare well with gestational age. A number of conditions found in high-risk pregnancies may cause a poor correlation between L/S ratios and gestational age.
   a. For example, a mature lung (L/S ratio greater than 2:1) is seen before 35 weeks' gestation with conditions associated with prolonged rupture of membranes (PROM), early onset of maternal toxemia, maternal infections, and narcotic addiction of the mother.
   b. Conversely, infants greater than 35 weeks' gestation with immature lungs (L/S ratio less than 2:1) are associated with diabetic mothers, with Rh disease, with hydrops fetalis, and with a smaller identical twin.
5. Another test that helps determine lung maturity is the shake test.
   a. A mixture of amniotic fluid, saline, and alcohol is placed in a test tube and shaken for a given period of time and then let stand.
   b. A complete ring of bubbles around the tube indicates an appropriate fetal production of surfactant.
   c. These results can be compared to an L/S ratio of greater than 2:1.
   d. The absence of bubbles indicates that surfactant production is incomplete.
   e. Blood or meconium may cause inaccurate results.
6. Other phospholipids such as phosphatidylglycerol (PG) are useful in pregnancies complicated by diabetes mellitus. PG is reliable, even when contaminated by blood or fluid, and eliminates determining a false maturity by using L/S ratio.

TABLE 4–3. ***Antepartum Risk Factors***

| *Antepartum Risk Factors* | | | |
|---|---|---|---|
| **Cardiovascular/Renal** | **Metabolic** | **Previous History** | **Miscellaneous** |
| Toxemia<br>Hypertension<br>Pre-eclampsia (toxemia of pregnancy with hypertension; edema, if untreated, results in eclampsia).<br>History of eclampsia (a true toxemia that is life-threatening, characterized by hypertension, edema, and proteinuria). | Diabetes<br>Family history of diabetes<br>Family history of genetic disorder | Previous stillbirth<br>Postterm greater than 42 weeks<br>Previous premature infant, neonatal death, cesarean section (para—previous viable offspring; gravida—pregnant women) | Multiple pregnancy<br>Severe anemia<br>Maternal age >40 or <15<br>Use of drugs, smoking, or alcohol<br>Pulmonary disease<br>Emotional problems<br>Congenital and genetic disorders |

TABLE 4–4. ***Intrapartum Risk Factors***

| *Intrapartum Risk Factors* | |
|---|---|
| **Maternal** | **Placental** |
| Hydramnios (>2 L of amniotic fluid) | Placenta previa—Implantation in the lower uterine segment |
| Oligohydramnios (reduced level of amniotic fluid, normal amount of amniotic fluid is about 1 L by 34–36 weeks' gestation). | Abruptio placentae—Premature detachment of a normally situated placenta. |
| Premature rupture of membranes (PROM) >12 h | Meconium-stained amniotic fluid |
| Prolonged labor >20 h | Post-term >42 weeks |
| Maternal bleeding | |

C. Tocolytic therapy for premature labor.
   1. A significant proportion of overall morbidity and mortality is directly related to preterm births.
   2. Several drugs are used to inhibit labor (Table 4–5).

## IV. Anatomy of the newborn infant

A. Head
   1. Approximately one-fourth of the body length (head-to-heel measurement, 19 to 22 in).
   2. Normal head circumference is approximately 34 cm.
   3. Molding may occur with vaginal delivery. This is temporary asymmetry of the skull.
   4. The skull is not completely closed and fontanelles exist. Anterior and posterior fontanelles are normal at birth and will fuse with growth.

B. Tongue
   1. In the newborn, the tongue is relatively large as compared to the oral cavity. Because of this, infants are considered to be obligate nose breathers.
   2. If the nares are blocked, the infant may exhibit some form of respiratory distress. Patency of nares may be checked by occluding either nostril and feeling for air passage. Also a soft catheter may be passed into the nostril and observed for signs of obstruction.
   3. Choanal atresia causes blockage of the posterior nares, thus increasing resistance to airflow. In this situation, inserting an oropharyngeal airway may be indicated to prevent the tongue from obstructing the oropharynx.

C. Larynx
   1. The newborn larynx is approximately 2 cm long and is funnel-shaped. The cricoid cartilage is the smallest opening of the upper airway.
   2. The opening of the vocal cords is found between the third and fourth cervical vertebrae and is higher in the oropharynx of the newborn than in that of the adult. As a result of this position, the infant struggling for air will hyperextend the neck.

TABLE 4–5. ***Tocolytic Drugs for Premature Labor***

| **Drug** | **Action** | **Administration** | **Fetal Side Effects** |
|---|---|---|---|
| Terbutaline sulfate (Brethine) | Selective $B_2$ receptor; relaxes uterine smooth muscle | Oral, subcutaneous, IV | Transient tachycardia, hypoglycemia, hyperinsulinemia |
| Magnesium sulfate ($MgSO_4$) | Inhibits uterine contractility by inhibiting acetylcholine release and decreases calcium available for contraction of smooth muscle | IV and oral | High dose—Decrease muscle tone, drowsiness, breathing rate, and variability of fetal heart rate (term infants take 40 h to excrete $MgSO_4$; preterm infants take longer) |
| Calcium channel blocker (nifedipine) | Inhibits uterine contractions by blocking calcium influx, thereby reducing contractile state of smooth muscle | Oral, sublingual | In animal studies, decreases $PaO_2$ and pH |

3. The larynx contains loosely adhered columnar epithelium, which may develop edema from irritation or infection. Swelling in this region can lead to partial or complete airway obstruction.

D. Epiglottis
   1. The newborn epiglottis is a U- or V-shaped organ lying at the level of the first cervical vertebra. In the adult, the epiglottis is at the level of the fourth cervical vertebra.
   2. The epiglottis becomes more erect as the tongue descends with growth.

E. Cricoid cartilage
   1. The cricoid cartilage, the smallest opening in the upper airway, is located at the third to fourth cervical vertebrae.
   2. In adults, it is approximately at the sixth cervical vertebra.
   3. Cricothyroid membrane connects cricoid cartilage with thyroid cartilage.

F. Trachea and mainstream bronchi
   1. The newborn trachea is 4 cm long, or one-third of the adult trachea (adult length is 11 to 13 cm), with an internal diameter of 3 to 5 mm.
   2. Bifurcation occurs at the third to fourth thoracic vertebrae, whereas in the adult, it occurs at the sixth thoracic vertebra.
   3. The right main-stem bronchus comes off the trachea at an angle of 30 degrees.
   4. The left main-stem bronchus comes off the trachea at an angle of approximately 47 degrees.

G. Thoracic cage
   1. The newborn thoracic cage has little musculature and short expansion range. The ribs are fixed in a horizontal position (as seen in adults following a full inspiration).
   2. Respiratory movement is almost completely diaphragmatic.
   3. The diaphragm is also limited to the level of descent because of a relatively large liver, stomach (partially filled with air), and abdominal organs.
   4. The diaphragm lies at the inferior level of the seventh rib and is rounded on the anteroposterior and lateral aspects.

## V. Body growth and measurements

A. Body measurements include the following:
   1. Weight
   2. Head circumference
   3. Length

B. An intrauterine growth curve is a way of assessing growth and maturity. A chart plots birth weights against gestational age.

C. Birth population is divided into three groups:
   1. Small-for-gestational-age (SGA) newborns have slow intrauterine growth but are delivered at, or later than, term. Factors contributing to the SGA infant include uteroplacental insufficiency (onset at more than 24 weeks' gestation), environmental contributions such as drugs and smoking, and multiple gestation.
   2. Appropriate-for-gestational-age (AGA) newborns have normal intrauterine growth occurring at the end of 37 weeks.
   3. Large-for-gestational-age (LGA) newborns are above the 90th percentile on the growth curve. Infants who tend to be LGA include infants of diabetic mothers and infants with hydrops fetalis.

D. An infant is considered to be preterm if birth has occurred before 37 weeks, regardless of birth weight.

## VI. Physical assessment

A. Following birth, the newborn infant goes through four stages of activity.
   1. Stage 1: Within the first 30 minutes of birth, the heart rate drops from a rate of more than 160 beats/min to 110 to 120 beats/min. There are irregular respirations, and periods of apnea and tachypnea.
   2. Stage 2: Over the next 90 min, the infant is sleeping and irregular respirations are still present.
   3. Stage 3: Over the next few hours, the infant goes through periods of being awake, of sleep, and of high activity.
   4. Stage 4: Finally the infant settles down and is ready to eat or sleep.

B. Color
   1. In the normal-term infant, skin and mucous membranes should be pink.
   2. Capillary refill should occur in less than 2 s, indicating good peripheral perfusion. Poor capillary refill occurs when extremities are cold. Extremities may show mottled skin, ashen or pallor color, or cyanosis.

3. Two types of cyanosis that occur in the newborn include acrocyanosis and general cyanosis.
   a. Acrocyanosis is present initially following birth. This is cyanosis of the hands and feet.
   b. General or central cyanosis, which is found in the lips and mucosal lining of the mouth, is an indication of respiratory distress with hypoxia (see Chapter 5).
4. Pallor is a loss of color that may be associated with low hemoglobin.
5. Plethora is a reddish color caused by the congestion of blood.
6. A slate gray color is associated with methemoglobin.
7. Preterm infants have differences from term infants that may affect color assessment.
   a. Preterm infants have a heavy coating of a cheeselike substance called vernix caseosa, whereas the term infant has only a small amount.
   b. The skin of the preterm infant is thin and transparent and venules may be seen in the abdominal area. The term infant's skin is pale and opaque.

C. Respiratory rate
   1. Normal respiratory rate is 30 to 60 breaths per minute (bpm). When observing respiratory rate, also observe for respiratory pattern, periodic breathing, and periods of apnea. Look for chest symmetry and retractions.
   2. Infants with respiratory illness may have a respiratory rate of greater than 60 bpm. This may be the result of pulmonary disorders such as transient tachypnea (delayed lung fluid absorption) and pneumonia. Nonpulmonary causes such as fever, cold stress, or infection may also cause tachypnea.
   3. A decreased rate, less than 30 bpm, may be associated with periodic breathing. Periodic breathing is recognized as a pattern of alternating breaths and pauses that lasts less than 20 s. This is seen within the first few weeks of life. This is considered non–life-threatening as long as the infant's heart rate and $SpO_2$ do not fall and the color remains pink.

D. Apnea
   1. Apnea is often accompanied by bradycardia, desaturation, and/or cyanosis.
   2. Apnea may require stimulation by gently shaking or rubbing the newborn, or breathing may return spontaneously. Two forms of apnea include the following:
      a. Primary apnea may last for 30 s to 1 min. Generally, the newborn will resume breathing following stimulation.
      b. Secondary apnea is present if the newborn does not resume breathing after 1 min. This may require positive-pressure ventilation (PPV) with a bag and mask and 100% oxygen.

E. Inspiratory effort
   1. Retractions, which are present during an increased inspiratory effort, are visible around the sternum and intercostal and supraclavicular spaces. There is a decrease in effective ventilation and an increase in dead-space ventilation (volume may decrease). Increased respiratory rates may lead to seesaw breathing, which is asynchronous between the abdomen and chest. The chest sinks and the abdomen rises during fast breathing. The sinking chest reduces volume, and the abdomen pushes up on the diaphragm, also reducing volume.
   2. Grunting is a sound heard on expiration as air passes through a partially closed glottis. In a newborn, grunting is created to establish an end-expiratory pressure in the lungs to maintain alveolar stability (small alveoli). Grunting increases oxygen consumption and uses more energy, leading to fatigue and weight loss because of the consumption of calories. Grunting is an indication of respiratory distress.
   3. Nasal flaring occurs as the infant increases airflow into the lungs. Nasal flaring is normally seen during crying episodes. The nares may stop flaring once crying stops. In a noncrying infant, nasal flaring may be indicative of respiratory distress.

F. Abdomen
   1. Note the shape of the abdomen. A flat scaphoid-shaped (football shaped) abdomen may indicate loss of abdominal contents to the chest.
   2. The umbilical cord is examined for the proper number of vessels, irregular-appearing vessels, and color.

G. Heart rate
   1. The normal heart rate is 120 to 160 beats/min. Heart rate is a sensitive indicator of hypoxia. Outside stimuli such as noise, cold, and heat can affect the heart rate. Transient increases in heart rate may occur during crying or other activity, such as the infant being handled or other procedures. Bradycardia, a heart rate less than 100 beats/min, may occur from vagal stimulation (suctioning), with apneic episodes or hypoxia.

TABLE 4–6. ***Blood Pressure for Infants Weighing 1000 to >3000 gm***

| Blood Pressure | 1000–2000 gm | 2001–3000 gm | >3000 gm |
|---|---|---|---|
| Systolic (mm Hg) | 49–59 | 59–64 | 65–70 |
| Diastolic (mm Hg) | 26–30 | 32–37 | 39–44 |
| Average systolic/diastolic (mm Hg) | 60/30 | 65/40 | 70/45 |
| Mean blood pressure (mm Hg) | 35–40 | 40–45 | 50–54 |

2. The point of maximal impulse is found by auscultating between the midclavicular line of the fifth intercostal space. This apical pulse may shift from normal location because of mediastinal shift caused by pneumothorax or diaphragmatic hernia.
3. Peripheral pulses are found by palpating the brachial, radial, and femoral arteries.

H. Body temperature
1. The newborn's normal core temperature is between 36.5 and 37.5°C (97.7 to 99.5°F). Surface temperature is 36.0 to 36.5°C.
2. The infant should always be monitored for proper temperature during the time when procedures are performed. Alarms should be set to prevent skin temperature from dropping below the set temperature level. An overhead portable heating device should be employed for procedures requiring an open bed. Also monitor the infant during this period to prevent overheating the infant.

I. Blood pressure (Table 4–6)
1. Blood pressure (BP) is measured by either the indirect or the direct method. The indirect method requires placing a BP cuff on the arm at heart level. The size of the cuff is important for accurate pressure measurements.
2. The direct method requires cannulation of a major artery such as the umbilical artery. This method is used for critically ill infants requiring constant monitoring.

J. Breath sounds
1. Checking for breath sounds is best performed with the infant in the prone position. Warm the stethoscope before applying it to the skin of the infant. Compare one side to the other.
2. Crackles
   a. Crackles are commonly present immediately following birth because of lung fluid still present in the lungs. In the normal term infant, crackling will disappear as lung fluid moves out of the lung. Crackles present 24 to 48 h after birth may indicate either pneumonia caused by bacterial infection or pulmonary edema caused by hyaline membrane disease.
3. Low-pitched wheeze (rhonchi)
   a. Rhonchi are heard in larger airways as air passes over loosely adhered secretions.
   b. The presence of rhonchi may be an indication for the need to suction to remove secretions from an intubated infant. Often rhonchi may be felt by palpating the chest of the infant. This is called tactile fremitus.
4. High-pitched wheeze
   a. A high-pitched wheeze is a sound created as gas flows and passes through narrow airways. Wheezing may be heard during inspiration and/or during expiration. Infants who develop wheezing may require bronchodilators and/or steroids.
5. Diminished breath sounds
   a. Diminished breath sounds are the result of reduced gas flow into the lung. This may be caused by airway blockage from meconium aspiration, secretions, mucus plugging, or atelectasis.
   b. Diminished sounds may be unilaterally heard following intubation. This may indicate right main-stem bronchus intubation. The complete absence of breath sounds may indicate esophageal intubation. In either situation, the tube will need to be repositioned until bilateral breath sounds are heard.

## VII. Apgar scoring method

A. Following birth, the newborn is evaluated at 1- and 5-min intervals. The evaluation assesses five factors (Table 4–7).

TABLE 4–7. *Apgar Scoring Method*

| Factor | 0 | 1 | 2 |
|---|---|---|---|
| **A**ppearance—color | Blue, pale | Body pink, extremities blue | Completely pink body |
| **P**ulse—heart rate | Absent | <100 | >100 |
| **G**rimace—reflex irritability | No response | Grimace | Cough, sneeze |
| **A**ctivity—muscle tone | Flaccid | Some flexion of extremities | Well flexed |
| **R**espirations—breathing effort | Absent | Weak, irregular | Good, crying |

B. The newborn is given a score of 0, 1, or 2 in all categories at 1 min and 5 min (further Apgar assessments may be taken until the score is 7 or above or the infant's condition deteriorates and requires intubation). The total score determines the need for resuscitation at 1 min. In general, Apgar scoring is useful for infants who are not critical and do not require immediate resuscitation. Therefore, do not delay or stop resuscitation to obtain an Apgar score.

C. Example of 1-min Apgar scoring:
   1. **A**ppearance: Body pink, blue extremities = 1 (in many infants, 1 is commonly deducted in the first minute for acrocyanosis).
   2. **P**ulse: 138 beats/min = 2.
   3. **G**rimace: Cough, sneeze = 2.
   4. **A**ctivity: Well-flexed extremities = 2.
   5. **R**espirations: Breathing effort is weak; irregular cry = 1.
   6. Total 1-min score = 8.

D. Level of asphyxia associated with Apgar scores:
   1. Score of 7 to 10: No asphyxia present (no treatment necessary).
   2. Score of 4 to 6: Moderate asphyxia present (blow-by oxygen and stimulation).
   3. Score of 0 to 3: Severe asphyxia present (intubation, PPV, and 100% oxygen).

## VIII. Assessment of gestational age

A. Dubowitz scoring method
   1. The Dubowitz scoring method determines the gestational age of the newborn and is assessed within the first day of life. It is accurate to within 2 weeks of the newborn's gestational age.
   2. The are 11 external signs and 10 neurological signs. The higher the score assigned, the greater the gestational age of the newborn.

B. Ballard score
   1. The Ballard score is similar to the Dubowitz scoring method, but includes only six neuromuscular and six physical signs.
   2. It assesses the most useful items from the Dubowitz scoring system. Accuracy is ± 2 weeks.

## IX. Neutral thermoregulation

A. Body temperature is a balance between the amount of heat produced and heat lost. A neutral thermal environment is best for the infant. This is an environment where there is minimal oxygen consumption and minimal metabolic demands. Neutral thermal temperatures vary, but in general the lower the birth weight, the greater neutral thermal temperature will be required to maintain the appropriate core temperature. For example, a normal newborn with a birth weight of greater than 3000 gm may require a neutral thermal temperature of 33°C, whereas a 1000-gm newborn requires 35°C.

B. Hypothermia
   1. Problems associated with a cold-stressed hypothermic infant include the following:
      a. Increased oxygen consumption
      b. Metabolic acidosis
      c. Depletion of glycogen stores and hypoglycemia
      d. Weight loss
   2. Mechanisms of heat loss
      a. Radiation: Heat loss from the body surface to cooler objects without being in contact with the object (isolette walls, outside wall, nursery ambient temperature, etc.). Therefore, use a radiant warmer, avoid exterior windows and walls, and use a double-walled isolette or body shields. At minimum, keep ambient temperatures at 24°C (75°F).

b. Conduction: A loss of heat from the body to a colder surface (such as a mattress or weighing scales). Therefore, cover all surfaces and prewarm. Warm hands and stethoscope; prewarm incubator.
c. Evaporation: Conversion of water on the surface of the body to water vapor. Term infants have little heat loss by this method because of the stratum corneum (outer layer of skin), which acts as a barrier. In infants less than 28 weeks' gestation and VLBW infants, evaporative heat loss exceeds all other sources of heat loss. Heat loss occurs in this way after birth (amniotic fluid). Therefore, dry the newborn immediately, remove damp blankets and clothes, and cover the head with a stocking cap (the head has a larger surface area compared to rest of body).
d. Convection: A loss of heat from cool air passing over the body. Temperature and velocity of a gas will determine heat loss. Therefore, warm all therapeutic gases, use appropriate flowrates, use a transport isolette, and avoid drafts. Also, a low incubator temperature, an incubator that is not prewarmed, and servo control dysfunction, such as with an unshielded temperature probe, can lead to heat loss through convection.

3. Normal mechanisms for heat production include shivering, voluntary muscle activity, and nonshivering thermogenesis.
4. The newborn uses nonshivering thermogenesis to produce heat. This requires the metabolism of brown fat, which when broken down produces heat, as opposed to yellow fat, which is primarily an insulator. The majority of brown fat is deposited during the last half of the third trimester. Two percent of the total body weight is brown fat, found in the greatest amount in areas that include the renal–adrenal area of the neck, clavicles, axilla area, mediastinum, and trapezius and deltoid muscles. Preterm infants have a limited amount of brown fat; therefore, maintaining a neutral thermal environment is essential.
5. Breakdown of brown fat
   a. The breakdown of brown fat to produce heat is initiated by thermal receptors in the skin and face.
   b. Norepinephrine is released (sympathetic nervous system) and activates adipose tissue lipase, which breaks down brown fat and produces heat.
   c. The increased utilization of oxygen and glucose may cause hypoxia and hypoglycemia in preterm infants. Metabolic acidosis may result from anaerobic metabolism (lactates enter blood, forming lactic acid and reducing pH).
6. The infant's response to cold-stress hypothermia includes the following:
   a. Signs of respiratory distress
   b. Hypoglycemia
   c. Failure to thrive
   d. Metabolic acidosis
7. Cardiopulmonary changes resulting from hypothermia (Table 4–8)
8. Infants at risk for hypothermia
   a. All infants, but specifically preterm infants, are at greater risk because of less white fat.
   b. Infants affected by RDS have an increased risk because of increased oxygen requirements.
   c. Infants who are unable to position themselves to conserve heat.
   d. Infants receiving constant therapy requiring specialized equipment. Improper equipment monitoring (improper temperature setting on a humidifier). Personnel (opening up the bedding too often without maintaining proper neutral thermal environment).

TABLE 4–8. ***Cardiopulmonary Changes Resulting from Hypothermia***

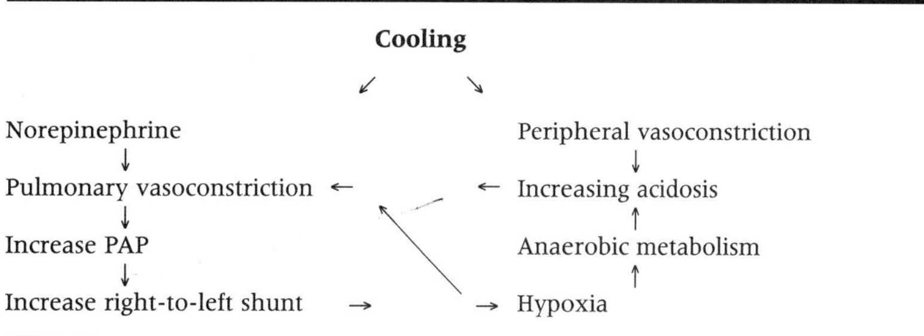

C. Equipment used to maintain neutral thermoregulation
   1. The isolette or incubator has servo-controlled temperature controls that are used to regulate the output of heat. A number of these controls are available on these units.
      a. Skin servo control: Heat output automatically adjusts to the temperature of the infant's skin thermistor.
      b. Air temperature servo control: Same as skin servo control, except the controlling variable is the temperature of the air.
      c. Manual control: Requires the health practitioner to maintain desired level.
   2. An isolette is used to maintain a neutral thermal environment.
      a. Temperature is monitored and maintained with a skin probe attached to the newborn's skin. Probe location is very important for accurate temperature. Abdominal areas have a higher skin temperature than distal sites (arms and legs). Placement of the probe on these distal sites will result in greater temperature output and hyperthermia. Also, placement of probes over areas with a high content of brown fat will cause a decrease in heater output.
      b. Newer isolettes are double-walled, which reduces radiant heat loss. These monitor the inner surface of the isolette and the patient's skin. If either of these temperatures falls below a preset value, the incubator responds by increasing heat production.
      c. Access to the newborn is provided by hand holes on the side of the hood, or the hood can be lifted for complete exposure. This reduces convective heat loss.
      d. The disadvantages of the isolette are that the device cannot achieve a specific fractional concentration of oxygen ($FIO_2$) and that humidification is provided by a system that blows air over standing water. Reduced relative humidity and infection are potential problems of these devices.
      e. Oxygen and humidity are delivered to an oxygen hood or tent placed inside the isolette. Adding humidity increases the relative humidity and reduces evaporative heat loss, especially in VLBW infants.
   3. Radiant warmer
      a. The radiant warmer is an open bed system that provides infrared heat from an overhead source. This device allows procedures to be performed on the newborn as well as allowing greater accessibility during treatment.
      b. The amount of infrared heat is determined by a probe attached to the skin. The probe has a reflective patch that prevents inappropriate temperature adjustments.
      c. Heat loss can occur from evaporation and convection.
      d. Side shields can be raised around the bed to prevent convection and insensible water loss, or a plastic sheet (Saran wrap) can be used to cover the newborn.

## X. Hyperthermia

A. Hyperthermia occurs either because environmental factors bring about overheating or because the infant generates heat from a disorder.
B. Environmental conditions causing hyperthermia:
   1. Blankets
   2. Sunlight in isolette
   3. Excessive clothing
   4. Lost contact with the skin by the thermistor probe
C. Hyperthermia can be caused by infection.
D. Dehydration, acidosis, hyperelectrolytemia, and brain damage can result from hyperthermia.
E. Diagnosis of environmental and disease state hyperthermia (Table 4–9)

## XI. Hyperbilirubinemia

A. There are two forms of bilirubin:
   1. Direct or conjugated, and indirect or unconjugated
B. Formation of bilirubin
   1. The most important source of bilirubin is catabolism of red blood cells (RBCs). Each gram of hemoglobin produces 34 to 35 gm of indirect bilirubin. When the RBC is lysed, hemoglobin is released, then reduced to heme and globin. Heme is broken down to biliverdin and carbon monoxide by various enzymes. Biliverdin reductase reduces biliverdin to unconjugated bilirubin (fat-soluble). This bilirubin enters plasma, combines with albumin, and enters the liver. Albumin combines with glucuronic acid and forms conjugated bilirubin.

TABLE 4–9. ***Differences between Environmental and Disease State Hyperthermia***

| Environmental | Disease State |
|---|---|
| Infant does not appear ill.<br>↓<br>Is there excessive clothing?<br>↓<br>Is the probe disconnected from the baby?<br>↓<br>Both abdomen and extremities are warm (<2° F difference. Skin temperature initially higher than core temperature). | Infection<br>↓<br>Mother had infection during labor.<br>↓<br>Extremities are cooler than abdomen (>2° F difference. Core temperature higher than skin temperature initially). |

2. Conjugated bilirubin enters the bile (water-soluble) and is brought to the small intestine. Intestinal bacteria convert it to urobilinogen, which forms orange-red–colored urobilin. Either this will move out with feces, or it will be reabsorbed by the colon and leave the body in the urine.

C. Noninvasive measurement of bilirubin
   1. Visual inspection may allow determination of whether jaundice is present (Table 4–10). The initial appearance of jaundice starts in the head and neck region.
   2. As levels of bilirubin increase (greater than 5 mg/dL), other parts of the body may take on a yellowish discoloration (bilirubin has a yellow color), otherwise known as jaundice. Infants develop jaundice following birth because the life of the RBC is shorter in the infant than in the adult (60 to 90 days versus 120 days in the adult). Consequently, more bilirubin is formed and may stay in the infant. The type of jaundice may be classified into physiological jaundice (normal appearing jaundice) and pathological jaundice.
      a. Physiological jaundice criteria include (1) that serum bilirubin levels are not greater than 12 mg/dL; (2) that jaundice appears after 24 h of life; and (3) that serum bilirubin levels exceed 5 mg/dL/day.
      b. Pathological jaundice occurs when the normal pathways for producing bilirubin and/or for removing bilirubin are affected. Consequently, greater levels of bilirubin are measured as compared to the levels in physiological jaundice.

D. Laboratory assessment
   1. Measurement of bilirubin is done by the following techniques:
      a. Serum bilirubin levels
      b. Transcutaneous bilirubin
      c. Coombs' test (direct and indirect bilirubin levels)

E. Management and treatment of jaundice
   1. Early feeding of the infant will help decrease bilirubin. Early feeding increases intestinal motility and establishes normal bacterial flora. This aids in decreasing bilirubin from returning to the liver to reconjugate.
   2. Phototherapy provides a major pathway for the removal of bilirubin from the body. Bilirubin is removed from the body by photoisomerization. Photoisomerization converts indirect bilirubin to photobilirubin and lumirubin, which are secreted in bile.
   3. In general, infants weighing less than 1500 gm have phototherapy initiated with levels at 5 to 8 mg/dL. Infants in the range of 1500 to 2000 gm have

TABLE 4–10. ***Approximating the Level of Bilirubin within Various Regions of the Body***

| Region or Zone of the Body (each zone includes the previous one) | Level of Bilirubin (mg/dL) |
|---|---|
| From head to neck (at the level of the clavicles) | 5 |
| Clavicles to umbilicus | 6–8 |
| Umbilicus to knees | 9–12 |
| Knees to ankles | 13–15 |
| Palms and soles | >15 |

phototherapy initiated with levels at 8 to 12 mg/dL. Healthy term infants (greater than 34 weeks) start phototherapy greater than 24 hours.

4. Dangerously high levels of bilirubin (greater than 25 mg/dL) can cause brain damage. Called kernicterus, this may require blood transfusion if the bilirubin levels do not drop following phototherapy.
5. Infants are placed under phototherapy lights for a prescribed period of time. Eye shields protect the eyes, and plastic sheeting may be used to prevent insensible water loss.
6. In general, jaundice resolves within 7 days in the term infant, and within 14 days for preterm infants.

## XII. Glucose

A. Glucose is principally derived from the mother through the placenta during fetal development. Glucose is important for energy and growth. Glucose is converted to glycogen and stored for use after birth.

B. It is important for the infant to have enough stores of glycogen after birth. Premature infants may not have the last trimester to store glycogen; therefore, there are few stores available for use after birth.

C. Glucose utilization is higher in the preterm infant than in the term infant and the adult. This is because the brain has a high requirement for glucose. In the preterm infant, the ratio of brain tissue to body weight is greater as compared to that in the term infant and adult.

D. Hypoglycemia.

1. Hypoglycemia is defined as serum glucose levels measuring less than 40 mg/dL.
2. The following are symptoms of hypoglycemia:
    a. Tremors
    b. Irregular respirations
    c. Jitteriness
    d. Weak cry
    e. Convulsions (brain is deprived of glucose)
    f. Apnea
3. Infants at risk for hypoglycemia include the following:
    a. Those with IUGR
    b. Infant of a diabetic mother (IDM)
    c. Infants receiving inadequate administration of exogenous glucose
    d. Septic infants
    e. Hypothermic infants
4. Diagnosis
    a. Dextrostix or chemstrip
    b. Blood sample sent to laboratory
    c. Colorimeter
5. Treatment
    a. Monitor blood glucose levels closely.
    b. If the infant has symptoms of hypoglycemia, then give IV glucose and monitor glucose levels every 30 min until normoglycemic.

## XIII. Systematic inspection and assessment of the newborn chest radiograph

A. Type of radiograph

1. The most common radiograph is the anterior-posterior (A-P). For viewing pulmonary disease, endotracheal tube placement, lines, catheters, and so on, it is best to have the infant supine.
2. The cross-table radiograph is used to diagnose pneumothorax. The patient is supine, and the radiograph plate is placed against the lateral side of the chest.
3. The lateral decubitus radiograph is used to determine pleural fluid or pleural air changes. For diagnosis of air, the suspected chest is up; for fluid, the suspected chest is down.

B. Degree of exposure

1. With proper exposure, the intervertebral disk spaces are visualized through the heart.
2. Pulmonary vessels are seen in the upper third of the lung.
3. The heart borders are distinct.
4. The diaphragm is clearly outlined, except for the left portion, which is close to the heart.
5. The newborn's lungs tend to be hyperlucent because of soft tissue, small hila lymph nodes, and pulmonary vessels that are smaller and thinner at this age.
6. The premature infant's cellular structure is different (cuboidal versus squamous); therefore, the lungs show a slight haziness and perihilar streaking (mostly from lung fluid).

C. Overexposure—radiolucent
   1. The heart appears darker than normal.
   2. The radiograph lacks contrast and sharpness of organs.
   3. The intervertebral spaces are difficult to see through the heart.
   4. The lungs appear dark, and pulmonary vasculature is more difficult to see.
D. Underexposure—radiopaque
   1. The lungs appear light and hazy.
   2. The pulmonary vasculature is more prominent.
E. Expansion of the chest.
   1. A good inspiratory film is one in which one can count at least six anterior ribs above the diaphragm (starting at the top of the lungs).
   2. Fewer than six ribs may indicate that there was reduced volume in one lung or that the radiograph was not taken during expiration.
   3. An overexpanded chest (caused by mechanical ventilation) has ribs that appear horizontal or flat, rather than oblique. There are 10 or more anterior ribs above the diaphragm.
F. Bones
   1. Inspect the ribs and look for any irregularities or fractures. A fracture appears as a dark line in any portion of the bone where air or tissue settles in between the bone fragments. Ribs, clavicles, or the humerus may have been fractured or broken during delivery.
G. Trachea, carina, and bronchi
   1. The air-filled trachea is easily seen on radiograph. This tends to shift because of the location of the aortic arch. The trachea shifts opposite to the location of the aortic arch.
   2. The carina is at the level of thoracic vertebrae 3 to 4.
   3. Right and left main-stem bronchi are also easily seen.
   4. Air bronchograms may be seen past the bifurcation. These are air-filled bronchi surrounded by collapsed alveoli.
H. Lung fields
   1. Following birth, the lungs appear opaque because of lung fluid. As fluid is removed, the lungs become radiolucent, except in the hilum, where thoracic structures are located.
   2. Premature lungs may appear hazy because of underinflation.
   3. An atelectatic lung has the following changes:
      a. Structure bounding affected lungs are displaced toward the lung.
      b. Reduced vascular markings
      c. Radiopaque appearance of the affected lung
I. Pulmonary vasculature
   1. Pulmonary arteries and veins should be sharp. Hazy or indistinct vasculature may indicate pulmonary interstitial edema.
J. Mediastinum, thymus, and heart
   1. Mediastinum contains esophagus, trachea, bronchi, ascending aorta, aortic arch, main pulmonary artery, the heart and its major vessels, and the thymus. This area appears opaque because of these tissues and structures. These structures are easily displaced.
   2. Thymus
      a. The thymus is a thin, bilobed organ located at the superior mediastinum. It varies in shape and size. It is visible on radiograph at birth and up to 2 years of age. Because of its location, it may cause the heart to appear larger than normal.
      b. The gland in the older child is proportionately smaller than in the newborn. On A-P film, because the thymus is found in the superior mediastinal area, it blends in with the cardiac silhouette bilaterally. On lateral, the thymus fills the anterosuperior mediastinal area. The "sail sign" appearance is the right lobe of the thymus extending into the right hemithorax. It resembles a saillike structure.
      c. The thymus may appear to have a "wavy" appearance, which is caused by overlying ribs, which indent the soft organ.
   3. Heart
      a. The loss of distinct heart borders may indicate fluid from the surrounding lung.
      b. On A-P film, the heart may appear larger. The heart may be tilted upward because of a high diaphragm as compared to that in the adult.
      c. Determining heart size.
         (1) Using a piece of paper, measure the width of the chest at its widest portion.
         (2) Fold the paper in half.
         (3) Align the paper with the widest portion of the heart.

(4) The width of the heart should equal that of the folded paper. Normal width is 50% of the transthoracic profile.

K. Diaphragm
  1. One may not see the costophrenic angles of the diaphragm because of lung fluid in the newborn.
  2. The right side of the diaphragm is higher than the left, and the left may have an air bubble beneath it.
  3. Look for proper level, shape, and contour. For example, a flat or depressed diaphragm may be caused from hyperaeration from meconium aspiration. An elevated diaphragm may result from abdominal distension or diaphragmatic hernia.

L. Stomach
  1. With A-P film, the stomach is usually seen below the left diaphragm sheath.
  2. The stomach contains air following delivery. Air may not be present because of intubation or a paralyzing agent.
  3. One should see air in the stomach within 30 to 60 min following the birth of a spontaneously breathing infant. If not, suspect esophageal atresia without a fistula.

M. Tubes and catheters
  1. Endotracheal tube (ETT) placement
     a. Proper placement of the ETT is at the level of, or just below the level of, the clavicles (in general, below the thoracic inlet and above the carina).
     b. High placement of the ETT is above the clavicles, whereas low placement may be in the right main-stem bronchus or at the level of the carina.
     c. Tube displacement may occur with hyperextension of the neck or with the head flexed forward. With hyperextension of the neck, the tube is pulled downward. When the head is flexed forward, the tube is displaced lower. Ensure a midline position of the head prior to taking a radiograph because this may alter the position of the ETT.
  2. Umbilical catheters.
     a. The umbilical artery catheter (UAC) is positioned either low (at lumbar vertebrae 3 to 4) or high (below ductus arteriosus between thoracic vertebrae 7 and 11).
     b. Umbilical venous catheter (UVC) is placed just above the level of the diaphragm, or it may be placed in the right atrium.
     c. The difference between the UAC and UVC on radiograph is that, upon entering the umbilicus, the UAC turns downward toward the pelvis and then turns upward through the iliac artery, the common iliac artery, and into the aorta. Upon entering the umbilicus, the UVC turns upward immediately.
     d. On A-P radiograph, the UAC is on the left side of the vertebrae (with respect to the patient) and the UVC is on the right side of the vertebrae.
  3. The central venous pressure (CVP) catheter is in the superior vena cava just proximal to RA.
  4. To drain air, the chest tube should be placed high anterior in the chest, and, to drain fluid, low posterior.
  5. The naso-orogastric tube should be placed downward, below the diaphragm, into the third portion of the duodenum.

N. Motion, positioning, and rotation
  1. Motion causes blurring of the cardiac silhouette, hemidiaphragms, and pulmonary structures. A skin fold may appear on radiograph as a result of patient moving.
  2. Positioning the patient
     a. A poor radiograph will result if the patient arches back or if the x-ray beam is centered over the abdomen. The anterior arc of the rib projects toward the head, above the posterior rib. This is a lordotic view.
     b. Heart size looks bigger (may be boot-shaped in appearance) than normal because of an increase in transverse diameter.
  3. Rotating the patient.
     a. In a properly aligned frontal chest, from the spine to the end of the anterior ribs is equal in distance when the right and left side are compared.
     b. The good quality of a radiograph might be impaired because of improper position such as rotation of the infant. Changes in the structures of the thorax and lung occur, such as the cardiac image appears enlarged, hyperlucency of one lung, ribs appear longer on one side, and asymmetry of the clavicles where one is higher than the other. For example, rotation to the left findings include the following: asymmetry of the ribs and clavicles,

ribs on the right appear longer than the ribs on the left, and the right lung appears hyperlucent.

c. A simpler way of determining rotation is to compare clavicular shadows. Both should be equal in size. Rotation is present if one clavicle is smaller than the other or if one is higher or lower than the other.

d. The lateral x-ray rotation can be seen by the amount of offset between the anterior tips of the right and left sets of ribs.

O. Other findings

1. Pleural fissures: Interlobe fissures may be seen in newborns because lung fluid is still present. As fluid clears, this fissure will become less distinct.
2. Skin folds: Common in premature infants because of rotation or folding of skin. May be interpreted as a pneumothorax. The differences between a skin fold and a pneumothorax include the following:
   a. A skin fold line extends beyond the lungs and pleura. A skin fold line is more oblique.
   b. A pneumothorax lung line does not travel beyond the lungs. Lines are more vertical. Hyperlucency is present past the outline of the lung.
3. Air bronchograms: Air contained within bronchi surrounded by atelectasis (fluffy white appearance). The bronchi appear as dark, lateral projections. Bronchograms may be seen in disease states such as hyaline membrane disease.
4. Identify electrodes, probe sensors, and port hole in incubator (if present). Metal density in area of the heart may be surgical clip to ligate PDA.
5. Atelectasis shows up as opaque, small lungs. With resuscitation, air enters trachea and stomach.
6. Pleural fluid shows up as opacification on the affected side and blunting of the costophrenic angles. If there is enough fluid in the pleural cavity, there may be a mediastinal shift away from the affected side.

P. Choanal atresia is an obstruction of the nasal passage by outward projection of the posterior nasal septum (choana). The lateral radiograph is helpful in identifying the choanal atresia.

Q. Pierre Robin syndrome is hypoplasia of the mandible. When the infant lies down, the tongue may occlude the posterior pharynx. Lateral x-ray shows a recessed mandible, which compromises the upper airway.

R. Summary of radiographic patterns in pulmonary disease (Table 4–11)

## XIV. Normal laboratory values following term birth

A. Blood gas values (Table 4–12)

B. Other laboratory values (Table 4–13)

TABLE 4–11. ***Summary of Radiographic Patterns in Pulmonary Disease***

| Radiological Findings | Pulmonary Disease |
|---|---|
| Pleural fluid | Chylothorax, empyema, hemothorax |
| Air trapped in pleural space | Pneumothorax |
| Large, bubbly (unilateral) | Diagphragmatic hernia |
| Small, bubbly (unilateral); reduced lung volume; bilateral granular lungs; uniform in appearance; no pleural effusion | Hyaline membrane disease (HMD) |
| Bilateral bubbly lungs—large appearance | BPD (advanced stages); Pulmonary interstitial emphysema (PIE) |
| Bilateral bubbly lungs—small appearance | BPD (early), PIE (early) |
| Bilateral congested lungs—fluid | TTN, amniotic fluid aspiration (no meconium) |
| Reticulonodular (a network of nodules) | Meconium aspiration, pneumonia, large amount of amniotic fluid aspirated |
| Streaky lungs—bilateral | TTN |
| Hazy lungs—bilateral | HMD (5–7 days post birth, healing), hypoventilation in premature lungs |
| Opaque—bilateral | Atelectasis, hypoventilation—premature infant |
| Respiratory distress—clear lungs | Cardiac disease, persistent fetal cirulation |
| Extensive granular confluent infiltrates, nonuniform, pleural fluid, normal lung volume | Pneumonia (group B streptococcus) |
| Obliteration of costophrenic angle | Pleural fluid |

TABLE 4–12. ***Blood Gas Values of a Normal Term Newborn***

| *Blood Gas Values of the Normal Term Newborn* | | | | |
|---|---|---|---|---|
| | **Umbilical Vein** | **Umbilical Artery** | **Within 5 Min After Birth** | **24 h to 7 Days After Birth** |
| pH | 7.32 | 7.24 | 7.20–7.34 | 7.20–7.34 |
| $PCO_2$ (mm Hg) | 38 | 49 | 46–35 | 33–35 |
| $PO_2$ (mm Hg) | 27 | 16 | 49–73 | 72–73 |
| $HCO_3$ (mEq/L) | 20 | 11 | 16–19 | 20 |
| $SaO_2$ (%) | 80 | 60 | >80 | >90 |

TABLE 4–13. ***Laboratory Values for the Term Infant's First Day of Life***

| | | | |
|---|---|---|---|
| Sodium | 147 mEq/L | Total $CO_2$ | 19 mEq/L |
| Potassium | 5.6 mEq/L | Glucose | 40–120 mg/dL |
| Calcium | 9.3 mEq/L | Red blood cells | 5.0 $mm^3$ |
| Chloride | 103 mEq/L | Hematocrit | 61% |
| Hemoglobin | 20 gm/dL | White blood cells | 18,100 |
| Phosphorus | 5.6 mEq/L | Platelets | 151,000 $mm^3$ |

4

# REVIEW QUESTIONS

1. What is the primary predictor of infant survival?

2. What one effect does maternal smoking, alcohol ingestion, and cocaine ingestion have on fetal outcome?

3. Describe one action of the following drugs that are used to inhibit premature labor:

   a. Magnesium sulfate

   b. Terbutaline sulfate

   c. Nifedipine

4. How many gestational weeks is considered premature for a newborn infant?

5. What is the weight of a newborn infant who is classified as low birth weight?

6. Compare the difference between early deceleration, late deceleration, and variable deceleration of fetal heart rate.

   a. Early deceleration

   b. Late deceleration

   c. Variable deceleration

7. What does an L/S ratio of <2:1 indicate?

8. Define the following:

   a. Para

   b. Gravida

   c. Eclampsia

   d. Preeclampsia

   e. Placenta previa

   f. Abruptio placentae

9. Where does the main-stem bronchus bifurcate in the newborn?

10. What is the approximate length of the newborn trachea?

11. What is the difference between small for gestational age, appropriate for gestational age, and large for gestational age?

    a. Small for gestational age (SGA)

    b. Appropriate for gestational age (AGA)

    c. Large for gestational age (LGA)

12. What is the normal respiratory rate in the newborn infant?

13. What is the difference between periodic breathing and apnea?
    a. Periodic breathing
    b. Apnea

14. Describe the changes in inspiratory effort when a newborn develops respiratory distress.

15. What is the normal heart rate of a newborn infant? What is bradycardia?
    a. Normal heart rate
    b. Bradycardia

16. Within the first 12 to 24 h of life, what is the normal blood pressure for an infant in the following weight groups:
    a. 1000 to 2000 gm
    b. 2000 to 3000 gm
    c. More than 3000 gm

17. What scoring method approximates the newborn infant's gestational age?

18. How does the Ballard scoring method differ from the Dubowitz scoring method for approximating gestational age?

19. List the five observations of the Apgar scoring method.
    a.
    b.
    c.
    d.
    e.

20. Given the following Apgar assessment, determine the 1-min score:

    Body pink, extremities blue
    Pulse 136/min
    Coughing and sneezing following bulb suctioning
    Well-flexed extremities
    Good cry and good breathing effort
    1-min Apgar score =

21. Give an example of how heat loss can occur by the following mechanisms:
    a. Radiant
    b. Conduction
    c. Convection
    d. Evaporation

22. How does nonshivering thermogenesis generate heat in the newborn infant?

23. What is the importance of oxygen and glucose in the maintenance of thermal stability in the newborn infant?

24. What therapy is used to reduce serum bilirubin levels in the newborn infant?

25. Describe the importance of monitoring serum glucose concentration in the newborn receiving mechanical ventilation.

26. Fill in the normal laboratory values in the accompanying table.

| | | | |
|---|---|---|---|
| Potassium | | Hemoglobin | |
| Calcium | | Platelets | |
| Sodium | | Hematocrit | |
| Total $CO_2$ | | Glucose | |
| Chloride | | White blood cells | |

27. On chest radiograph, where should a properly placed endotracheal tube be located?

28. A proper inspiratory chest radiograph should have how many ribs above the diaphragm?

29. In the accompanying table, fill in the blood gas values.

| | **Umbilical Vein** | **Umbilical Artery** | **Within 5 Min After Birth** | **24 h to 7 Days After Birth** |
|---|---|---|---|---|
| pH | | | | |
| $PCO_2$ (mm Hg) | | | | |
| $PO_2$ (mm Hg) | | | | |
| $HCO_3$ (mEq/L) | | | | |
| $SaO_2$ (%) | | | | |

30. Fill in the radiological findings for each disease listed in the accompanying table.

| **Disease** | **Radiological Finding** |
|---|---|
| Transient tachypnea of the newborn | |
| Meconium aspiration syndrome | |
| Pneumothorax | |
| Pneumopericardium | |
| Pneumomediastinum | |
| Pulmonary Interstitial Emphysema | |
| Respiratory distress syndrome (HMD) | |
| Air bronchograms | |
| Pleural fluid | |
| Congenital diaphragmatic hernia | |
| Pneumonia (group B streptococcus) | |
| Bronchopulmonary dysplasia (advanced stages) | |

## BIBLIOGRAPHY


Avery, G. (1986). *Neonatology Pathophysiology and Management of the Newborn,* ed 3. Philadelphia: J. B. Lippincott.

Blackburn, S. (1995). Hyperbilirubinemia and neonatal jaundice. *Neonatal Network* 14:15.

Burgess, W., and Chernick, V. (1986). *Respiratory Therapy in Newborn Infants and Children,* ed 2. New York: Thieme Medical Publishers, Inc.

Carlo, W., and Chatburn, R. (1988). *Neonatal Respiratory Care.* Chicago: Year Book Medical Publishers.

D'Allessandro, M. P. (1996, September 10). Virtual Hospital Paedipedia: *Neonatal Chest Diseases* [WWW document]. URL http://indy.radiology.uiowa.edu/html

Fanoroff, A., and Martin, R. (1987). *Neonatal-Pediatric Medicine Disease of the Fetus and Infant.* St. Louis: Mosby.

Gerdes, J. S. (1996). Assessment of lung maturity. In Spitzer, A. R. *Intensive Care of the Fetus and Newborn.* St. Louis: Mosby-Year Book.

Gomella, T., and Cunningham, M. (1988). *Neonatology Basic Management: On Call Problems, Diseases, Drugs.* Norwalk, CT: Appleton & Lange.

Harwood, R. Intrauterine development and comparative respiratory anatomy. In Kacmarek, R. M., Mack, C., and Dimas, S. (1990). *The Essentials of Respiratory Care,* ed 3. St. Louis: Mosby-Year Book.

Harwood, R. Embryology and growth of the respiratory system. In Pierson, D., and Kacmarek, R. (1992). *Foundations of Respiratory Care.* New York: Churchill Livingstone.

Johnson, T. R. B. Perinatal monitoring. In Seidel, H. M., Rosenstein, B. J., and Pathak, A. (1997). *Primary Care of the Newborn,* ed 2. St. Louis: Mosby-Year Book.

Johnson, T. R. B. High-risk pregnancy. In Seidel, H. M., Rosenstein, B. J., and Pathak, A. (1997). *Primary Care of the Newborn,* ed 2. St. Louis: Mosby-Year Book.

Klans, M., and Fanaroff, A. (1986). *Care of the High-Risk Neonate,* ed 3. Philadelphia: W. B. Saunders.

Klein, A. (1996, May 17). *Management of Hyperbilirubinemia in the Healthy Full-Term Infant* [WWW document]. CSMC Neonatology on the WEB. NICU Files. URL http://www.CSMC.edu

Korones, S. (1986). *High-Risk Newborn Infants: The Basis for Intensive Care Nursing,* ed 4. St. Louis: Mosby.

Maisels, M., et al. (1988). Jaundice in the healthy newborn infant: A new approach to an old problem. *Pediatrics* 81:505.

Murenstein, G., and Gardner, S. (1995). *Handbook of Neonatal Intensive Care,* ed 3. St. Louis: Mosby.

Schreiner, F., and Bradburn, N. (1988). *Care of the Newborn,* ed 2. New York: Raven Press.

Seidel, H. M. Physical examination of the newborn. In Seidel, H. M., Rosenstein, B. J., and Pathak, A. (1997). *Primary Care of the Newborn,* ed 2. St. Louis: Mosby-Year Book.

Sehgal, S. (1996, October 1). *Kernicterus* [WWW document]. CSMC Neonatology on the WEB. NICU Teaching Files. URL http://www.CSMC.edu

Solof, A., Hunt, J., and Jain, A. (1996, July 1). *Hypoglycemia Monitoring Guidelines* [WWW document]. Vineland Pediatrics Homepage. URL http://www.acy.digex.net/~vpeds/vp/lga-prot.html

Wapner, R. F., Trauffer, P. M. L., and Johnson, A. Amniocentesis. In Spitzer, A. R. (1996). *Intensive Care of the Fetus and Neonate.* St. Louis: Mosby-Year Book.

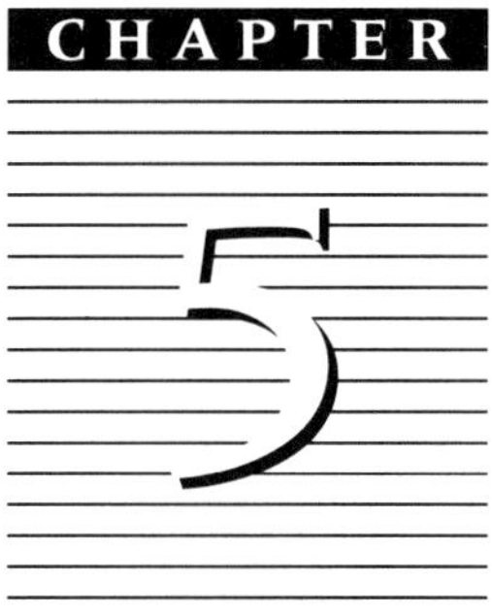


# Resuscitation of the Newborn Infant

## I. Neonatal asphyxia

A. Following normal birth, lungs expand, and blood flow increases to the lungs. Normal circulatory shunts close; these include the ductus arteriosus, ductus venosus, and foramen ovale.

B. Problems that occur in the newborn and that may have begun in utero may be the result of interruptions in the normal exchange of oxygen and carbon dioxide between the fetus and mother. These problems cause asphyxia, which is a deficiency in oxygen and an increase in carbon dioxide in blood and tissues.

C. Asphyxia may carry over into the newborn period if lung fluid remains in alveoli because of weak respiratory movement or apnea. Low partial pressure of alveolar oxygen ($PAO_2$) vasoconstricts pulmonary vasculature, increasing pulmonary artery pressure. As a result, right-to-left shunting continues through the ductus arteriosus and foramen ovale. Hypoxia and acidosis continue.

D. The mildly asphyxiated newborn develops the following:
   1. Bradycardia from hypoxemia
   2. Other signs include the following:
      a. Pallor
      b. Cyanosis (late)
      c. Irregular respirations
      d. Hypotension
   3. If adequate ventilation and oxygen are initiated immediately and the asphyxia is not severe, the heart rate improves and perfusion improves (in newborns, cardiac output is heart rate–dependent).

E. The severely asphyxiated newborn may not respond to oxygen and ventilation, and thus hypoxemia continues (Table 5–1). As a result:
   1. Continuous deterioration of the infant occurs.
   2. Metabolic acidosis occurs.
   3. Medications may be required to reverse asphyxiated state.

F. Primary versus secondary apnea
   1. An asphyxiated infant may present with either primary apnea or secondary apnea following birth.
   2. Primary apnea is present when rapid gasping occurs, respirations cease, and heart rate falls. Infants respond to tactile stimulation and exposure to oxygen by increasing heart rate and blood pressure (BP).
   3. If asphyxia continues, the infant develops deep, gasping respirations, heart rate continues to decrease, and the BP falls. Respirations become weaker, until a last gasp is taken by the infant. This period of time following the last gasp is secondary apnea. Heart rate, blood pressure, and partial pressure of

TABLE 5–1. ***Response by the Fetus and Newborn to Hypoxemia***

| Fetal Response | | Newborn Response |
|---|---|---|
| Reduced heart rate | → | Reduced heart rate |
| ↓ | | |
| Reduced CNS activity | | |
| ↓ | | |
| Reduced muscle activity | → | Poor muscle tone |
| Reduced response to stimulation | → | Decreased to absent reflexes |
| Poor respiratory effort | → | Apnea |

TABLE 5–2. ***Response by the Fetus and Newborn to Maternal Anesthesia and Analagesia***

| **Fetal Response** | | **Newborn Response** |
|---|---|---|
| Decrease CNS activity ↓ | | Heart rate may not be affected initially |
| Neuromuscular activity decreased | → | Poor muscle tone, flaccid |
| Response to stimuli decreased | → | Absent reflexes |
| Respiratory effort decreased | → | Apnea with bradycardia possible |

arterial oxygen ($PaO_2$) continue to fall. The infant is unresponsive to tactile stimulation and oxygen. The longer the delay in starting positive pressure ventilation (PPV), the longer it will take for the infant to initiate spontaneous respirations. Therefore, initiate PPV immediately. Studies show that without PPV with 100% oxygen, the $PaO_2$ can drop to 0 mm Hg; partial pressure of arterial carbon dioxide ($PaCO_2$) can rise 8 mm Hg/min; pH can drop 0.04 units/min; and sodium bicarbonate can drop 2 mEq/L/min within 5 min.

4. Since infants may be asphyxiated in utero, it may be difficult to differentiate between primary and secondary apnea at birth. Therefore, assume secondary apnea is present when an asphyxiated infant is presented at birth.

G. Causes of neonatal asphyxia
   1. Anesthetics, analgesics, and narcotics agents can cause asphyxia. Responses to these agents are listed in Table 5–2.
   2. Physical and mechanical hemorrhage (prolapsed cord, ruptured cord, and abruptio placentae)
   3. Developmental abnormalities (congenital heart disease, diaphragmatic hernia)
   4. Environmental (hypothermia)
   5. Postmaturity (meconium aspiration)
   6. Iatrogenic (excessive airway pressure during resuscitation)

**II. Initial steps in resuscitation. On receiving the newborn at birth, do the following:**

A. Bring the infant to a preheated radiant warmer, dry the infant, and discard wet towels. This will help prevent heat loss.

B. Open the infant's airway
   1. Make sure that the infant's neck is in a neutral, or sniffing, position with the head down.
   2. Suction the mouth and then the nose with a bulb syringe and continue evaluating during this procedure. Monitor the infant closely during oropharyngeal and nasopharyngeal suctioning because of potential vagal stimulation, which causes bradycardia and apnea.
   3. If thin, watery, meconium-stained fluid is present without particulate matter, then suction the mouth and nose with a bulb syringe. If particulate matter is thick, this requires that the trachea being viewed be suctioned past the vocal cords with a meconium aspirator or meconium suction device. NO PPV IS ADMINISTERED UNTIL TRACHEAL SUCTIONING IS COMPLETED. Continue suctioning until there is clear return through the catheter; then begin PPV with 100% oxygen.

C. Evaluate infant
   1. Normal respiratory rate is 30 to 60 breaths per minute (bpm) with good rhythm and depth. If these are present, then evaluate heart rate next.
   2. If the patient is apneic, then begin PPV with 100% oxygen.
      a. Bag the patient at a rate of 40 to 60 bpm.
      b. Apply appropriate pressure to open the lungs. Initially, this may require greater than 20 cm $H_2O$ because of the reduced lung compliance. As the lungs open and the lung compliance increases, reduce the peak pressure to 15 to 20 cm $H_2O$.
      c. Use of a 1-s inspiratory pause with PPV may help open the lungs and improve lung compliance. Studies show both pressure and inspiratory hold are effective in achieving spontaneous respirations. Of these two, pressure stimulation is more effective in stimulating an inspiratory effort by the newborn. Because of the wide variation in positive pressure during resuscitation, it is important to monitor these pressures with a manometer to minimize the incidence of pneumothorax.

3. Heart rate
   a. Palpate the umbilicus or auscultate the chest to determine heart rate.
   b. If more than 100 beats/min, then evaluate color.
   c. If less than 100 beats/min but greater than 80 beats/min, start PPV with 100% oxygen. After 15 to 30 s, re-evaluate and continue PPV if the heart rate is less than 100 but above 80 beats/min. If there is still no change after 2 min, intubate.
4. Color
   a. Acrocyanosis, which is normal immediately after birth, may be present in the hands and feet. If no central cyanosis is present and heart rate is greater than 100 beats/min with normal respiratory effort, then begin routine care.
   b. If central cyanosis is present (lips, mucous membranes, and ears) with spontaneous breathing, begin free-flowing oxygen. This can be delivered by the following:
      (1) Oxygen tubing or bag-mask over the mouth and nose.
      (2) Oxygen tubing with a liter flow of 5 to 8 L/min provides 80 to 100% oxygen within 1/2 in of the nose and mouth. Bag and mask flowrate should be sufficient to provide a flow from the bag. Generally, 8 to 10 L/min is sufficient with appropriate adjustment of the pressure relief device.
   c. Whenever possible, oxygen should be heated. Cold oxygen can cause breath holding and deceleration of heart rate, leading to bradycardia and apnea.

## III. Resuscitation bag

A. Flow-inflating resuscitation bag
   1. A flow-inflating resuscitation bag should have the following:
      a. Volume of 500 mL or less (the Vt of a newborn is 20 to 30 mL or 5 to 7 mL/kg of body weight).
      b. Able to deliver 100% oxygen
      c. Manometer attachment
      d. Pressure control or relief system
   2. Prior to administering positive pressure, the amount of pressure should be determined by squeezing the bag and observing the manometer. If appropriate pressure is not being achieved, two adjustments can be made. Flowrate can be adjusted, and the pressure relief device can be adjusted. It is easier to keep flowrate constant while adjusting the pressure relief device to maintain a specific pressure.

B. Self-inflation bag
   1. A reservoir is required to deliver a high fractional concentration of oxygen ($FIO_2$). Without a reservoir, the bag may only deliver a $FIO_2$ less than 0.50.
   2. The bag self-inflates and does not need an oxygen flow to inflate.

## IV. Bag and mask ventilation

A. Indications for bag and mask ventilation include the presence of apnea or a heart rate less than 100 beats/min.

B. A cushioned mask provides an appropriate seal when applied correctly.

C. Determine effective ventilation by:
   1. Looking for bilateral chest excursion
   2. Listening to breath sounds
   3. Improvement in heart rate, respirations, and color.
      a. Keep ventilating as heart rate increases. When the heart rate is greater than 100 beats/min, stop ventilating but continue giving oxygen by flow-by and monitor.
      b. When spontaneous breathing and heart rate are acceptable, provide gentle stimulation and monitor to determine if the infant has achieved acceptable rate and depth of breathing.
      c. Continue monitoring the infant for appropriate color change.

D. Inadequate chest expansion may occur because of the following:
   1. An inadequate mask seal. This will require repositioning of the mask.
   2. A blocked airway. Check for appropriate neutral or sniffing neck position. Check mouth, nasopharynx, and oropharynx for obstruction.
   3. Increase the pressure to achieve better chest expansion.

E. When bag-mask ventilating, insert an orogastric tube. This will prevent gastric and abdominal distension and remove gastric contents, preventing aspiration. After insertion and aspiration, leave open to room air and secure.

## V. Tracheal intubation

A. The upper airways of infants and adults differ structurally. The structure of the upper airway in infants predisposes them to obstruction caused by the narrowness of the nasal passages, glottis, and trachea. The larynx is situated higher in the neck at the level of the third or fourth cervical vertebra. The presence of highly vascular connective tissue predisposes the infant to development of subglottic edema caused by tracheal intubation.

B. Indications for intubation
   1. Ventilation: Intubation is needed if an infant has been on prolonged PPV with bag-mask ventilation.
   2. Obstruction: Intubation is needed when obstructive lesions of the airway decrease efficient ventilation from bag and mask ventilation. These problems may include, but are not limited to, the following:
      a. Tracheomalacia
      b. Laryngeal paralysis
      c. Webbing
      d. Stenosis
   3. Diaphragmatic hernia: An infant suspected of diaphragmatic hernia is intubated to prevent air from entering the bowel and compromising lung expansion.
   4. Suctioning: Tracheal suctioning is required for an infant born with thick or particulate meconium in the amniotic fluid.

C. Hazards and complications of endotracheal intubation
   1. Bradycardia: Provide oxygen and PPV with bag-mask. Monitor heart rate and oxygen saturation by pulse oximetry ($SpO_2$).
   2. Hypoxia: Ensure that the tube is properly placed, that the tube is not obstructed, and that the tube is not kinked. Provide oxygen and PPV with bag-mask. Monitor heart rate and $SpO_2$.
   3. Trauma to the lips, gums, pharynx, trachea, and vocal cords: Ensure use of an appropriately sized laryngoscope blade and endotracheal tube.
   4. Infection: Ensure the observation of clean, sterile technique, as possible.
   5. Pneumothorax: Main-stem intubation causing overinflation of one lung from PPV with bag-mask.

D. Equipment for intubation
   1. Endotracheal tube (ETT) (Table 5–3)
   2. Laryngoscope handle and blade. Blade—Miller No. 0,00 (premature) or No. 1 (term infant). Extra batteries and extra bulb
   3. Suction catheters, Nos. 5, 6, and 8 French
   4. Resuscitation bag and masks
   5. Oxygen source
   6. Tape or tube holder
   7. Benzoin
   8. Stylet
   9. Orogastric tube
   10. Oxygen tubing and flowmeter
   11. Stethoscope
   12. Bulb syringe

E. Route of intubation and procedure
   1. An infant being orally intubated should be on a flat surface with the head in midline position and the neck in a neutral or sniffing position. It may be helpful to place something under the baby's shoulders to maintain a slight extension of the neck.
      a. Hold the laryngoscope in left hand.
      b. Open the mouth with the fingers of the right hand.
      c. Insert the blade and sweep the tongue to the left.

TABLE 5–3. *Endotracheal Tube Size and Depth of Insertion*

| Weight of Infant (gm) (gestational age in weeks) | Endotracheal Tube Size (mm) | Depth of Insertion (cm) |
|---|---|---|
| <1000 (<28) | 2.5 | 6 |
| 1000–2000 (28–34) | 3.0 | 7, 8 |
| 2000–3000 (34–38) | 3.5 | 9 |
| 3000–4000 (>38) | 3.5–4.0 | 10 |

TABLE 5–4. ***Mainstem Bronchus vs. Esophageal Intubation***

| Mainstem Bronchus Intubation | Esophageal Intubation |
|---|---|
| Unilateral breath sounds—right greater than left.<br>No air entering stomach.<br>No gastric distention.<br>**What to Do?**—Pull tube back 1 cm; then listen for bilateral and equal breath sounds. Obtain chest radiograph to confirm location. | No breath sounds heard.<br>Air entering stomach.<br>Gastric distension; stomach contents may be seen in ETT.<br>**What to Do?**—Remove tube, bag-mask ventilate with oxygen. When infant is stabilized (heart rate and $SpO_2$) proceed with tracheal intubation. Confirm with chest radiograph. |

d. Advance the blade tip to just below the base of the tongue.
e. Lift the blade slightly to expose the pharyngeal area. (DO NOT use a rocking motion or pull the handle toward you.)
f. Once the glottic opening is identified, pass the ETT through the vocal cords using the vocal cord guide on the ETT as a reference for insertion depth.
g. Intubation should be completed within 20 s. If, after 20 s, the infant is not intubated, then stop intubating, and bag-mask ventilate with appropriate levels of oxygen to maintain heart rate, color, and $SpO_2$. Then reattempt the intubation.
h. Once the tube has been correctly placed, determine the correct depth of insertion (see Table 5–3).
i. Stabilize the tube and order a chest radiograph.

F. Determination of tube placement
1. Auscultation: Bilateral breath sounds should be evident.
2. Inspection: Symmetrical chest movement should be visible on inspiration.
3. Chest radiograph: The tip of the tube should be approximately at the level of the clavicles and/or above the carina.
4. Determination of incorrect placement of ETT: The main-stem bronchus intubation versus esophageal intubation (Table 5–4)

## VI. Chest compressions

A. Indications: After 15 to 30 s of PPV with 100% oxygen and the heart rate is less than 60 beats/min, or a heart rate between 60 to 80 beats/min and not increasing
B. Compression rate: 90/min
C. Compression depth: 1/2 to 3/4 in
D. Location of fingers: Fingers below nipple line over bottom third of sternum. Two methods can be used: (1) two-finger method on sternum, or (2) side-by-side method, where the hands are wrapped around the chest of the infant and the thumbs are located side by side on the sternum.
E. Ventilations: 30/min; interpose one breath every three compressions.
F. Heart rate situations
1. Check heart rate 30 s after compressions are initiated.
2. Check for 6 s by palpating the umbilicus.
   a. Example: 5 beats in 6 s = 50 beats/min.
3. Heart rate is 50 beats/min. You should do the following:
   a. Continue compressions, ventilate with 100% oxygen, and continue to check heart rate.
4. 30 s later, if the heart rate is 68 beats/min and not increasing, you should do the following:
   a. Continue compressions and check heart rate.
   b. If heart rate does not improve, medications may be administered (Tables 5–5 to 5–7).
5. 30 s later, the heart rate is 98 beats/min and rising. You should do the following:
   a. Stop compressions
   b. Continue ventilation until the heart rate is greater than 100 beats/min and the infant is breathing spontaneously. If the newborn is not intubated, provide oxygen by flow-by at 5 to 8 L/min and continue to monitor patient. If the patient is intubated, continue with PPV and transport to the neonatal intensive care unit (NICU).

TABLE 5–5. ***Indications, Action, and Desired Effects of Resuscitation Drugs***

| Drugs | Indications | Action | Desired Effects |
|---|---|---|---|
| Epinephrine | Heart rate remains below 80/min despite at least 30 s of PPV with 100% $O_2$ and chest compressions; or, heart rate is zero. | Cardiac stimulant: (+) inotropic (+) chronotropic | Increase heart rate over 100 beats/min within 30 s. Can be given every 5 min. |
| Volume expanders: Whole blood (O-negative blood cross-matched with mother's) | Pallor persisting after oxygenation. Weak pulses, good heart rate. Poor response to resuscitative effects. | Increases vascular volume. Improves tissue perfusion. | Increases BP. Strong pulse. Pallor improves. If no improvement, then consider metabolic acidosis (administer sodium bicarbonate). |
| 5% albumin/saline solution or other plasma substitute | Decreased or absent BP. | | |
| Normal saline Ringer's lactate | | | |
| Sodium bicarbonate | Documented metabolic acidosis pH < 7.10, base deficit > 15 mEq/L. | Buffers acids to bring pH back within normal range. Volume expander. Increases pH, which increases myocardial contractility. | Heart rate should increase >100 within 30 s. If no change, consider giving epinephrine, volume expander, and chest compressions (if not already started). |
| Naloxone hydrochloride (Narcan) | Respiratory depression and a history of the mother receiving a narcotic within the last 4 h. | Narcotic antagonist. | Spontaneous respirations. Readminister if respiratory depression continues or recurs. |

6. PPV requires an orogastric tube to be inserted to decompress the stomach with evidence of gastric insufflation. To determine the length of the tube, measure the tube from the infant's nose to the ear, and then from the ear to the xiphoid process. Attach a 20-mL syringe to the orogastric tube. After the tube is inserted, aspirate air and then leave the orogastric tube open to room air.

**VII. Management and care of the airway following intubation**

A. Suctioning
   1. Indications
      a. Course breath sounds by auscultation or "noisy" breathing
      b. Reduced tidal volume (pressure-limited, time-cycled ventilator); increased peak inspiratory pressure (PIP) (volume-cycled ventilator).
      c. Visible secretions in the airway
      d. Deterioration of $SpO_2$ or arterial blood gas values
      e. Radiologic changes consistent with retention of pulmonary secretions
   2. Hazards and complications
      a. Hypoxia and hypoxemia
      b. Cardiac dysrhythmia
      c. Infection
      d. Bronchospasm
      e. Elevated intracranial pressure
      f. Alteration in blood pressure
      g. Tissue trauma to trachea or bronchus
      h. Interruption of mechanical ventilation
   3. Assessment of outcome
      a. Breath sounds improved
      b. Improved $SpO_2$ and arterial blood gas value
      c. Pulmonary secretion removal
      d. Decreased PIP with narrowing of PIP-plateau pressure (volume-cycled ventilator), increased tidal volume (pressure-limited, time-cycled ventilator), decreased airway resistance, and increased dynamic compliance.

TABLE 5–6. ***Preparation of Resuscitation Drugs***

| | Epinephrine | Volume Expanders | Sodium Bicarbonate | Naloxone Hydrochloride |
|---|---|---|---|---|
| Prepare this amount of drug | 1 mL | 40 mL | 20 mL or two 10-mL prefilled syringes | 1 mL |
| Concentration | 1:10,000 | Whole blood; 10% albumin; NaCl; Ringer's lactate | 0.5 mEq/mL (4.2% solution) | 0.4 mg/mL or 1.0 mg/mL |
| Administer the drug via | ETT | IV | IV | Preferably by ETT or IV. IM or SQ response slower. |
| How much drug is given? | 0.1–0.3 mL/kg | 10 mL/kg | 2 mEq/kg | 0.1 mg/kg (for the 0.4 mg/mL concentration, give 0.25 mL/kg. For the 1.0 mg/mL concentration, give 0.1 mL/kg). |
| How fast is the drug given? | Fast | Over 5–10 min | Slow, at least 2 min. | For either concentrations, administer fast. |
| Special considerations | Dilute 1:1 with NaCl if giving down the ETT. Solution can be given through a No. 5 feeding tube inserted within the ETT. | Give by syringe or IV drip. | Patient must be ventilated because of $CO_2$ by-product formed from $NaHCO_3$ breakdown. Intracranial hemorrhage from fluid shifts and ↑ ABP. May worsen intracellular acidosis. | May have to give more than 1 dose because narcotic is longer lasting than Narcan dose. Seizures may occur in the infant of a narcotic-addicted mother. |

4. Monitor before, during, and after suctioning.
   a. Breath sounds
   b. Oxygen saturation, heart rate, and blood pressure
   c. Skin color
   d. Respiratory pattern and rate
   e. Sputum characteristics including volume, color, consistency, and odor
   f. Ventilator parameters including tidal volume, PIP, pressure, flow, and volume graphics
5. Vacuum pressure less than 100 mm Hg
6. Endotracheal tube size and appropriate catheter size (Table 5–8)
7. Administer a $FIO_2$ to maintain $SpO_2$ greater than 90%. Generally, the same $FIO_2$ is used during suctioning, unless the infant is desaturating below 90%. If the infant is desaturating, a higher $FIO_2$ is administered, either through the ventilator or by manual ventilation, to raise the saturation to greater than 90%. PEEP levels should be maintained for infants requiring greater than 5 cm $H_2O$.
8. Instill normal saline when thick secretions are present.
9. Use sterile technique and wear goggles, mask, and gloves according to universal precautions.
10. Suction methods.
    a. Insert the catheter with no suction until obstruction is felt, then withdraw the catheter 0.5 cm. Note the centimeter mark on the suction catheter at the top of the ETT. For future suctioning, the catheter will be advanced to this mark.
    b. Another method of estimating suction catheter insertion requires taking the centimeter mark at the top of the ETT and lining this up with 1-cm unit greater on the suction catheter. For example, if the top of the ETT centimeter mark is 13, then the catheter centimeter mark of 14 cm is

TABLE 5–7. ***Calculation of Dosage of Commonly Administered Resuscitation Drugs***

| Drug | Dosage | Infant's Weight | Dosage Calculation |
|---|---|---|---|
| Epinephrine | 0.1–0.3 mL/kg | 3250 gm (3.25 kg) | Infant's weight × drug dosage<br>3.25 kg × 0.1 mL = 0.325 mL<br>3.25 kg × 0.3 mL = 1.1 mL |
| Sodium bicarbonate | 2 mEq/kg (0.5 mEq/mL solution) | 3250 gm (3.25 kg) | Infant's weight × 2 mEq × 2 (converts mEq to mL)<br>3.25 × 2 × 2 = 13 mL of a 0.5 mEq/mL solution |
| Naloxone HCl (Narcan) | 0.1 mg/kg of a 0.4-mg/mL solution | 3250 gm (3.25 kg) | Infant's weight × 0.1 mg/kg<br>Conversion from mg to mL:<br>0.1 mg = 0.25 mL/kg<br>0.2 mg = 0.50 mL/kg<br>0.3 mg = 0.75 mL/kg<br>0.4 mg = 1.00 mL/kg<br>3.25 kg × 0.1 mg/kg = 0.325 mg<br>Convert 0.325 mg to mL<br>3.25 kg × 0.25 mL/kg = 0.8 mL |

lined up with the ETT centimeter mark of 13, giving a 1-cm distance beyond the end of the ETT.

11. Apply intermittent suction and withdraw. Suction should not be applied for any longer than 3 to 5 s.

TABLE 5–8. ***Endotracheal Tube Size and Catheter Size***

| ETT Size (mm) | Catheter Size (French) |
|---|---|
| 2.5 | 5–6 |
| 3.0 | 6 |
| 3.5 | 6–8 |
| 4.0 | 8 |

5

# REVIEW QUESTIONS

1. What are two causes of hypoxia in the fetus?

   a.

   b.

2. What is the difference between primary and secondary apnea?

   Primary apnea:

   Secondary apnea:

3. Why is it important to initiate immediate resuscitation efforts in the newborn recognized as having secondary apnea?

4. Describe the initial steps of resuscitation upon receiving a newborn following delivery.

5. In a normal newborn, why should a bulb syringe be used to remove secretions instead of a suction catheter?

6. What are the first three evaluations used to assess a newborn immediately following delivery?

   a.

   b.

   c.

7. Describe the sequence of events that should be followed if any of the 3 evaluations (in Question 6) are out of normal range.

8. What are two indications for bag-mask resuscitation?

   a.

   b.

9. Describe the difference between a flow-inflating resuscitation bag and self-inflating resuscitation bag.

   a. Flow-inflating resuscitation bag:

   b. Self-inflating resuscitation bag:

10. What is the importance of a pressure manometer and pressure-relief device found on a resuscitation bag?

11. List the appropriate ventilating rate and inflating pressure given the following situations.

    a. Newborn with normal compliant lungs immediately following delivery:

    Ventilating rate: Inflating pressure:

    b. Newborn with low compliant lungs immediately following delivery:

    Ventilating rate: Inflating pressure:

12. Describe the technique used to determine proper inflation pressure prior to administration of bag and mask ventilation.

13. List three signs in a newborn that would indicate effective bag-mask ventilation.

    a.

    b.

    c.

14. What actions should be taken if the infant is not responding to bag and mask resuscitation?

15. List and describe four indications for tracheal intubation.

    a.

    b.

    c.

    d.

16. List four hazards or complications of tracheal intubation and describe how these can be avoided.

    a.

    b.

    c.

    d.

17. List the equipment that should be available for tracheal intubation.

18. Fill in the accompanying table.

| Weight of Infant (gm) | Gestational Age (weeks) | Endotracheal Tube Size (mm inside diameter [ID]) | Depth of Insertion (cm) |
|---|---|---|---|
| <1000 | | | |
| 1000–2000 | | | |
| 2000–3000 | | | |
| 3000–4000 | | | |

19. How much vacuum pressure is used for suctioning an endotracheal tube? How long should suction be applied?

20. List three indications and three contraindications to suctioning.

| Indications | Contraindications |
|---|---|
| a. | a. |
| b. | b. |
| c. | c. |

21. List two assessments of outcome for suctioning.

    a.

    b.

22. What should be monitored before, during, and after suctioning an infant on mechanical ventilation (list three responses)?

    a.

    b.

    c.

23. Fill in the accompanying chart with the appropriate indications, actions, and desired effects of the listed medications.

| Drugs | Indications | Actions | Desired Effects |
|---|---|---|---|
| Epinephrine | | | |
| Volume expanders<br>Whole blood<br>5% albumin/saline solution or other plasma substitute<br>Normal saline<br>Ringer's lactate | | | |
| Sodium bicarbonate | | | |
| Naloxone hydrochloride (Narcan) | | | |

24. In the accompanying table, given the size of the endotracheal tube, list the size suction catheter used for suctioning.

| Endotracheal Tube (mm inside diameter [ID]) | Suction Catheter Size (French) |
|---|---|
| 2.5 | |
| 3.0 | |
| 3.5 | |
| 4.0 | |

## BIBLIOGRAPHY

American Association Respiratory Care Clinical Practice Guideline. (1993). Endotracheal suctioning of mechanically ventilated adults and children with artificial airways. *Respiration Care* 38:500.

American Heart Association. (1994). *Textbook of Neonatal Resuscitation*. Dallas.

Bhat, R., and Zikos-Labropoulou, E. (1986). Resuscitation and respiratory management of infants weighing less than 1000 grams. *Clinics in Perinatology* 13:285.

Brown, W., et al. (1976). Newborn response to oxygen blow over the face. *Anesthesiology* 14:535.

Field, D. J., Milner, A. D., and Hopkin, I. E. (1986). Intrathoracic pressure and volume changes during onset of respiration. *Archives of Disease in Childhood* 61:300.

Goldsmith, J., and Karotkin, E. (1997). *Assisted Ventilation of the Neonate*, ed 3. Philadelphia: W. B. Saunders.

Goldstein, B., et al. (1985). The role of manometers in minimizing peak and mean airway pressure during hand-regulated ventilation in newborn infants. *Lancet* 1:207.

Gomella, T., Cunningham, M., and Eyal, F. (1994). *Neonatology: Management, Procedures, On-Call Problems, Diseases and Drugs*, ed 3. Norwalk, CT: Appleton & Lange.

Hoskyns, E. W., et al. (1987). Endotracheal resuscitation of preterm infants at birth. *Archives of Disease in Childhood* 62: 663.

Koff P., Eitzman, D., and Neu, J. (1993). *Neonatal and Pediatric Respiratory Care*, ed 2. St. Louis: Mosby-Year Book.

Merenstein, G., and Gardener, S. (1993). *Handbook of Neonatal Intensive Care,* ed 2. St. Louis: Mosby.
Milner, A. D. (1991). Resuscitation of the newborn. *Archives of Disease in Childhood* 66:66.
Pawlak, R., and Herfert, L. A. (1988). *Drug Administration in the NICU.* Petaluma, CA: Neonatal Network.
Upton, C. J., and Milner, A. D. (1991). Endotracheal resuscitation of neonates using a rebreathing bag. *Archives of Disease in Childhood* 66:39.
Zaritsky, A. (1989). Drug therapy of cardiopulmonary resuscitation in children. *Drugs* 37:356.

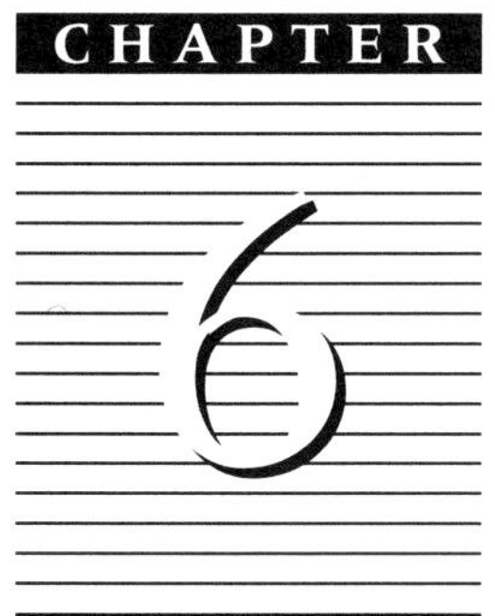

# Newborn Diseases

**I. Transient tachypnea in the newborn (TTN)**

A. Description
   1. TTN is also known as wet lung or type II respiratory distress syndrome (RDS).
   2. Seen in near term, term, and large premature infants.
   3. Respiratory distress shortly after birth. The disease is self-limiting and generally resolves within 3 days after birth.

B. Etiology and pathophysiology
   1. In TTN, there is delayed absorption of lung fluid at birth.
   2. Infants have normal surfactant development.
   3. Lecithin-sphingomyelin (L/S) ratio is normal.
   4. High-risk factors for development of TTN include the following:
      a. Maternal analgesia
      b. Asphyxia while in utero
      c. Prolonged labor greater than 18 h
      d. Prolapsed cord
      e. Cesarean section
      f. Infant of diabetic mother

C. Clinical presentation
   1. Good Apgar scores at birth, but within hours the newborn develops the following:
      a. Nasal flaring
      b. Grunting
      c. Retractions
      d. Cyanosis
      e. Tachypnea
   2. Respiratory rates may rise as high as 150 breaths per minute (bpm).
   3. Decreased lung compliance, increased respiratory rate, and decreased tidal volume.
   4. In general, the infant improves over the next 3 days, whereas the RDS infants worsen.

D. Laboratory findings
   1. Arterial blood gases (ABGs) while breathing room air show metabolic acidosis with hypoxemia and mild hypercarbia.
   2. Complete blood count (CBC) and differential are done to rule out infection.

E. Radiographic findings
   1. Pulmonary congestion and patchy infiltrates
   2. Enlarged anterior–posterior diameter and flattened diaphragms
   3. Prominent vascular markings (perihilar streaking)
   4. Fluid in minor fissure
   5. Chest radiographic findings may mimic neonatal sepsis, pneumonia (group B streptococcus) or cardiac problems, but conditions resolve within 24 to 48 h with TTN.

F. Treatment
   1. Supplemental oxygen to maintain the partial pressure of arterial oxygen ($PaO_2$) between 50 and 70 mm Hg and pulse oximetry greater than 90%. Generally, these infants respond to the administration of a fractional concentration of oxygen ($FIO_2$) of 0.40 to 0.50 by way of an oxygen hood. If no response to oxygen, cardiac abnormalities may be present.
   2. Continuous positive airway pressure (CPAP) may be used if there is no response to supplemental oxygen.

3. Generally, mechanical ventilation is not required because resolution occurs within 3 days. If the infant does not respond to oxygen and CPAP, then the infant is placed on mechanical ventilation and another disease should be suspected.

## II. Meconium aspiration syndrome (MAS)

A. Description
   1. Eleven to 22% of births present with meconium aspiration. Of these, 35% have meconium below the vocal cords. Newborns aspirating thick meconium are at greatest risk for developing MAS. In severe cases, pulmonary hypertension or pneumothorax leading to persistent pulmonary hypertension of the newborn develops requiring mechanical ventilation.
   2. MAS is seen in full-term and post-term newborns and is rarely seen in newborns less than 37 weeks' gestational age.
   3. White males have a higher incidence of MAS.

B. High-risk factors
   1. Post-term pregnancy
   2. Excessive maternal smoking
   3. Small for gestational age infants
   4. Maternal diabetes mellitus
   5. Oligohydramnios
   6. Abnormal fetal heart rate tracing (late deceleration pattern)

C. Etiology and pathophysiology
   1. MAS is associated with infants who aspirate meconium into the lungs.
   2. Meconium develops in the small intestines at about the fourth week of gestation. Meconium is found in the colon late in gestation because of the following:
      a. The consistency of meconium is highly viscous.
      b. The tone of the anal sphincter is constricted.
      c. Peristalsis is lacking (because of fetal gut vasoconstriction).
      d. Meconium is made up of undigested amniotic fluid and epithelial cells, pancreatic juice, mucus, and bile. Initially meconium is a viscous liquid. With further fetal development, meconium becomes thicker as water is absorbed by the fetus.
   3. With intrauterine hypoxia, apnea occurs initially. However, as hypoxia worsens, respiratory effort increases along with gasping. As a result of intrauterine hypoxia, redistribution of blood flow to vital organs causes relaxation of the anal sphincter and increased peristalsis. As meconium is passed into the amniotic fluid, aspiration of meconium into fetal lungs occurs. Further meconium may be aspirated into the lungs during birth. Respiratory distress develops following birth.
   4. Newborn infants with thin, watery meconium consistency have fewer respiratory problems than those with thick green "pea-soup" meconium.
   5. In the distal airway, a ball-valve obstruction may develop, leading to hyperinflation and atelectasis (in the nonaffected areas). Alveolar edema and mucosal damage result.
   6. Over the next few hours following birth, hypercarbia, hypoxia, and metabolic acidosis develop. The ductus arteriosus and foramen ovale may open, causing persistent fetal circulation. Consequently, a right-to-left shunt occurs, causing refractory hypoxia. Persistent pulmonary hypertension may also be present in these infants.
   7. If mechanical ventilation is required, barotrauma and pneumothorax may complicate the recovery.

D. Radiologic findings
   1. Coarse, irregular densities
   2. Diminished aeration
   3. Air bronchograms and consolidation in more severe cases
   4. Hyperexpansion with air trapping

E. Clinical presentation
   1. At birth, the infants appear yellow- or green-stained (especially at the nail beds) from the meconium.
   2. The newborn presents with the following:
      a. Low Apgar score
      b. Tachypnea
      c. Grunting
      d. Cyanosis
      e. Nasal flaring
      f. Hypoxia

3. Hyperexpanded chest from air trapping
4. Coarse rhonchi and rales
5. Prolonged expiration

F. Laboratory values
1. ABG values associated with mild meconium aspiration show respiratory alkalosis from hypoxia.
2. For infants with severe meconium aspiration who experienced severe intrauterine asphyxia and hypercarbia, combined respiratory acidosis and metabolic acidosis develops.

G. Treatment (Table 6–1)
1. Upon presentation of the newborn's head and before presentation of the thorax, the mouth, nose, nasopharynx, and oropharynx are suctioned. In spite of vigorous suctioning, the newborn infant may still have meconium below the vocal cords.
2. The infant is taken to the preheated radiant warmer, and the posterior pharynx is suctioned. If the meconium is thick or the infant is depressed, direct endotracheal tube suctioning with a meconium aspirator is performed (see Chapter 5). A vigorous infant with thin meconium may not need endotracheal suctioning.
3. Clearing of meconium by suction is performed before bag or mask positive-pressure ventilation (PPV) is administered. This will facilitate removal of meconium in the lungs and will prevent distal movement of meconium. Generally, good suctioning before the first breath will decrease the incidence of tracheal intubation. Tracheal intubation can be reserved for depressed infants requiring PPV.
4. Supplemental oxygen is provided to raise the $PaO_2$ above 50 mm Hg.
5. Vigorous chest physiotherapy may be performed once the infant is stabilized.
6. Newborns who do not respond to increased $FIO_2$ may require CPAP or mechanical ventilation. These infants tend to have a lower 1-min Apgar score at birth.
7. CPAP may help some infants to maintain $PaO_2$ greater than 50 mm Hg. Watch for hyperinflation from air trapping.
8. Those infants not responding to CPAP require mechanical ventilation. The following are ABG indications for mechanical ventilation:
   a. pH less than 7.20
   b. Partial pressure of arterial carbon dioxide ($PaCO_2$) greater than 70 mm Hg
   c. $PaO_2$ less than 50 mm Hg
   d. $SpO_2$ less than 90%
9. Goals of mechanical ventilation
   a. Maintain $PaCO_2$ less than 50 mm Hg
   b. Maintain $PaO_2$ greater than 50 mm Hg
   c. Maintain pH greater than 7.30
10. Ventilator settings
   a. Short inspiratory times and long expiratory times to prevent air trapping.
   b. Lowest peak inspiratory pressure necessary to achieve good chest excursion and adequate tidal volume.

TABLE 6–1. ***Mild, Moderate, and Severe Meconium Aspiration Syndrome (MAS)***

| **Mild (+1)** | **Moderate (+2, +3)** | **Severe (+4)** |
|---|---|---|
| Tachypnea<br>Mixed acidosis with mild hypoxemia. Patient is stable.<br>Treatment: Head hood with an $FIO_2$ of 0.30–0.40. Goals for ABGs: pH > 7.30, $PaO_2$ > 50 mm Hg, $PaCO_2$ < 50 mm Hg. Generally, symptoms resolve with 48–72 h following birth. | Initially, symptoms resemble mild MAS.<br>Infant worsens. ABGs: Mixed acidosis and worsening hypoxemia.<br>Treatment: Initially may use a head hood at $FIO_2$ of 0.40. If no improvement (ABGs same goal as in mild MAS), then initiate CPAP or mechanical ventilation. Generally, this is short term if the newborn does not develop PPHN or sepsis (3–7 days of therapy). | Severe respiratory acidosis within hours after birth.<br>Severe mixed acidosis with profound refractory hypoxemia. Presence of PPHN and PDA. Potential pneumothorax.<br>Treatment: Refractory hypoxemia requiring initiation of mechanical ventilation. May be unresponsive to ventilatory care. High-frequency ventilation, ECMO may be required. |

c. Minimal positive end-expiratory pressure (PEEP) (5 cm $H_2O$ or less).
d. $FIO_2$ to maintain $PaO_2$ greater than 50 mm Hg and $SpO_2$ greater than 90%. If the infant is diagnosed with persistent pulmonary hypertension in the newborn (PPHN), high $FIO_2$s are required to keep the $PaO_2$ greater than 80 to 90 mm Hg.
e. The oxygenation index (OI) has been used to predict those infants requiring extracorporeal membrane oxygenation (ECMO) (see Chapter 15). The OI formula is ($\bar{P}aw$) $FIO_2 \times 100/PaO_2$. Infants with an OI above 40 have a greater than 80% chance of mortality. Therefore, ECMO is required for survival.

11. Broad-spectrum antibiotics
12. High-frequency oscillation (HFO)
13. ECMO
14. Surfactant administration

## III. Pulmonary air leaks (PAL)

A. Description of PAL
1. Rupture of overdistended alveoli where visceral and parietal pleura join. A spontaneous pneumothorax results when air enters the pleural space. With further accumulation and pressure within this cavity, a tension pneumothorax will develop. Air can dissect along perivascular or interstitial spaces, causing pulmonary interstitial emphysema (PIE). Air may dissect into the mediastinum, causing a pneumomediastinum. Air can also dissect into the pericardium sac from the mediastinum, causing pneumopericardium.

B. Pneumothorax
1. Description
a. Commonly, pneumothorax develops from rupturing of blebs from excessive pressure or volume. These pressures may be from PPV during vigorous resuscitation.
b. Infants with pulmonary disease who are on mechanical ventilation are also at high risk for pneumothorax. Infants breathing asynchronously with the ventilator can develop pneumothoraces from increased intrathoracic pressures.

2. Etiology and pathophysiology
a. Compliant alveoli adjacent to atelectatic alveoli may be overdistended from high intrapulmonary pressure.
b. There may be ruptured alveoli blebs from uneven distribution of air in premature lungs.
c. Noncompliant lungs become more compliant while on mechanical ventilation following surfactant administration.
d. Pneumothorax may develop from thickened secretions, resulting in air trapping if inspired temperatures of gases are not kept in the appropriate range of 35 to 37°C. This will provide appropriate water content to the lung (greater than 36 mg/L).

3. Clinical presentation
a. Hypertension precedes a small pneumothorax
b. Hypotension precedes a large pneumothorax
c. Tachypnea
d. Tachycardia
e. Cyanosis
f. Pallor
g. If an infant is on mechanical ventilation, there may be increased respiratory efforts.
h. There will be a change in cardiac impulse shifting away from the affected side (with tension pneumothorax).
i. There will be decreased chest excursion and breath sounds on affected side.

4. Diagnosis
a. Perform a rapid radiologic interpretation. When this is not available, use transillumination. The transilluminator is placed superior, and then inferior, to the newborn's nipple bilaterally in a darkened room. If the chest "lights up," this suggests that there is an abnormal amount of air in the chest cavity. The unaffected lung appears darker.
b. Pneumopericardium or pulmonary interstitial emphysema may accompany pneumothorax.

5. Management and treatment
a. For infants on mechanical ventilation who are in distress, prompt decompression with tube thoracostomy is required. The chest tube is placed

between the second and third intercostal space lateral to the midclavicular line.

b. The chest tube is connected to an underwater seal drainage unit with an appropriate amount of suction. Improvement of the newborn's condition is immediate, unless other pneumothoraces occur or other conditions limit the improvement of the infant.

C. Pneumomediastinum
   1. Often this is asymptomatic and is found during inspection for a pneumothorax.
   2. Clinical presentation
      a. Tachycardia
      b. Increased anteroposterior chest diameter
      c. Decreased heart sounds
      d. Symptoms of respiratory distress
      e. Subcutaneous emphysema
      f. Severe pneumomediastinum associated with distended neck veins and decreased BP
   3. Radiographic appearance
      a. Anterior air causes the bilobed thymus to be pushed upward away from the heart.
   4. Treatment and management
      a. Commonly no treatment is required—just observation. Rarely does the condition become severe enough to cause clinical deterioration.
      b. If treatment is required, using 100% oxygen with an oxygen hood may be helpful to resolve the pneumomediastinum. With further deterioration, insertion of a chest tube is recommended.

D. Pneumopericardium
   1. This can be anywhere in the range of asymptomatic to life threatening.
   2. Clinical presentation
      a. Cardiac tamponade
      b. Initially, there is increased cardiac output and tachycardia. As the pneumopericardium becomes more severe, decreased cardiac output, hypotension, and bradycardia develop.
   3. Radiologic appearance
      a. Hyperlucent ring around the heart
   4. Treatment and management
      a. Asymptomatic infants who are not on mechanical ventilation require monitoring and intervention only when clinical deterioration develops.
      b. Infants receiving ventilatory assistance require placement of pericardial tubes.

E. Pulmonary interstitial emphysema (PIE)
   1. Predisposing factors
      a. Infants on mechanical ventilation
      b. Lung immaturity
      c. RDS
      d. Aspiration syndromes
      e. Infection
      f. Pulmonary anomalies such as lung hypoplasia or diaphragmatic hernia
   2. The earlier the appearance of PIE following birth, the greater the mortality rate.
   3. Etiology and pathophysiology
      a. As a result of PPV, a small rupture in the alveoli occurs, allowing air to move outside of the lungs. As air moves out, it dissects along peribronchial and perivascular sheaths, interlobular septa, visceral pleura, alveoli ducts, and lymphatics. This results in air-filled cysts.
      b. The alveoli-capillary membrane widens, causing diffusion problems.
      c. Pneumomediastinum and/or pneumothorax may result from rupturing alveoli. This process may be localized or diffuse.
      d. A high $\bar{P}$aw increases the incidence of PIE. Ventilator settings that lead to an increased $\bar{P}$aw include the following:
         (1) Peak inspiratory pressure (PIP) greater than 25 cm $H_2O$.
         (2) PEEP greater than 5 to 10 cm $H_2O$.
         (3) Inspiratory time greater than 0.3 s.
         (4) Expiratory time less than 0.3 s.
         (5) Reverse inspiratory-expiratory (I/E) ratio.
         (6) Inadvertent PEEP from the following:
            (a) Increased rate
            (b) Small ETT less than 3 mm internal diameter (ID)

(c) Increased airway resistance
(d) Prolonged time constants
(7) Asynchronous breathing will increase intrathoracic pressures, leading to PAL.

4. Radiologic appearance
   a. The chest radiograph will have a bubble appearance because of cyst formation.
   b. Progression of the disease causes cysts called pneumatoceles to enlarge, which decreases diffusion.
5. Management and treatment
   a. Reduce $\bar{P}aw$
   b. Maintain low mechanical ventilator settings while keeping blood gas values within ranges as acceptable as possible.
   c. Maintain PIP at less than 25 cm $H_2O$.
   d. Maintain PEEP at 5 cm $H_2O$ or less.
   e. Check for inadvertent PEEP levels.
   f. Perform selective intubation of the uninvolved lung.
   g. Place the affected side in a dependent position (unless very small premature infant).
   h. HFO

## IV. Persistent pulmonary hypertension in the newborn (PPHN)

A. Description
1. In spite of lung expansion and increased $PaO_2$, the pulmonary vascular resistance (PVR) fails to decrease. The PVR is the same or greater than systemic pressure. As a result, persistent opening of the ductus arteriosus and foramen ovale occurs. This causes right-to-left shunting that is secondary to pulmonary hypertension.
2. Refractory hypoxemia and severe systemic hypoxemia develop.
3. There are three forms of PPHN:
   a. PPHN associated with pulmonary parenchymal disease, such as hyaline membrane disease, and meconium aspiration. In this type, PVR is the result of decreased alveolar oxygen tension.
   b. PPHN with radiographically normal lungs, frequently called persistent fetal circulation (PFC).
   c. PPHN associated with hypoplasia of the lungs in the form of diaphragmatic hernia where the number of capillary vessels is reduced and obstructed from the reduced lung size.

B. Etiology
1. No etiology can be found in many cases of PPHN. Conditions in infants at high risk for developing PPHN include the following:
   a. Sepsis
   b. Meconium aspiration
   c. RDS
   d. Diaphragmatic hernia
   e. Idiopathic PPHN
   f. Congenital heart disease
   g. Maternal factors such as diabetes or cesarean section

C. Pathophysiology
1. In infants who die of PPHN, there is an increase in muscle within the blood vessels from the small pulmonary arteries down to the arteries within the alveolar walls. This muscularization reduces the internal diameter of the vessel, which increases the PVR. Blood flow tends to stagnate or be completely reduced, as a result reducing the cross-sectional area of the pulmonary vasculature. Formation of pulmonary emboli within these vessels as a result of stagnation of blood flow further reduces the vascularity. Larger arteries are also affected. Smooth muscle is thicker, and this occludes the lumen and reduces the number of small arteries.
2. The elevation of PVR in PPHN may also be from a decreased release of vasodilator substances, an increased release of vasoconstrictor substances, altered smooth-muscle-cell responsiveness to birth-related stimuli, and vasoactive mediators.

D. Clinical presentation
1. The disease is noted in term and post-term infants. Within 12 h following birth, the infant presents with cyanosis, tachypnea, and signs and symptoms of respiratory distress. A large right-to-left shunt is seen through the ductus arteriosus and the foramen ovale.

2. ABGs show hypoxemia and hypercarbia.
3. There is a heart murmur.

E. Diagnosis
1. PPHN can occur in conjunction with pulmonary, cardiovascular, or other generalized disorders.
2. Consider PPHN with any hypoxic infant.
3. When diagnosing PPHN, remember the history of pregnancy, labor, and delivery as well as risk factors.
4. Infants with congestive heart disease (CHD) do not have these risk factors.
5. Perform tests to differentiate between parenchymal lung disease, PPHN, and cyanotic CHD.
   a. Hyperoxia test
      (1) Place infant in 100% oxygen for 5 to 10 min.
      (2) Determine $PaO_2$. If $PaO_2$ is greater than 100 mm Hg, lung disease is probable. If $PaO_2$ is less than 50 mm Hg, either PPHN or cyanotic congenital heart disease is present (a right-to-left shunt is present).
   b. To determine if shunting is present, do a preductal and postductal comparison.
   c. Perform a preductal and postductal gas sample comparison (simultaneous gases).
      (1) Infant breathes 100% oxygen.
      (2) Measure blood gases from preductal arteries: right radial, right brachial, and temporal. For postductal arteries, use the left radial, posterior tibial, and umbilical artery.
      (3) Preductal and postductal transcutaneous oxygen measurements can be obtained by placing an electrode on the postductal position of the left lower quadrant of the chest and on the preductal position of the right upper quadrant of the chest.
      (4) Results: A preductal and postductal $PaO_2$ difference of greater than 15 mm Hg indicates ductal shunting (in some cardiac problems, ductal values may be normal). For example, ductal shunting is present if the preductal value is 60 mm Hg and the postductal value is 30 mm Hg. Reduced ductal shunting is present if the preductal value is 200 mm Hg and the postductal value is 90 mm Hg. Although the value difference is greater than 15 mm Hg, the postductal value is normal. Differences between preductal and postductal $SpO_2$ also are helpful in determining shunting. For example, a preductal value of 96% and a left lower extremity value of 80% indicates shunting.
   d. Hypoxemia-hyperventilation test.
      (1) Most definitive to determine PPHN.
      (2) Performed on intubated and nonintubated infants.
      (3) Patient is hyperventilated either by face mask and resuscitation bag or connected to an endotracheal tube with an $FIO_2$ of 1.0.
      (4) Watch rise and fall of chest, and listen to breath sounds to determine ventilation.
      (5) Results: PPHN is diagnosed if the postductal $PaO_2$ increases. By hyperventilating, $PaCO_2$ will decrease, pH becomes alkalotic, and the $PaO_2$ will increase, thus reducing pulmonary vascular resistance, pulmonary hypertension, and right-to-left shunting.
   e. Right-to-left shunting is also diagnosed by contrast echocardiography or color Doppler imaging.

F. Management and treatment
1. Mechanical ventilation
   a. Set peak inspiratory pressures and rate to hyperventilate. Maintain ABGs as follows:
      (1) $PaCO_2$ between 25 and 30 mm Hg (critical $PCO_2$ level).
      (2) pH greater than 7.50 to 7.55 (alkalosis has greatest effect on reducing pulmonary vasoconstriction).
      (3) $PaO_2$ at greater than 60 mm Hg (use as low an $FIO_2$ as possible to achieve this).
2. Conservative approach—ventilator settings adjusted to achieve the following:
   a. $PaCO_2$ at 35 to 45 mm Hg
   b. $PaO_2$ at 60 to 80 mm Hg
   c. pH at 7.50
   d. Sodium bicarbonate is infused to cause systemic alkalosis, thus reducing the degree of hyperventilation and barotrauma. Monitor serum sodium levels.

3. Pharmacology
   a. The alpha-adrenergic antagonist tolazoline (Priscoline) vasodilates the pulmonary arteries to reduce PAP. Side effects include pulmonary hemorrhage, GI bleeding, and systemic hypotension.
   b. Volume expanders, dopamine, and dobutamine may be used to treat systemic hypotension and reduce right-to-left shunting.
   c. Prostaglandin $I_2$ ($PGI_2$) is a major vasodilator of the lungs. It is produced by the lungs when they are in a constricted state, thereby relaxing pulmonary vasculature. Side effects include systemic hypotension.
4. Induce muscle paralysis and sedation.
5. Institute fluid therapy, transfusions, and antibiotics as indicated.
6. Institute nitric oxide (NO) therapy.
   a. NO is found in the airway cells and endothelium of the pulmonary vasculature. The normal quantity of NO exhaled from the lung is 6 to 8 parts per million (ppm).
   b. In the perinatal lung, there is a marked increase in NO activity, leading to a dramatic decrease in PVR and PAP and an increase in blood flow during the transition to an adult circulation. Stimulation of NO occurs by shear stress of tissue as breathing movements and ventilation begin. NO activity remains high up to 2 weeks after birth.
   c. NO, which has been identified as an endothelium-derived relaxing factor (EDRF), performs functions such as neurotransmission, regulation of vascular tone, and bronchodilation.
   d. In the newborn, PVR and PAP decrease because of an increase in oxygen tension. This vasorelaxation is mediated by NO through the pathway shown in Figure 6–1. Endothelial cell production of NO is dependent on an amino acid in the blood (L-arginine), which is synthesized by the enzyme nitric oxide synthase. NO then activates guanylate cyclase in vascular smooth muscle and increases intracellular cyclic guanosine monophosphate (cGMP) levels.
   e. As a gas, NO rapidly diffuses across lipid membranes into underlying vascular smooth muscle, activating soluble guanylate cyclase, increasing cGMP levels and causing vasorelaxation. Some of the NO that enters the intravascular space quickly binds with hemoglobin, forming nitrosyl hemoglobin (bioactivity is reduced and prevents systemic activity), which then forms nitrate, nitrite, and methemoglobin. Nitrate and nitrite are

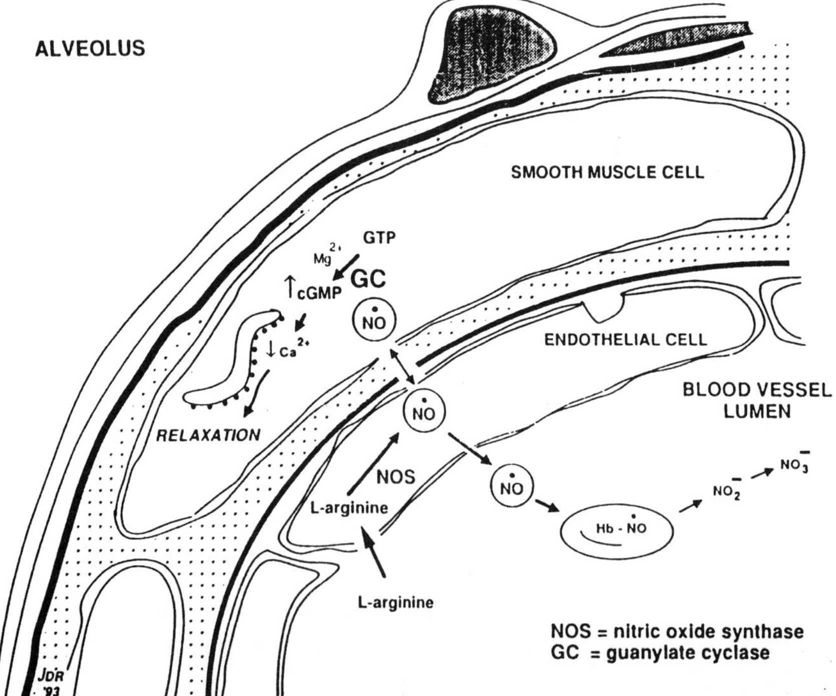


**FIGURE 6–1** Illustration of nitric oxide synthesis and action. (Fratacci, MD, Frostell, CG, and Chen, TY, et al. [1991]. Inhaled nitric oxide: A selective pulmonary vasodilator of heparin-protamine vasoconstriction in sheep. *Anesthesiology* 75:990, with permission.)

TABLE 6–2. ***Summary of Treatments and Rationale for PPHN***

| Treatment | Rationale |
|---|---|
| Hyperventilation | Decrease pulmonary vascular resistance and pulmonary artery pressure by making the infant alkalotic. |
| Sodium bicarbonate | Decrease pulmonary vascular resistance and pulmonary artery pressure by making the infant alkalotic. |
| Tolazoline | Decrease pulmonary vascular resistance and pulmonary artery pressure by vasodilating the pulmonary vascular bed. |
| Dopamine, dobutamine | Increase systemic blood pressure and decrease right-to-left shunt. |
| Nitric oxide | Reduce PVR, PAP, and right-to-left shunting and increase $PaO_2$. |
| Oxygen | Reduce PVR, PAP, and right-to-left shunting. |
| Fresh frozen plasma, saline | Increase systemic blood pressure and decrease right-to-left shunt. |

released in the urine. Methemoglobin is converted back into hemoglobin by methemoglobin reductase, which is found in erythrocytes. Methemoglobin levels should be measured periodically.

f. Since infants are on mechanical ventilation or high-frequency ventilation, NO is delivered through the inspiratory side of the patient circuit. A hazard of delivering NO within the ventilator circuit is that it may convert to $NO_2$, which is toxic to the body. Therefore, NO and $NO_2$ must be analyzed as close to the patient as possible. The analyzer records the level of NO in parts per million. Also, the ventilator must be attached to a scavenger system to collect exhaled NO gas.

g. NO is delivered in variable concentrations. In studies, low doses of NO (as low as 5 ppm) and high doses (as high as 80 ppm) delivered over a period from a few hours up to 72 h have sustained vasodilation; furthermore, the lower doses were as effective as the higher doses. Selecting the optimal dose is critical, since the higher dose may have a greater potential for toxicity from $NO_2$ formation and methemoglobinemia.

G. Summary (Table 6–2)

**V. Infant respiratory disease syndrome (IRDS); hyaline membrane disease**

A. Incidence
1. Occurs in 60% of premature infants weighing less than 1500 gm at birth.
2. Occurs in those with a gestational age of less than 35 weeks (5% of newborns).
3. Occurs in those with risk factors for RDS, which include the following:
   a. Cesarean section delivery
   b. Maternal hemorrhage
   c. Maternal diabetes
   d. Asphyxia at birth
   e. Multiple births
   f. Prematurity
      (1) Surfactant deficiency (Table 6–3)
      (2) Compliant chest wall
      (3) Incomplete lung structure, resulting in severely reduced compliance (Fig. 6–2).
      (4) Patent ductus arteriosus, which causes a right-to-left shunt.
      (5) Increased pulmonary perfusion from left-to-right shunt, causing pulmonary edema (Table 6–4).

B. Clinical presentation (onset of symptoms may be present at birth or a short time after birth)
1. Low Apgar score
2. Expiratory grunting
3. Nasal flaring
4. See-saw breathing
5. Tachypnea
6. Compliant chest wall sinks in during inspiratory phase and reduces alveolar ventilation.
7. Oxygen requirements differ. Severely affected infants require 100% immediately following birth, whereas less severe cases may require increased concentrations a few hours following birth.

C. Radiologic findings
1. Classic appearance in the untreated newborn is reticulogranular infiltrates 12 to 24 h after birth.

TABLE 6–3. ***Hyaline Membrane Formation***

**Pulmonary Complications from Surfactant Deficiency—Hyaline Membrane Formation**

Premature infant with hypoxia and acidosis
(Reduced surfactant production)

↙ ↘

| | |
|---|---|
| Capillary permeability<br>↓<br>Fluid/fibrin exudate (plasminogen)<br>↓<br>Hyaline membrane formation (lines terminal bronchioles and alveolar ducts)<br>↓<br>Increased diffusion gradient (↑ $AaDO_2$)<br>↓<br>Further reduction of surfactant production because of changes in blood pH, perfusion, and temperature)<br>↓<br>Within 72 h of formation of hyaline membrane, macrophages begin eliminating the membrane by means of phagocytosis. | Pulmonary vasoconstriction<br>↓<br>Pulmonary hypertension<br>↓<br>Pulmonary hypoperfusion and extra pulmonary right-to-left shunt. |

2. "Ground-glass" appearance
3. Air bronchograms
4. Decreased lung volume

D. Diagnosis based on the following:
1. History
2. Clinical assessment
3. Radiologic findings
4. Lab evaluation

E. Laboratory findings
1. ABGs
   a. Initially: pH less than 7.30, $PaCO_2$ less than 40 mm Hg, and $PaO_2$ less than 50 mm Hg.
   b. Progression of disease: pH less than 7.25, $PaCO_2$ greater than 45 mm Hg, and $PaO_2$ less than 40 mm Hg.
2. Urine output low from lack of peripheral perfusion before second day of life. If spontaneous diuresis occurs on the second or third day, respiratory

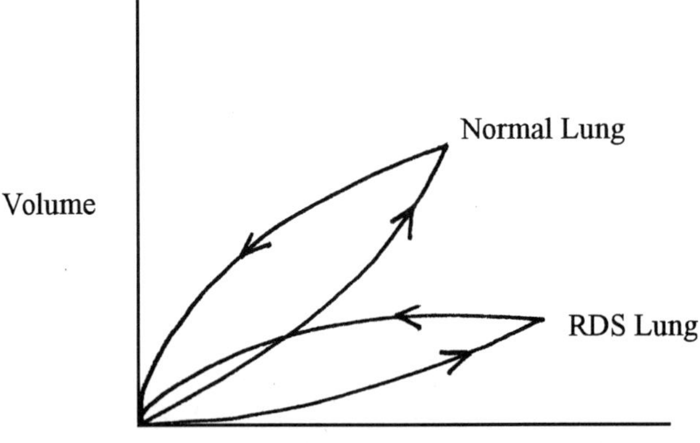


**FIGURE 6–2** Graphic illustration showing a normal volume-pressure curve (V-P) and a V-P that reflects RDS. Notice the amount of pressure that is generated to create a volume change in the RDS lung as compared to the normal lung.

TABLE 6–4. ***Formation of Pulmonary Edema from Surfactant Deficiency***

**Hemodynamic Complications from Surfactant Deficiency—Pulmonary Edema**

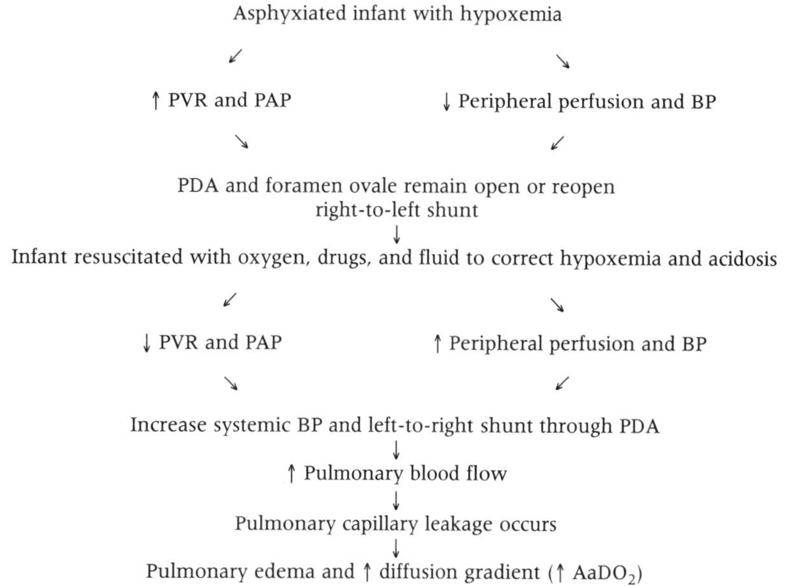


improvement occurs (urine output greater than 80% of fluid intake) and alveolar-arterial diffusion gradient and arterial-alveolar ratio improve.

F. Treatment and management
1. Prevent birth as long as possible to allow lungs to mature.
2. Administer glucocorticoids.
   a. Evidence suggests that antenatal administration of corticosteroids administered prior to preterm delivery is associated with a substantial reduction in the incidence of neonatal death, as well as in RDS, intraventricular hemorrhage, and necrotizing enterocolitis. Administration of corticosteroids has been shown to stimulate both production of surfactant and structural development of the lungs. In addition to surfactant secretion, glucocorticoids increase lung compliance and maximal volume independent of surface-active material. Furthermore, protein leak from the pulmonary vasculature is reduced, which accelerates the removal of lung fluid before delivery. Beneficial effects are greatest more than 24 h after beginning treatment, although treatment less than 24 h in duration also improves outcome. Dexamethasone and beclomethasone are preferred for antenatal therapy.
3. Avoid hypoxemia and hypercapnia and improve gas exchange after birth.
4. Indications for exogenous surfactant replacement include the following:
   a. An infant who weighs less than 1300 gm or is less than 32 weeks' gestational age.
   b. A L/S ratio or bubble stability test that shows immature lungs.
   c. The absence of phosphatidylglycerol.
   d. Results of surfactant administration include improved survival, improved gas exchange (increased $PaO_2$), improved pulmonary mechanics, and significant reduction in pulmonary air leak and barotrauma. The $\bar{P}aw$ and respiratory rate decrease, and there is a greater ability to change more quickly from mechanical ventilation to CPAP. The mortality rate of BPD decreased (although the incidence did not change) because of rapid weaning and a reduced incidence of volutrauma.
   e. Two methods of administering surfactant include prophylaxis and rescue.
      (1) Prophylaxis is administered two ways. In the first, it is given in the delivery room to an intubated infant immediately following birth. The advantages of this method include that the optimal distribution of surfactant occurs with a fluid-filled lung and surfactant is administered before PPV is initiated. The disadvantage of giving surfactant this way is that the infant must be intubated and the position of the ETT

may not be confirmed by chest radiograph. If the ETT is in the right main-stem bronchus, surfactant is put into the right lung. This will overdistend that lung, potentially leading to an air leak if positive pressure by mechanical ventilation is administered. The left lung is still atelectatic. The second method administers surfactant after a short period of resuscitation (5 to 30 min).

(2) Rescue therapy of surfactant is given after a diagnosis of RDS has been made using clinical and radiologic criteria. Surfactant is administered when the infant is receiving a $FIO_2$ of 0.30 to 0.40 and the $\bar{P}aw$ is 7 cm $H_2O$. The advantage of this method is that only RDS infants who are stabilized in the neonatal intensive care unit (NICU) are treated. The disadvantage is that lung damage and atelectasis may have occurred secondary to hyperoxia and mechanical ventilation.

f. Hazards and contraindications
   (1) Plugging of the endotracheal tube
   (2) Desaturation and increased need for supplemental oxygen
   (3) Bradycardia from hypoxia
   (4) Tachycardia from agitation
   (5) Deposition of surfactant in one lung
   (6) Inaccurate dosing from miscalculation of drug
g. Indication of improvement following dosing
   (1) Decreased $FIO_2$ requirement
   (2) Decreased work of breathing
   (3) Increased lung volumes and lung field, as noted by chest radiograph
   (4) Improved pulmonary functions, specifically dynamic compliance, airway resistance, tidal volume, and minute ventilation.
   (5) Reduction in PIP, PEEP, and $\bar{P}aw$
   (6) Increase in $a/AO_2$ and oxygen index
h. Monitor the following when administering surfactant:
   (1) Proper placement of endotracheal tube and position
   (2) $FIO_2$ and ventilator settings
   (3) Chest wall movement
   (4) Saturation by pulse oximeter
   (5) Heart rate, respiratory rate, and skin color
i. The following are indications for the multiple administration of surfactant:
   (1) Failure of clinical improvement after initial dose
   (2) Increased ventilator requirements
   (3) Deterioration of clinical states

5. Dosing
   a. Exosurf (Burroughs/Wellcome): Administer 5 mL/kg, which is 100 mg of phospholipid per kilogram.
   b. Beractant (Survanta, Ross Laboratories): Administer 4 mL/kg, which is 100 mg of phospholipid per kilogram. The 100 mg of phospholipid per kilogram dose was established showing this was the quantity of surfactant in the premature infant's lungs.
   c. Dosing procedures are different for Beractant and Exosurf (Table 6–5).
   d. During dosing, the infant is continually monitored. While maintaining the ETT in the midline position, monitor pulse, oxygen saturation, chest wall movement, breath sounds, and blood gases. Ventilator settings may require adjustment as the infant's compliance improves to prevent possible pneumothorax. If mucus plugging occurs, immediate reintubation may be necessary if the suction catheter cannot clear the ETT.
   e. Single dosing improves gas exchange and decreases pneumothorax. Multiple dosing reduces the need for increased oxygen, reduces the incidence of pneumothorax, and significantly reduces mortality as compared to single dosing. Up to four doses within 48 h can be given if an infant still requires a $FIO_2$ of 0.30 to 0.40 and a $\bar{P}aw$ of greater than 7 cm $H_2O$. Not all infants require four doses. Infants may not respond to a lower number of doses because of the following factors:
      (1) Pulmonary hemorrhage where proteins in the blood inhibit surfactant function.
      (2) CHD, pulmonary hypoplasia, PDA, inactivation by hyperoxemia, and inflammation.
6. Prevention of neonatal lung injury.
   a. Acute physiological effects include increased $PaO_2$ and increased static compliance.
   b. Lung volume and functional residual capacity (FRC) are increased. One study showed an increase in FRC from 11.4 to 19.6 mL/kg.

TABLE 6–5. *Comparison of Dosing Procedures for Beractant and Exosurf*

| Beractant Dosing Procedure | Exosurf Dosing Procedure |
|---|---|
| 1. Administer into an ETT through a No. 5 Fr. catheter, extending beyond the ETT and above the carina. Only the amount of dose should be in the syringe. Discard extra surfactant.<br>2. Suction the ETT and determine proper placement of the ETT.<br>3. Administration will be divided into quarter doses. With the administration of each quarter dose, the infant is positioned prior to dosing in the following positions (each dose takes 2–3 s to administer down the ETT):<br>**First 1/4 dose**—head and body down,* head turned to right.<br>**Second 1/4 dose**—head and body down, head turned to left.<br>**Third 1/4 dose**—head and body up, head turned to right.<br>**Fourth 1/4 dose**—head and body up, head turned to left.<br>After each quarter dose is administered, remove the catheter from the ETT and ventilate the infant for 30 s or until stable. Then reposition the infant for the next quarter dose. Do not suction the infant for up to 1 h after dosing, unless significant signs of airway obstruction are present. Repeat dosing no sooner than 6 h after the preceding dose and, if the infant remains intubated on a $FIO_2$ of at least 0.30, to maintain a $PaO_2$ of at least 80 mm Hg and chest radiograph indicating RDS. To ventilate, following repeat dosages, use the mechanical ventilator and adjust settings as needed. | 1. The full dose is drawn into the syringe and is given in 2 equal doses. Prior to dosing, select an adapter appropriate for the size ETT. Switch this dosing adapter with the universal adapter that is currently on the ETT. The side port of the dosing adapter will facilitate administration of surfactant down the ETT. With the appropriate amount of Exosurf, attach the syringe to the Luer-Lock sideport. Prior to administration, position the infant for the following:<br>**First 1/2 of dose**: Midline position. Instill Exosurf with the inspiratory breath from the ventilator over 1–2 min or 30–50 mechanical breaths. After this first half dose is given, rotate the infant 45° to the right and hold in this position for 30 s.<br>**Second 1/2 of dose**: Return the infant to midline position and instill the second half of the dose over 1–2 min during the inspiratory breath of the ventilator. After this second half dose has been given, rotate the infant 45° to the left, holding this position for 30 s. After this time, return the infant to midline position and recap the Luer-Lock on the adapter. Do not suction infant for up to 1 h following dosing, unless significant respiratory distress from airway obstruction is present. |

*Infants may be administered surfactant in flat bed to reduce the incidence of increased intracranial pressure.

   c. Lung compliance may decrease in some cases because an increase in FRC occurs in the face of constant ventilator settings. Without any ventilator setting changes, the infant is being ventilated at the top of the compliance curve.
   d. Reduced incidence of BPD in infants less than 1250 gm birth weight with RDS. However, infants still develop BPD, possibly because of sepsis, and the release of inflammatory cells. In spite of surfactant administration, these infants remain on mechanical ventilation and develop BPD.

7. The following are goals of mechanical ventilation:
   a. $PaO_2$—greater than 50 mm Hg
   b. $PaCO_2$—less than 50 mm Hg
   c. pH—greater than 7.25
   d. $SaO_2$—greater than 90%
8. CPAP may initially be used under the following conditions:
   a. $PCO_2$—less than 50 mm Hg, $PO_2$—less than 50 mm Hg on $FIO_2$ of 0.60 or more, and pH—greater than 7.30.
   b. Initiate at levels of 4 to 6 cm $H_2O$. Monitor with $SpO_2$ and ABGs.
   c. Hypercarbia, hypoxemia, acidosis, and increased episodes of apnea and bradycardia indicate the need for mechanical ventilation.
9. Mechanical ventilation settings include rates up to 60 bpm, a low PIP of less than 25 cm $H_2O$, a PEEP of 4 to 6 cm $H_2O$, and an inspiratory time of 0.3 s. Adjust ventilator settings to treat hypoxemia and acidosis rather than administering sodium bicarbonate. An improvement in oxygenation is seen by an increase in the $a/AO_2$ ratio and a decrease in the $A\text{-}aDO_2$.
10. Maintain appropriate inspiratory gas temperature.
11. Maintain appropriate fluid and electrolyte balance.
12. Maintain appropriate hematocrit and glucose levels.
13. Watch for acute problems such as pneumothorax. When compliance starts to improve, there is a danger of pneumothorax.
14. Watch for infections or the development of sepsis.

15. Infants who are not recovering and who are on mechanical ventilation with excessive ventilator settings may require HFO or ECMO.

G. Prognosis
1. In general, recovery occurs within 10 to 14 days with minimal complications in infants weighing more than 1500 gm. Infants weighing less than 1500 gm may require a longer mechanical ventilator course.
2. If mechanical ventilation progresses longer than 2 weeks, bronchopulmonary dysplasia (BPD) may develop.

## VI. Bronchopulmonary dysplasia (BPD)

A. Definition
1. BPD is defined as oxygen dependence for greater than 28 days of life to keep normal or near normal $SpO_2$ following treatment of neonatal respiratory failure.

B. Multifactorial risk factors implicated in the development of BPD include the following:
1. Immature lungs from low birth weight (LBW) (less than 1500 gm)
2. Low gestational age (less than 34 weeks)
3. Race (Caucasian)
4. Gender (males)
5. Lung injury from mechanical ventilation
6. Oxygen toxicity ($FIO_2$ greater than 0.50)
7. Infection

C. Etiology and pathophysiology
1. Significant lung injury occurs early from overdistension of the tracheobronchial tree and atelectasis. Over time, this leads to increased ventilatory support. Continuation of overdistension and atelectasis leads to ventilation-perfusion (V/Q) mismatching. Pneumothorax and pulmonary interstitial emphysema may develop. High PIPs and large tidal volumes are particularly harmful to the lungs.
2. Oxygen toxicity causes endothelial cell damage, creating pulmonary edema. Proteins inactivate surfactant, and surface tension increases, leading to atelectasis, decreased compliance, and increased V/Q mismatching. Oxidant stress from increases in inspired oxygen breaks down lung tissue (antioxidants vitamin E and superoxide dismutase help fight this stress). Inflammatory cells such as neutrophils and macrophages cause further damage and impair healing.
3. The common maternal genital *Mycoplasma* agent found in the tracheal aspirants of infants within the first 48 h after birth that causes pneumonia and pulmonary disease in premature infants is *Ureaplasma urealyticum* (Uu). Infants weighing less than 1000 gm have twice the death rate or development of BPD as compared to infants weighing more than 1000 gm. This agent may also show up in blood cultures, causing sepsis.

D. Radiography
1. Acute phase: 2 to 3 days after birth
   a. Classic RDS picture
   b. Ground-glass appearance of chest radiograph and air bronchograms
2. Stage II: Up to 10 days
   a. A hyaline membrane forms
   b. There are changes in lung structure
   c. Necrosis develops
   d. Pulmonary edema and patent ductus arteriosus develop
3. Stage III: Up to 20 days (increased oxygen requirements, hypercarbia, and increased ventilator requirements).
   a. Cysts form (although this may be pulmonary interstitial emphysema and may clear in a few days).
   b. Alveolar emphysema and interstitial fibrosis develop.
4. Stage IV: Over 1 month
   a. Severe hyperinflation develops.
   b. There is increased density because of collapse or fibrosis.
   c. Cardiomegaly caused by cor pulmonale develops.

E. Clinical presentation
1. Initially, typical appearance of an infant with respiratory distress who needs assisted ventilation and oxygen.
2. No improvement clinically, requiring prolonged mechanical ventilation from complications such as intracranial hemorrhage, pulmonary infection, and PDA. These complications may increase the need for higher concentrations of

oxygen and airway pressures. This begins the vicious cycle in which required therapy further aggravates pulmonary damage.

3. Although some infants start with low pressure, a mild increase in oxygen requirements, infection, or heart failure from PDA causes the infant's condition to deteriorate.
4. Pneumothorax and PIE complicate the case because of high inflation pressures and reduced compliance.
5. Changes in ventilatory parameters indicate poor response to ventilatory support. Not one aspect by itself is the cause of BPD but a combination of factors.
   a. Increase in PIP: Greater than 25 cm $H_2O$.
   b. Rate: Greater than 60 bpm.
   c. $FIO_2$: Greater than 0.50 for long periods.
6. Infants may develop heart failure, which is secondary to pulmonary hypertension. Signs of heart failure include cardiomegaly, hepatomegaly, and fluid retention.

F. Management and treatment
1. Avoid lung overdistention.
   a. Use of patient-synchronized ventilation with pressure-limited, time-cycled ventilator. This helps reduce or prevent a controlled inspiratory breath delivered on top of the exhaled breath.
   b. Ability to measure inspired and exhaled tidal volumes
   c. Volume-controlled ventilation with synchronized intermittent mandatory ventilation (SIMV) mode and pressure-support ventilation mode
   d. High-frequency oscillation (HFO)
2. Achieve a low $FIO_2$ and PIP and a long expiratory time to avoid air trapping.
3. Tracheostomy is the preferred method of ventilation because it reduces airway scarring; it allows for greater comfort clinically, as seen by decreased cyanotic spells and irritability; it produces fewer oral secretions; and it allows for a better interaction between patient and caregiver.
4. Pharmacological therapy goals include the following:
   a. To minimize the biochemical and physical trauma to the lungs associated with hyperoxic exposure and mechanical ventilation.
   b. To prevent the occurrence of hypoxemic-related cellular damage.
   c. To reduce the tissue diffusion gradient for oxygen and improve lung compliance by decreasing interstitial edema.
   d. To reduce airway resistance by causing airway bronchodilation.
   e. To improve effective vascular perfusion and thus improve the V/Q matching.
   f. To prevent and minimize biochemical trauma resulting from oxygen therapy. These goals are approached with the following drugs.
5. Pharmacological therapy
   a. Diuretic therapy—Furosemide to help reduce pulmonary interstitial edema. Also chlorothiazide and spironolactone have been used in combination.
   b. Bronchodilator therapy—Terbutaline, metaproterenol, and albuterol are all employed as bronchodilators. These drugs are delivered with a small-volume nebulizer (SVN) and metered-dose inhaler (MDI) with spacer device. A longer inspiratory time should be provided to ensure a good deposition of drugs. Adjust the inspiratory time during the treatment; then readjust it to the setting prior to the treatment. Theophylline is used to help achieve diaphragm contraction and smooth-muscle relaxation.
   c. Infants with a tracheostomy will benefit from a tracheostomy collar to administer the drug, or the MDI with spacer can be attached directly to the tracheostomy.
   d. Anti-inflammatory therapy—Corticosteroids are used extensively to control inflammation. Studies show improvements in the diffusion gradient and in lung compliance, as well as a reduction in ventilator settings in terms of pressure, rate, and $FIO_2$. Unfortunately, there are many side effects from long-term steroid use, which include hypertension, hyperglycemia, disruption of body growth and development, adrenal insufficiency, and infection.
   e. Vasodilator therapy—Used to reduce vascular resistance. Drugs used include tolazoline, nitroprusside, nitroglycerin, $PGE_1$, and $PGE_2$.
   f. Sedative-hypnotic therapy—Used to reduce sudden, intense periods of hypoxia and cyanosis caused by agitation. Drugs used include chlorpromazine.

g. Vitamin E and antioxidants—Help reduce oxygen-induced lung injury and injury to the surfactant system.
h. Exogenous surfactant

6. Bronchial hygiene; suctioning, percussion and postural drainage, and humidity
7. Nutrition
8. In spite of these therapies, infants may remain on mechanical ventilation for a long term.
   a. Respiratory problems include the following:
      (1) Ventilatory drive impairment
      (2) Respiratory muscle fatigue
      (3) Abnormal pulmonary mechanics
      (4) Localized atelectasis
   b. Other problems not related to respiratory problems include the following:
      (1) Nutritional compromise
      (2) Neurologic problems
      (3) Intercurrent infection
      (4) Congestive heart failure

G. Weaning
1. Infections interrupt the weaning process.
2. Decrease ventilator settings slowly and watch for intolerance to weaning. Weaning may occur after a period of steady improvement, which may take from weeks to months. Infants may be on volume-controlled ventilation. Use of CPAP and PSV may assist the infant and allow support to minimize the ventilator settings.
3. After extubation, infants may still have retractions, tachypnea, rales, and rhonchi on auscultation, all of which may require oxygen delivery. Use of nasal cannula with a blender will provide specific oxygen delivery. Maintain $SpO_2$ between 92 and 94%. Lobar and segmental atelectasis results from retained secretions, requiring good bronchial hygiene to avoid airway obstruction.

H. Outcome
1. Infants with moderate BPD for more than 3 years showed increased lung volumes and increased compliance near normal levels. However, later in life the infant may have such problems as airway hyperactivity.
2. Some have persistent problems even into their 20s. The main problems are airflow limitation and decreased alveolar surface area.

## VII. Diaphragmatic hernia

A. Diaphragmatic hernia is a congenital condition in which there is a herniation of the abdominal organs into the thoracic cavity.

B. Diaphragmatic hernia occurs 1 in 3000 births, with 70% of these occurring on the left side. One possible reason for fewer occurrences on the right side is that the liver may partially block the defect, thereby preventing herniation.

C. Etiology and pathophysiology
1. The diaphragm, which is made up of four parts, begins to develop between 3 and 5 weeks' gestation. Each part begins to form and move inward to the pleuroperitoneal canals. Closure of the diaphragm occurs at approximately the ninth week of gestation. At the same time, the stomach, intestines, and midgut are forming. If these organs form prior to the closure of the diaphragm, herniation occurs.
2. Common herniation (or eventration) is a left Bochdalek, or posterolateral, hernia.
3. Lungs on both the affected and unaffected side are often hypoplastic or aplastic. This is caused by the intestines and/or heart, which are occupying the space, preventing appropriate lung development.
4. At the time of delivery, adequate lung inflation cannot occur because of the intrusion of the intestinal organs into the area normally occupied by the lungs. This leads to a respiratory distress that is usually seen immediately or soon after delivery. A mediastinal shift toward the unaffected side occurs. This often inhibits adequate inflation of lung tissue on the unaffected side.
5. Increased pulmonary vascular resistance may lead to PPHN.

D. Clinical manifestations (usually seen at delivery or soon after birth)
1. Respiratory distress that does not respond to oxygen or resuscitation with PPV.
2. A scaphoid (football-shaped) abdomen, caused by the intrusion of part of the abdominal contents into the thoracic cavity.
3. Point of maximal impulse may be shifted to unaffected side.

4. Breath sounds that are decreased over the affected side; bowel sounds may also be heard over the affected side.

E. Radiologic appearance

1. Air-filled bowels are seen in the thoracic cavity with a mediastinal shift away from the affected side.

F. Treatment

1. If a diaphragmatic hernia is suspected at birth, the infant should be intubated immediately. This prevents air from entering the stomach and gut, which will compress the available lung tissue.
2. Mechanical ventilation with as low a PIP as possible and a minimum PEEP, keeping the affected side down. Maintain low pressures to prevent barotrauma and pneumothorax.
3. Surgery to remove intestines

## VIII. Esophageal atresia (EA) with and without tracheoesophageal fistula (TEF)

A. General description

1. Approximately 10% of cases of EA are not associated with TEF.
2. Approximately 3% of cases of TEF exist without EA.
3. The most common anomaly is EA with distal TEF (Fig. 6–3).
4. Approximately 25% of the infants are premature and may be born with other anomalies including congenital heart disease, Down syndrome, tracheal malacia, and duodenal atresia.

B. Esophageal atresia with tracheoesophageal fistula

1. Clinical manifestations
   a. Initially at birth infants are asymptomatic.
   b. Infants develop respiratory distress because of aspiration of secretions from the upper pouch of the esophagus, reflux of gastric juices through

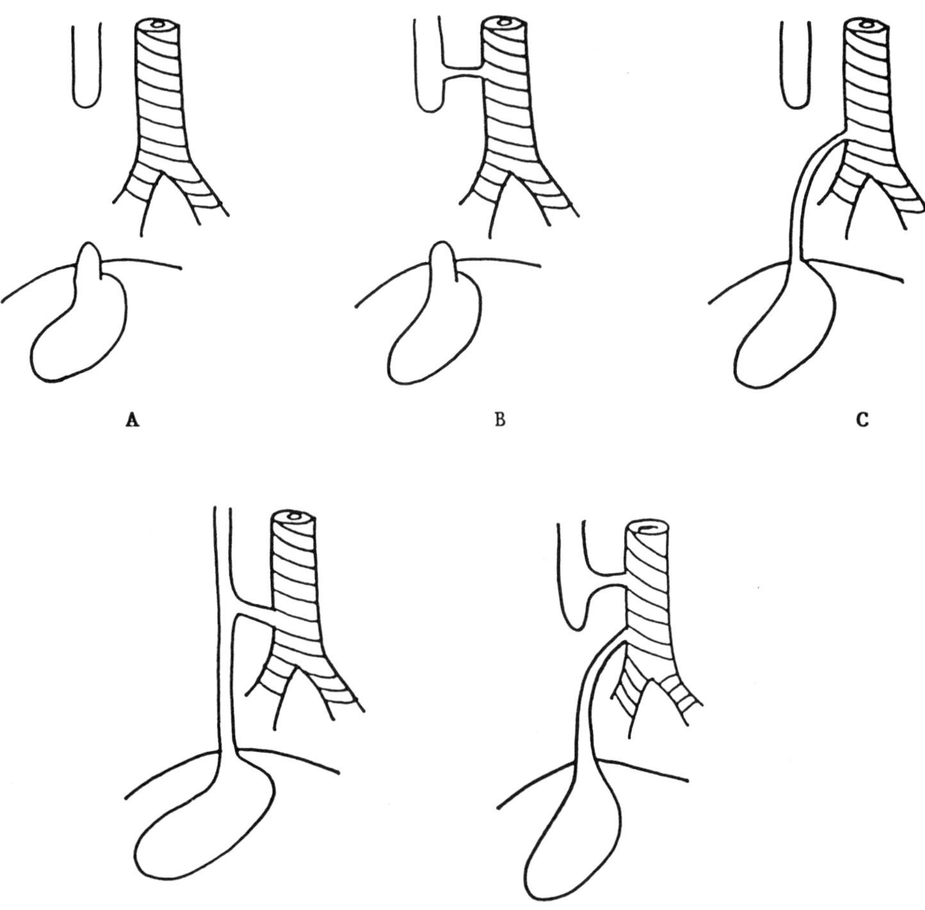


**FIGURE 6–3** Esophageal atresia with and without TEF. *(A)* EA without TEF, *(B)* EA with proximal TEF, *(C)* EA with distal TEF, *(D)* "H" type or TEF without EA, and *(E)* EA with proximal and distal TEF.

the TEF, and air entering the stomach through the TEF pushing up on the diaphragm and affecting pulmonary function.

2. Diagnosis
    a. Profuse oral, bubbly secretions in spite of continuous oropharyngeal suctioning
    b. Progression of tachypnea, dyspnea, choking, and cyanosis during feeding (this occurs very quickly with a EA with proximal TEF).
    c. Regurgitation of feeding as esophageal pouch fills and overflows.
    d. Nasogastric (NG) tube that stops 10–13 cm from the nose. On chest radiograph a radiopaque NG tube will be seen coiled in the esophageal pouch.
    e. Contrast injected into the NG tube fills the pouch and demonstrates the atresia on chest radiograph.
3. Chest radiograph
    a. Infants with EA with TEF exhibit aspiration pneumonia with air in the stomach and bowel (except with EA with proximal TEF as this will have an airless stomach).
4. Treatment
    a. Infants should be placed in an upright position.
    b. Infants with severe respiratory distress may have a gastrostomy to decompress the stomach and decrease gastroesophageal reflux from abdominal distention from air in the stomach.
    c. Surgery.

C. Esophageal atresia without tracheoesophageal fistula
1. Pathophysiology
    a. The connection between the esophagus and trachea is found in the neck below the larynx and thoracic inlet.
    b. The lungs get a continual insult from the esophagus and the infant develops significant infection.
2. Diagnosis
    a. Recurrent pneumonia
    b. Cough, choking, cyanosis following feeding.
    c. Gastric distention (from air entering stomach) from crying or coughing.
    d. Wet lungs following feedings.
    e. Esophagogram
3. Chest radiograph
    a. Aspiration pneumonia
    b. Air in the stomach and bowels.
4. Treatment
    a. Infants should be placed in an upright position.
    b. Surgery

## IX. Intraventricular-periventricular hemorrhage (IVH-PVH)

A. Incidence
1. In infants weighing less than 1000 gm, the incidence is 50 to 60%; in infants weighing more than 1500 gm, the incidence is 10 to 20%.
2. During the first 4 days of life, the VLBW infant is at greatest risk for IVH-PVH. Within the first 12 h of life, hemorrhage may be detected.

B. Intravascular factors causing IVH-PVH
1. Increases in cerebral blood flow—changes in blood flow from hypoxia, hypercarbia, abrupt systemic BP change, and apnea.
2. Alterations in cerebral blood flow—changes in blood flow from asphyxia accompanied by systemic hypotension. Reduced blood flow to the highly oxygenated germinal matrix may cause reperfusion in response to the asphyxia. This, along with volume replacement during resuscitation, may increase flow and pressure significantly enough to cause injury.
3. Increases in cerebral venous pressure—long labor with vaginal delivery compresses the compliant cranium, which obstructs cerebral venous blood flow and increases pressure. Mechanical ventilation contributes by reducing venous return by introducing positive pressure within the thoracic cavity. The addition of PEEP, a longer inspiratory time, and an inadvertent PEEP, as well as an infant's breathing out of synchrony with the ventilator, contribute to this process.

C. Etiology and pathophysiology
1. The underlying cause of IVH-PVH is the inability to regulate blood flow in the germinal matrix and choroid plexus.
2. In the term infant, bleeds often occur within the area called the choroid plexus, whereas in the premature infant, the germinal matrix is the most

TABLE 6–6. *Classification of IVH-PVH*

| GRADE I (MILD—40% OF SURVIVING INFANTS) | GRADE II (MILD—30% OF SURVIVING INFANTS) |
|---|---|
| Isolated periventricular hemorrhage | Intraventricular hemorrhage with normal ventricular size |
| **GRADE III (MODERATE—20% OF SURVIVING INFANTS)** | **GRADE IV (SEVERE—10% OF SURVIVING INFANTS)** |
| Intraventricular hemorrhage with acute ventricular dilation | Intraventricular hemorrhage with parenchymal hemorrhage |

common source of bleeding. In about 40% of the cases, PVH remains confined to the germinal matrix. In about 60% of the cases, bleeding ruptures through into the ventricular system. The severity of hemorrhaging is identified by a grading system (Table 6–6).

3. Large hemorrhages enter the ventricles, enlarging their size and compressing the brain parenchyma. If hemorrhaging extends into the brain tissue, further damage is done.

D. Clinical features—three basic syndromes
  1. The "catastrophic" syndrome—acute, severe, rapid onset of symptoms including the following:
     a. Stupor, coma
     b. Apnea
     c. Tonic seizures
     d. Decerebrate posturing
     e. Nonreactive pupils
     f. Falling hematocrit
     g. Bulging anterior fontanelle
     h. Systemic hypertension and bradycardia
     i. Metabolic acidosis
     j. Abnormal glucose
  2. The "saltatory" syndrome takes hours to days for symptoms to appear, which include changes in alertness, hypotonia, subtle abnormalities of eye movement and position, and subtle seizures.
  3. The clinically "silent" syndrome shows no abrupt deterioration and no clinical manifestations.

E. Diagnosis is made by real-time cranial sonography (head ultrasound).

F. General interventions to reduce IVH-PVH include the following:
  1. Prevent infant stress by reducing sound and light transmission in the area of the infant.
  2. Minimize heat and insensible water loss.
  3. Position the infant for optimal hemodynamic stability, which includes keeping the head midline; raise the head of bed to 30 degrees; minimize handling (coordinate treatment with other caregivers); reduce interventions that cause crying (obtain blood gases by umbilical artery catheter, perform pulse oximetry and transcutaneous monitoring, if possible).
  4. If sodium bicarbonate administration is given for documented metabolic acidosis, give slowly over 2 min to ventilated infant. Fast administration with undiluted solution (dilute 1:1 with sterile water) causes reduced cerebral blood flow.
  5. Maintain "low ventilator settings," as possible. Utilize a synchronous mode of ventilation or use muscle-paralyzing agents or sedatives to minimize fluctuating cerebral blood flow.

G. Prognosis
  1. Survival rate depends on the grade of the hemorrhage and hypoxic-ischemic cerebral injury. Mortality is greatest among infants with a grade IV bleed.

## X. Bacterial infections

A. Bacterial infections cause sepsis and are common in early neonatal life because of the immature host's reduced defenses.

B. The etiology of bacterial infections include group B *Streptococcus, Staphylococcus, Enterococcus, Escherichia coli, Klebsiella, Haemophilus,* and *Pseudomonas.*

C. Bacterial sepsis

TABLE 6–7. *Early versus Late Neonatal Sepsis*

| | **Early** | **Late** |
|---|---|---|
| Age | <7 days | >7 days |
| Common source of pathogen | Maternal genital tract | Environment—health-care personnel performing procedures on the infant. |
| Organism | Group B *Streptococcus* (GBS); *E. coli* (these are most common and account for 60–70% of bacterial sepsis). | *Staphylococcus aureus*<br>GBS<br>*E. coli*<br>*Klebsiella*<br>*Pseudomonas*<br>*Staphylococcus epidermis*<br>*H. influenzae* |
| Common condition caused by pathogen | Pneumonia | Meningitis |

1. In general, infant mortality rate is 10 to 40%. Infants weighing less than 1000 gm have a mortality rate of 25 to 30%.
2. Predisposing factors include the following:
   a. PROM greater than 24 h
   b. Premature labor
   c. Urinary tract infection
   d. Chorioamnionitis
   e. IV catheters
3. Neonatal sepsis is divided into early and late sepsis. Each has specific features (Table 6–7).
4. Most bacterial infections are present during the first week of life and as early as a few hours after birth. Bacteria that invade the infant colonize around the vaginal-anal region of the mother. Infection from the ascending, or anal, route follows the rupturing of the amniotic membrane, whereas colonization through the vaginal route occurs during birth, either by the infant aspirating bacteria or by bacteria colonizing the mucous membranes.
5. Routine procedures allow bacteria to invade the infant and cause an inflammatory response.
6. Clinical manifestations (from most common to less common) include the following:
   a. Hyperthermia
   b. Jaundice
   c. Respiratory distress
   d. Loss of weight
   e. Vomiting
   f. Cyanosis
   g. Apnea
   h. Abdominal distension
   i. Hypothermia
   j. Diarrhea
7. Laboratory studies
   a. White blood cell count (WBC)—More than 25,000 $mm^3$ (normal for the term infant is 10,000 to 26,000 $mm^3$; for premature infant, the WBC is 5,000 to 19,000 $mm^3$ for the first day of life).
   b. Differential—Neutropenia occurs when the absolute neutrophil count is less than 1800 $mm^3$ (normal for the term infant is 5,000 to 13,000 $mm^3$; for the premature infant, it is 2000 to 9000 $mm^3$). The neutrophil count is low because the infant is unable to replenish the neutrophil pool. The immature neutrophil count is increased.
   c. C-reactive protein (CRP)—An acute phase of globulin synthesized by the liver within 6 to 8 h of inflammatory stimulus. The normal value is less than 1.6 mg/dL for the first 2 days. It drops to less than 1.0 mg/dL after day 2.
   d. Platelets—Normal for the premature and the term infant is greater than 250,000 $mm^3$. Thrombocytopenia indicates infection.
   e. Cerebral spinal fluid specimen
   f. Tracheal aspirate from ETT following intubation
   g. Urine culture
   h. Chest radiograph

8. Treatment
   a. After cultures are obtained, begin empiric antibiotic therapy.

C. Group B *Streptococcus* (GBS)
   1. The highest incidence of bacterial infections causing pneumonia is from GBS.
   2. Pregnant women harbor GBS in the lower genital tract.
   3. The fetus becomes infected with GBS in the same way as with bacterial sepsis.
   4. Early-onset disease is the most common, where infants develop symptoms during the first week of life (as early as a few hours after birth).
   5. Predisposing factors include the following:
      a. Women identified prenatally as carriers of GBS
      b. PROM
      c. Premature delivery
      d. Previous delivery of an infant who had GBS
      e. Maternal fever (greater than 37.5°C)
   6. Clinical manifestations
      a. Temperature instability
      b. Cardiovascular changes including tachycardia, bradycardia, and hypotension.
      c. Respiratory irregularities including tachypnea, apnea, nasal flaring, grunting, and retractions.
      d. Feeding problems including increased glucose requirements, vomiting, diarrhea, and gastric distension.
      e. Hematologic problems including jaundice, bleeding, bruising, and petechiae.
      f. Blood gas changes causing lactic acidosis.
   7. Radiographic findings
      a. Resembles HMD and transient tachypnea of the newborn, especially in small infants.
      b. Granular infiltrates and atelectasia are evident but are less uniform than those of HMD.
      c. Lung volume is normal; may have a pleural effusion.
   8. Diagnosis
      a. Abnormal chest radiograph and complete blood count (CBC)
      b. Blood culture (repeat if positive)
      c. Lumbar puncture (if repeat blood culture is positive)
   9. Treatment
      a. Ampicillin or penicillin G, IV antibiotics

## XI. Congenital infections

A. TORCHS is an acronym for common infections—TO = toxoplasmosis, R = rubella virus, C = cytomegalovirus, and HS = herpes simplex virus.

B. Toxoplasmosis is maternally acquired either by the ingestion of oocytes in raw meat or by exposure to cat feces during pregnancy. The fetus is infected by transplacental passage of the organism.

C. Rubella is acquired through a nonvaccinated or rubella-susceptible mother. The fetus is infected by transplacental passage of virus.

D. Cytomegalovirus (CMV) is the most common congenital infection. It is vertically transmitted during pregnancy. Postnatally, the infant is infected by blood transfusion, breast-feeding, or nosocomial spread in the nursery.

E. Transmission of herpes simplex virus types 1 and 2 occurs at birth from direct contact with the recurrent lesions during birth or postnatally by contact with an infected caregiver.

F. Human immunodeficiency virus (HIV), although not a part of the acronym, is a congenital infection. Transmission may occur by the transplacental route or from exposure to maternal blood and secretions at delivery.

## XII. Nosocomial infection

A. Nosocomial infections occur at greater than 48 h of life. The infection was present in the newborn at birth or incubating in the fetus.

B. Infants exposed to a prolonged hospital stay and invasive supportive measures are at high risk for developing nosocomial infections.

C. The most common agent is coagulase-negative staphylococci. Others include *Staphylococcus aureus,* gram-negative enteric bacilli, respiratory syncytial virus (spread by droplet contamination), and methicillin-resistant *S. aureus* (MRSA).

D. Treatment includes empiric antibiotic therapy and isolation.

E. To prevent contamination of noninfected infants, handwashing, gloving, masking, and gowning are imperative. Health-care personnel working with infected infants should not work with noninfected infants.

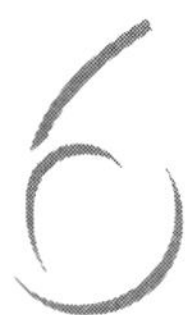

# REVIEW QUESTIONS

1. What are two high-risk factors for development of transient tachypnea of the newborn (TTNB)?

   a.

   b.

2. Describe the radiographic findings for TTNB.

3. Describe the treatment for TTNB.

4. What is meconium, and how is it formed in the fetus?

5. What causes meconium to pass from the fetus into the amniotic fluid?

6. Upon presentation of a newborn infant with thick meconium, what action should be taken?

7. In the accompanying table, list the treatment for each level of meconium aspiration.

| **+1 Meconium** | **+2, +3 Meconium** | **+4 Meconium** |
|---|---|---|

8. Fill in the accompanying table for pulmonary air leaks.

| | Pneumothorax | Pneumopericardium | Pneumomediastinum | Pulmonary Interstitial Emphysema |
|---|---|---|---|---|
| Description | | | | |
| Clinical presentation | | | | |
| Radiologic appearance | | | | |
| Management and treatment | | | | |

9. Define persistent pulmonary hypertension of the newborn (PPHN).

10. Give two reasons why PPHN occurs in the newborn infant.

    a.

    b.

11. In the accompanying table, compare and contrast the tests that differentiate between lung disease, PPHN, and cardiac heart disease.

| | Hyperoxia Test | Pre-Post Ductal Test | Hypoxemia-Hyperventilation Test |
|---|---|---|---|
| Description | | | |
| Diagnostic findings | | | |

12. Where should blood be drawn to determine ductal shunting? Where should the electrodes of a transcutaneous monitor be placed to determine ductal shunting?

13. Describe two ventilatory approaches to treat PPHN.

    a.

    b.

14. Describe how nitric oxide (NO) causes vasodilation.

15. Besides NO, what other pulmonary vasodilator may be used to reverse PPHN?

16. Why is NO a better agent to treat PPHN than the other pulmonary vasodilator listed in question 15?

17. How is hyaline membrane formed causing RDS?

18. In the accompanying table, give the rationale for each treatment for PPHN.

| Treatment | Rationale |
|---|---|
| Hyperventilation | |
| Sodium bicarbonate | |
| Tolazoline | |
| Dopamine, dobutamine | |
| Nitric oxide | |
| Fresh frozen plasma, normal saline | |

19. What is the classic radiologic appearance of the untreated newborn with RDS?

20. Give two reasons why administration of antenatal corticosteroid reduces the incidence of neonatal death associated with RDS?

    a.

    b.

21. List and describe two improvements in the lungs following the administration of exogenous surfactant.

    a.

    b.

22. List two hazards or contraindications to the administration of surfactant.

    a.

    b.

23. What should be monitored when administering surfactant to a newborn infant?

24. What is the difference between rescue and prophylactic administration of surfactant?

25. What is the definition of bronchopulmonary dysplasia (BPD)?

26. Describe the four radiologic phases of BPD.

    a. Phase I

    b. Phase II

    c. Phase III

    d. Phase IV

27. Describe how lung overdistention can be avoided, thus preventing BPD.

28. List two multifactorial risk factors implicated in the development of BPD.

    a.

    b.

29. In the accompanying table, fill in the rationale for the use of therapy to treat BPD.

| Therapy | Rationale for Use |
|---|---|
| Diuretic therapy | |
| Bronchodilator therapy | |
| Anti-inflammatory therapy | |
| Vasodilator therapy | |
| Sedative-hypnotic therapy | |

30. At birth, what clinical manifestations indicate that a newborn has diaphragmatic hernia?

31. Once the diagnosis of diaphragmatic hernia is made, what immediate treatment is suggested?

32. List the four grades of intraventricular-periventricular hemorrhage (IVH-PVH) and what occurs in each grade.

    a. Grade I

    b. Grade II

    c. Grade III

    d. Grade IV

33. List the types of esophageal atresia (EA) with tracheoesophageal fistula (TEF).

    a.

    b.

    c.

    d.

34. How would EA with TEF be diagnosed?

35. List three intravascular factors causing IVH-PVH.

    a.

    b.

    c.

36. What are three predisposing factors for bacterial infection in the fetus and newborn?

    a.

    b.

    c.

37. List clinical manifestations of bacterial sepsis.

    a.

    b.

38. What bacterium is the most common cause of pneumonia in the fetus and newborn infant?

## BIBLIOGRAPHY


American Association for Respiratory Care. (1994). Surfactant replacement therapy: Clinical practice guideline. *Respiratory Care* 39:824.

Abman, S., and Kinsella, J. (1994). Nitric Oxide in the Pathophysiology and Treatment of Neonatal Pulmonary Hypertension. *Neonatal Respiratory Diseases* 4:1.

Abu-Osba, Y. (1991). Treatment of persistent pulmonary hypertension of the newborn: Update. *Archives of Disease in Childhood* 66:74.

Alkalay, A. (7 August 1996). *Group B Streptococcal Infections in Newborns* [WWW document]. CSMC Teaching Files. URL http://www.csmc.edu/neonatology/syllabus/gbs.html

Allred, T., and Auten, R. (1995). Surfactant therapy in the newborn. *Seminars in Respiration and Critical Care Medicine* 16:39.

American Heart Association. (1992). Guidelines for cardiopulmonary resuscitation and emergency cardiac care: Recommendations of the 1992 national conference. JAMA 268:2171.

Ballard, R., and Ballard, P. (1994). Scientific basis for antenatal steroid use. In *Report of the Consensus Development on the Effect of Corticosteroids for Fetal Maturation on Perinatal Outcomes*. National Institutes of Health. NIH Publication No. 95-3784.

Berry, D. (1991). Neonatology in the 1990s: Surfactant replacement therapy becomes reality. *Clinical Pediatrics* 30:167.

Bhat, R., et al. (1990). Effect of a single dose surfactant on pulmonary function. *Critical Care Medicine* 18:590.

Centers for Disease Control. (17 May 1996). *Group B Streptococcal Infections* [WWW document]. URL http:www.cdc.gov/ncidod/diseases/bacter/strep_b.htm

Davis, J. (1993). *Surfactant Administration Strategies: How Fast, How Much, How Often in Surfactant Replacement Therapy, A Clinical Symposium*. Boston: Floating Hospital/Tufts University School of Medicine.

D'Alessandro, M. P. (9 October 1996). *Pneumonia, Neonatal (Group B* Streptococcus*)* [WWW document]. The Virtual Hospital. URL http:WWW.vh.org/

Dietch, J. (1993). Periventricular-intraventricular hemorrhage in the very low birth weight infant. *Neonatal Network* 12:7.

Emmanouilides, G., and Baylen, B. (1988). *Neonatal Cardiopulmonary Distress*. Chicago: Yearbook Medical.

Fox, W., and Duara, S. (1983). Persistent pulmonary hypertension in the neonate: Diagnosis and management. *Journal of Pediatrics* 103:505.

Gaston, B., et al. (1994). The biology of nitrogen oxides in the airways. *American Journal of Respiratory Critical Care Medicine* 149:538.

Goldberg, R., and Bancalari, E. (1986). Bronchopulmonary dysplasia: Clinical presentation and the role of mechanical ventilation. *Respiratory Care* 31:591.

Goldsmith, L., et al. (1991). Immediate improvement in lung volume after exogenous surfactant: alveolar recruitment vs. distention. *Journal of Pediatrics* 119:424.

Harwood, R. (1990). Respiratory disorders of the newborn. In Kacmarek, R., Mack, C., and Dimas, S. *The Essentials of Respiratory Care*, ed 3. St. Louis: Mosby-Year Book.

Hoffman, D. J., and Harris, M. A. (1996). Diagnosis of neonatal sepsis. In Spitzer, A. *Intensive Care of the Neonate*. St. Louis: Mosby-Year Book.

Hospital Infections. (1996). Staphylococcus aureus, *Methicillin Resistant* [WWW document]. URL http://www.cdc.gov

Kinney, J. S., et al. (1997). Infection. In Seidel, H. M., Rosenstein, B. J., and Pathak, A. *Primary Care of the Newborn*. St. Louis: Mosby-Year Book.

Kling, P. (1989). Nursing interventions to decrease the risk of periventricular-intraventricular hemorrhage. *JOGN Nursing* 18:457.

Korones, S. (1986). *High-Risk Newborn Infants*, ed 4. St. Louis: CV Mosby.

Lierl, M. (1993). Congenital abnormalities. In Hilman, B. C. *Pediatric Respiratory Disease*. Philadelphia: WB Saunders.

Maycock, D. (1997) *Persistent Pulmonary Hypertension in the Newborn* [WWW document]. University of Washington. URL http://weber.u.washington.edu/~neonatal/NICU-WEB/pphn.html

Pearlman, S., and Maisels, J. (1989). Preductal and postductal transcutaneous oxygen tension measurements in premature newborns with hyaline membrane disease. *Pediatrics* 83:98.

Puri, A. (1997). *IVH/PVH Management and Prophylaxis* [WWW document]. CSMC NICU Teaching Files. URL http://www.csmc.edu.neonatology.

Reidel, F. (1987). Long-term effects of artificial ventilation in neonate. *Acta Paediatrica Scandinavica* 76:24.

Roberts, J., and Shaul, P. (1993). Advances in the treatment of persistent pulmonary hypertension of the newborn. *Pediatric Clinics of North America* 40:983.

Salzberg, A. M., and Krummel, T. R. (1990). Congenital malformations of the lower respiratory tract. In Chernick, V. *Kendig's Disorders of the Respiratory Tract in Children*, ed 5. Philadelphia: WB Saunders.

Steele, R. (1994). *The Clinical Handbook of Pediatric Infectious Disease*. New York: Pantheon Publishing.

Stern, L. (1983). *Diagnosis and Management of Respiratory Disorders in the Newborn*. New York: Addison-Wesley Publishing.

Steinhorn, R., Milliard, S., and Morin, F. (1995). Persistent pulmonary hypertension of the newborn. *Clinics in Perinatology* 22:405.

Virtual Hospital. (21 February 1997). *The Neonate* [WWW document]. URL http://www.vh.radiology.uiowa.edu

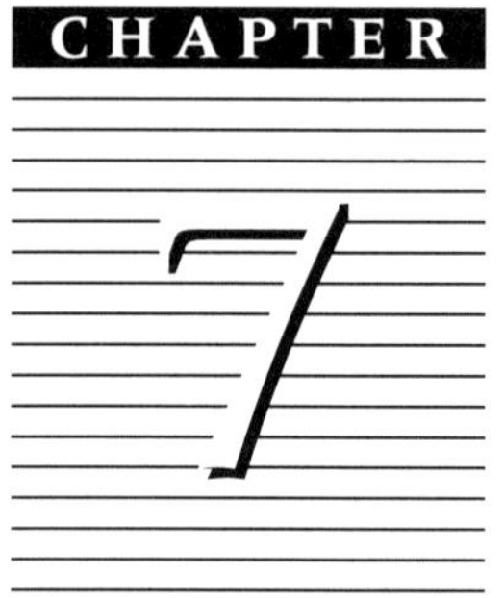

# Invasive and Noninvasive Monitoring

**I. Blood gas monitoring**

A. Respiratory acidosis
1. The primary cause of respiratory acidosis is hypercapnia.
2. In the newborn, uncomplicated respiratory acidosis is unusual because hypoxia accompanies respiratory acidosis. This leads to concurrent metabolic acidosis (see Metabolic Acidosis later in this chapter).
3. An acute rise in the partial pressure of arterial carbon dioxide ($PaCO_2$) of 10 mm Hg will drop the pH approximately 0.08 units.
4. Causes of respiratory acidosis (with normal lungs) include the following:
   a. Central nervous system (CNS) depression from sedatives or narcotics.
   b. Trauma, including to the chest, brain, and spinal cord.
   c. Neuromuscular disease, including myasthenia gravis and poliomyelitis.
5. Chronic respiratory acidosis is a result of chronic lung disease, such as bronchopulmonary dysplasia and cystic fibrosis.
   a. The body compensates for the accumulated carbon dioxide by retaining bicarbonate ($HCO_3$).
   b. Renal compensation masks the respiratory problem by preventing a serious drop in pH.
   c. Metabolic processes may cause the pH to become more acidic than the calculated pH.
   d. As the plasma bicarbonate level increases, the plasma $Cl^-$ level decreases.
6. To correct respiratory acidosis, the underlying cause should first be determined. In the acute phase, improving alveolar ventilation lowers the $PaCO_2$.

B. Respiratory alkalosis
1. The primary cause of respiratory alkalosis is hypocarbia.
2. An acute drop in $PaCO_2$ of 10 mm Hg will cause a rise in the pH of 0.08 units.
3. Factors other than respiratory disease that cause respiratory alkalosis include the following:
   a. Anxiety and/or fear
   b. Fever
   c. Pain
4. Diseases that cause respiratory alkalosis include the following:
   a. Exacerbation of asthma
   b. Pneumonia
   c. Any hypoxemic condition
   d. Stimulation of lung receptors (vagal)
5. Iatrogenic causes of respiratory alkalosis include ventilator-induced alveolar hyperventilation (in newborns this may be the treatment for persistent pulmonary hypertension in the newborn [PPHN]).
6. Compensation for respiratory alkalosis is by renal excretion of bicarbonate. Some potassium is excreted, which predisposes the body for development of hypokalemia.
7. Correction of respiratory alkalosis requires determining the underlying cause.
   a. Respiratory alkalosis may be induced by some procedure that causes the patient to hyperventilate. In this case, when the procedure is finished, the hyperventilation ceases.
   b. Hypoxemia may induce increased ventilation. Administration of oxygen would raise the $PaO_2$, reducing the stimulus to hyperventilate.
   c. Iatrogenic hyperventilation caused by mechanical ventilation requires the correction in minute ventilation to lower the pH, unless ventilation is

medically required, such as when there is PPHN or high intracranial pressure from head trauma.

8. Interpretation (Table 7–1)

C. Metabolic acidosis
1. To determine the degree of metabolic imbalance, after accounting for the respiratory component, look at the relationship between pH and the base change. A pH change of 0.15 units (not caused by $PaCO_2$) results in a base change of 10 mEq/L (for every 0.01 pH unit increase or decrease, there is a 2/3 mEq/L change in base excess).
2. The following are sources of added acids:
   a. Diet (increased level of dietary acid from food)
   b. Hypoxia
   c. Ketoacid (reduced level of glucose)
   d. Renal insufficiency
3. Bicarbonate is lost because of the following:
   a. Diarrhea
   b. Sepsis
   c. Renal failure
4. Drug-induced metabolic acidosis is caused by the following:
   a. Salicylate intoxication
   b. Acetazolamide (Diamox)
5. Other causes of metabolic acidosis include the following:
   a. Hypothermia or cold stress
6. Compensation
   a. Metabolic acidosis is also caused by an increased carbonic acid removal from the lungs in the form of $CO_2$. In general, the response by the body is quick; often, the $PaCO_2$ is low, unless there is a ventilatory disorder, in which case there would be a mixed respiratory and metabolic acidosis.
7. Severe metabolic acidosis
   a. Negative effects on the body
      (1) Depressed CNS
      (2) Impaired cardiovascular system. Elevated $H^+$ ion decreases cardiac contractility. Systemic hypotension as a result of peripheral vasodilation.
   b. Positive effects on the body
      (1) Oxygen transport improved from reduced systemic vascular resistance (SVR).
      (2) Increased loading of oxygen at tissue level (reduced pH).

D. Metabolic alkalosis
1. Base is increased by the following:
   a. Administration of $HCO_3^-$.
   b. Diuretic therapy (with bronchopulmonary dysplasia [BPD]).
2. Loss of $H^+$ ions, $Cl^-$, $K^+$ from the following:
   a. Vomiting
   b. Nasogastric (NG) tube drainage
   c. Corticosteroids
   d. Soybean infant feedings ($Cl^-$ deficit)

TABLE 7–1. ***Respiratory Acidosis and Respiratory Alkalosis Interpretation***

| | | ***Respiratory Acidosis*** | |
|---|---|---|---|
| | **pH** | **$PCO_2$ (mm Hg)** | **$HCO^-_3$ (mEq/L)** |
| Acute | <7.35 | >45 | Normal |
| Partly compensated | <7.35 | >45 | >26 |
| Compensated | >7.35 <7.40 | >45 | >26 |
| | | ***Respiratory Alkalosis*** | |
| | **pH** | **$PCO_2$ (mm Hg)** | **$HCO^-_3$ (mEq/L)** |
| Acute | >7.45 | <35 | Normal |
| Partly compensated | >7.45 | <35 | <22 |
| Compensated | <7.45 >7.40 | <35 | <22 |

TABLE 7–2. ***Metabolic Acidosis and Metabolic Alkalosis Interpretation***

| | | *Metabolic Acidosis* | |
|---|---|---|---|
| | **pH** | **$PCO_2$ (mm Hg)** | **$HCO^-_3$ (mEq/L)** |
| Acute | <7.35 | Normal | <22 |
| Partly compensated | <7.35 | <35 | <22 |
| Compensated | >7.35 <7.40 | <35 | <22 |
| | | *Metabolic Alkalosis* | |
| | **pH** | **$PCO_2$ (mm Hg)** | **$HCO^-_3$ (mEq/L)** |
| Acute | >7.45 | Normal | >26 |
| Partly compensated | >7.45 | >45 | >26 |
| Compensated | <7.45 >7.40 | >45 | >26 |

3. Long-term effects of metabolic alkalosis
   a. Muscle spasm
   b. Seizures accompanied by apnea
4. Compensation
   a. Hypoventilation (some increase in $PaCO_2$ may be seen as compensation).
   b. Restore normal fluid volume and electrolyte concentrations of potassium and chloride.
5. Interpretation (Table 7–2)

**II. Methods of obtaining blood for acid-base determination**

A. Capillary blood gases

1. Indications
   a. Estimate pH and $PaCO_2$ values at the same locations as where there are arterial punctures and indwelling catheters. Correlation of the capillary and arterialized blood is unreliable for administering oxygen therapy.
   b. Transcutaneous, pulse oximetry, and capnography are unreliable.
   c. Any change in modalities, assessment of initiation, or administration of modalities.
   d. History or physical assessment detecting changes in patient status.
   e. Monitoring and documenting a change in disease process.
2. Contraindications: Capillary puncture should not be performed at or through the following sites:
   a. Posterior curvature of the heel
   b. Fingers of the neonate
   c. Previous puncture sites
   d. Tissues that are edematous, swollen, or inflamed
   e. Any poorly perfused or cyanotic area
   f. On patients requiring assessment of oxygenation
   g. Sites of infection
   h. IV in foot
3. Relative contraindications
   a. Polycythemia (longer clotting times)
   b. Hypotension
   c. Clotting disorder
4. Factors affecting accuracy
   a. Inappropriate excess pressure applied to puncture site.
   b. Inadequate warming of site (poor correlation of pH and $PaCO_2$ values with arterial blood gas values).
   c. Air bubbles in capillary tube. Collect the sample aerobically and in anticoagulated form. Analyze within 10 to 15 min if left at room temperature, or chill the sample (sample can be chilled for over 60 min at 4°C).
5. Assessment of need
   a. Determine the need to obtain a capillary blood gas (CBG) by looking at the history and physical assessment.
   b. Compare noninvasive blood gas values, including transcutaneous, pulse oximetry, and capnography readings.
   c. Inability to obtain arterial blood.

6. Materials
   a. Puncture device
   b. Heparinized capillary tube
   c. Warming pad (42°C)
   d. Skin antiseptic
   e. Gauze and bandage
   f. Ice
   g. Gloves
   h. Sharps container
7. Obtaining capillary blood gases
   a. Use heel of foot.
   b. Warm area (5 to 10 min).
   c. Wipe site with appropriate solution (povidone-iodine, alcohol).
   d. Puncture site, wipe off first drop of blood.
   e. Collect sample (should not squeeze area).
   f. When collection is complete, use a bandage to maintain pressure at puncture site.
   g. Immediately run sample or place in ice bath.
8. Documentation and monitoring
   a. $FIO_2$ or oxygen flow
   b. Ventilator settings or oxygen delivery device
   c. Patient temperature, respiratory rate, heart rate, and clinical appearance
   d. Appearance of puncture site before and after blood sampling
   e. Problems obtaining the CBG (multiple sticks, poor bleeding, or excessive movement of patient)
   f. Date, time, and sampling site
9. Frequency
   a. Frequent CBGs may indicate the need for placement of an indwelling catheter because repeated punctures cause scarring, osteomyelitis, and cellulitis of the puncture site. If possible, alter the site for punctures.
10. Control of infection
    a. Aseptic techniques should be used.
    b. Universal precautions should be followed.
    c. Contaminated equipment should be disposed of properly.

B. Percutaneous arterial sample
1. Indications
   a. The need to assess pH, $PaCO_2$, partial pressure of arterial oxygen ($PaO_2$), hemoglobin, total hemoglobin, dyshemoglobin saturations, and intrapulmonary shunting.
   b. The need to quantify the response to therapy intervention and/or diagnostic intervention.
   c. Monitor the severity and progression of the disease state.
2. Contraindications
   a. Negative modified Allen test results.
   b. Vascular disease or infection of the involved site.
   c. Coagulopathy or medium- to high-dose anticoagulation therapy (heparin, streptokinase, or warfarin [Coumadin]).
   d. Improperly functioning analyzer.
   e. Lack of validation of function by commercially prepared control products or tonometered whole blood.
   f. Specimen containing air bubbles and not anticoagulated.
   g. Specimen that has been at room temperature for more than 5 min.
   h. Specimen has been chilled in an ice bath for ≥ 2 h or has not been properly chilled in an ice bath for ≤ 2 h.
3. Complications and hazards
   a. Hematoma
   b. Excessive bleeding
   c. Infection introduced by needle stick
   d. Air or clotted-blood emboli
4. Obtaining peripheral arterial blood gases (ABGs) (radial).
   a. Check chart and gather equipment.
   b. Determine the best site for the puncture. The best site for a puncture should be accessible, easy to palpate, and easily stabilized.
   c. The radial artery best fits this description. The branchial artery should be considered next if the radial artery is not accessible.
   d. Once the peripheral site has been determined, the patient is assessed for collateral blood flow. The modified Allen test best assesses collateral blood flow.

(1) The practitioner occludes both the radial and ulnar artery.
(2) The patient clenches the hand in a tight fist. This blanches the hand. If the patient is unable to perform this maneuver, the practitioner can blanch the hand by squeezing it several times.
(3) The clenched hand then is opened to a relaxed position and the practitioner releases the ulnar artery.
(4) If color returns to the blanched hand, then there is collateral blood flow by way of the ulnar artery. This represents good capillary refill (should take less than 2 s), and the puncture can be performed on that hand.
(5) If no blood flow has returned, then the puncture should not be performed on that hand. The other hand can then be evaluated in the same manner, and if good capillary refill is present, the puncture can be performed.

e. If a patient has been ordered to receive oxygen, it is important to perform the puncture while the patient is on oxygen. Any changes in the prescribed $FIO_2$ should include a 10- to 20-min period before obtaining the sample. This also includes any changes in ventilatory parameters such as tidal volume, rate, positive end-expiratory pressure (PEEP), continuous positive airway pressure (CPAP), synchronized intermittent mandatory ventilation (SIMV), intermittent mandatory ventilation (IMV), PIP, and so on.
f. A number of circumstances that may prevent a practitioner from obtaining a blood gas sample include the following:
   (1) Needle passes through the artery
   (2) Needle passes on either side of the artery
   (3) Low blood pressure
   (4) Constricted artery
   (5) Clot in the needle
g. The most common trauma that occurs from puncture is a hematoma. Following the puncture, pressure should be applied to the puncture site for 5 min and until the bleeding stops.
h. The sample should now have all the air bubbles removed. Air bubbles can cause a change in the values. The $PaCO_2$ may be lowered, which would affect the pH, and the $PaO_2$ may be higher than normal.
i. For newborns and small infants, a butterfly needle attached to a syringe may be used to obtain the sample. In cases where the artery cannot be felt, transillumination of the artery will identify the location of the vessel.

C. Peripheral arterial catheter (PAL)
1. Indications
   a. Frequent blood gas sampling
   b. Continuous blood pressure monitoring
   c. Inability to place an umbilical artery catheter
2. Fluid-filled monitoring system
   a. A fluid-filled system is used to maintain arterial access and provide arterial blood pressure values.
   b. This system consists of fluid system with heparinized saline, microdrip chamber, and infusion pump (for newborns) or pressurized bag (for adult system). The neonatal system uses an infusion pump with a maximum pressure of 100 mm Hg. This system is designed to deliver very small volumes and prevent fluid overload.
   c. After zeroing the transducer, the transducer must be leveled with the tip of the catheter. Circulating pressures are referenced to midchest level with the patient supine.
   d. A transducer below the catheter tip increases hydrostatic pressure on the transducer, resulting in a higher pressure reading. A transducer above the catheter tip decreases hydrostatic pressure on the transducer, resulting in a low pressure reading.
3. Inserting PAL
   a. Radial artery most often used.
   b. Perform Allen's test.
   c. Cleanse the site with appropriate solution (povidone-iodine, alcohol).
   d. Puncture artery, watch for blood flow.
   e. Flush catheter, then attach to a fluid-filled system.
   f. Secure catheter.
   g. Provide povidone-iodine to insertion site and stabilize arm.
4. Obtaining arterial blood for analysis from PAL.

a. Gather equipment.
   (1) Heparinized blood gas syringe
   (2) 3-mL syringe
   (3) Syringe of flush solution for neonates (Adult system will use the flush solution in the pressurized bag.)
   (4) Gloves
b. Insert 3-mL syringe.
c. Turn three-way stopcock toward transducer. The arterial waveform will disappear.
d. Withdraw appropriate amount of blood from the line. Turn stopcock off to the syringe.
e. Remove syringe and insert heparinized blood gas syringe.
f. Turn stopcock toward transducer and withdraw appropriate amount of blood for analysis. Turn stopcock off to the syringe. Remove any air bubbles from the sample and chill the sample in an ice bath if the sample cannot be analyzed within 5 min.
g. Insert 3-mL syringe with blood. Turn stopcock off to transducer. First aspirate for any air bubbles in stopcock; then inject blood into line. Observe for any air bubbles entering line. If bubbles enter the line, aspirate the line removing the bubbles; then inject blood.
h. Turn stopcock off to the syringe.
   (1) For neonatal systems, insert flush solution into the hub of the three-way stopcock. Turn the stopcock off to the transducer. First aspirate for any air bubbles; then inject flush until the line is clear of any blood. Leave the flush solution in the stopcock. Turn the stopcock off to the syringe. The arterial waveform should now be visible on the monitor.
   (2) Fluid-filled devices using a pressurized bag system utilize the fast flush device to clear the hub of the three-way stopcock and the line entering the patient.

D. Umbilical artery catheter (UAC)
   1. Indications
      a. Frequent blood gas sampling
      b. Continuous blood pressure monitoring
      c. Exchange transfusion
   2. The fluid-filled monitoring equipment is the same as for peripheral arterial line.
   3. Placement
      a. Two placements may be used:
         (1) Low-position catheter tip is at lumbar vertebrae 3 to 4.
         (2) High-position catheter lies above the diaphragm at thoracic vertebrae 6 to 9.
      b. Once the catheter is placed, aspirate and observe for blood return.
      c. A radiograph is taken to confirm placement (abdominal for low position, chest radiograph for high position).
      d. On a lateral radiograph look for a downward and then an upward turn in the catheter to confirm placements.
   4. Problems and complications
      a. Thromboembolus
      b. Air embolus
      c. Hemorrhage
      d. Infection
      e. Vessel perforation
   5. Indications for removal
      a. Access to umbilical artery no longer needed.
      b. Nonfunctioning catheter
      c. Infection

E. Umbilical venous catheter
   1. Indications
      a. Access for fluids and medications
      b. Blood sampling
      c. Central venous pressure monitoring
   2. Placement
      a. Insert 2 to 3 cm, withdraw blood, and then continue to advance for the prescribed distance and location.
      b. An inability to withdraw blood may mean there is a clot at the end of the catheter. The catheter should be removed.

TABLE 7–3. ***Umbilical Cord Blood Gas Values for Term Fetus***

| | Artery | Vein |
|---|---|---|
| pH | 7.26±0.08 | 7.33±0.07 |
| $PaCO_2$ (mm Hg) | 53±10.0 | 43±8.3 |
| $PaO_2$ (mm Hg) | 19±7.0 | 29±10 |

3. Obstruction to insertion may indicate that the catheter is wedged in the vein or has entered the portal system.
4. Once the catheter is properly placed, a radiograph is taken to verify catheter position. A lateral radiograph may be required for location if the anterior-posterior (A-P) radiograph does not verify location.

F. Umbilical cord blood gases
1. Objective measure of the newborn's condition immediately following birth
2. Determine the extent of hypoxia, hypercapnia, and acidosis.
3. This, in combination with physical assessment, is evidence of birth asphyxia.
4. No significant difference in mean values of infants of different gestational ages (24 to 36 weeks)
5. No significant difference in mean values between infants born vaginally and those born in the breech position
6. Cord gases can be left without ice for up to 1 h without a significant mean value change.
7. Normal umbilical cord blood gas values (Table 7–3)

## III. Hemodynamic monitoring

A. Pulmonary artery pressure and pulmonary vascular resistance (PVR)
1. PVR is the result of the tone or caliber of the vessels. PVR is low as compared to systemic vascular resistance (SVR). A change in PVR will alter blood flow.
2. Pressure gradient to determine blood flow equals inflow of blood and outflow of blood.
3. In the pulmonary system the pressure gradient is determined by the difference between the mean pulmonary artery pressure (mPAP) and left atrial pressure (LAP).
4. If PVR increases, blood flow into the lungs and out to the heart decreases. This puts a greater strain on the heart, specifically the right side of the heart, to maintain stroke volume (milliliters of blood per beat of the heart).
5. Factors that affect PVR
   a. Autonomic nervous system
   b. Vasoactive agents
   c. Atelectasis
   d. Other physical factors, including alveolar pressure from spontaneous breathing and mechanical ventilation and gravity
   e. Hypoxemia, hypercapnia, and acidosis (Table 7–4)
6. Determination of PVR and PVR index (PVRI)
   a. $$\text{PVR} = \frac{\text{mPAP} - \text{PCWP}}{\text{Cardiac output (CO)}} \times 80 = \text{dynes/s/cm}^{-5}$$

TABLE 7–4. ***Causes of PVR Change***

| Cause | Change |
|---|---|
| Hypoxemia from poor alveolar oxygenation | Increased PVR |
| Hyperoxemia | Decreased PVR |
| Hypercarbia | Increased PVR |
| Hypocarbia | Decreased PVR |
| Acidosis | Increased PVR |
| Alkalosis | Decreased PVR |
| Nitric oxide | Decreased PVR |
| Pain | Increased PVR |
| Hypothermia | Increased PVR |

b. $$PVRI = \frac{mPAP - PCWP}{\text{Cardiac index (CI)}} \times 80 = \text{dynes/s/cm}^{-5}/\text{m}^2$$

B. Systemic blood pressure (BP) and systemic vascular resistance
   1. Factors that control systemic blood pressure include the following:
      a. Local autoregulation: This regulates blood flow at the tissue level.
      b. Chemoreceptor: Changes in blood components (oxygen, $H^+$, and pH) alter blood blow.
      c. Chemical: ADH reduces fluid loss. Epinephrine increases the rate and contractility of the heart. It also constricts arterioles.
   2. Mean arterial pressure (MAP) represents the average pressure throughout the cardiac cycle (systole and diastole).
      a. $$MAP = \frac{\text{Systole} + (2 \times \text{diastole})}{3}$$
      b. MAP = Diastolic pressure + one-third pulse pressure (systolic pressure – diastolic pressure).
   3. Systemic vascular resistance and systemic vascular resistance index (SVRI)
      a. SVR = CO × BP, where CO = stroke volume × heart rate, and BP is developed from SVR, CO, and blood volume.
      b. $$SVR = MAP - \frac{CVP \times 80}{CO} = \text{dynes/s/cm}^{-5}/\text{m}^2$$
      c. $$SVRI = MAP - \frac{CVP \times 80}{CI} = \text{dynes/sec/cm}^{-5}/\text{m}^2$$

C. Clinical indicators of cardiac output
   1. Blood pressure. Decrease BP with reduced cardiac output after all compensating factors are utilized by the body, including increased heart rate, vasoconstriction, and decreased fluid output.
   2. Saturation of venous blood with oxygen ($SvO_2$) (normal is 70 to 75%) decreases as cardiac output decreases.
   3. Arterial oxygen concentration ($CaO_2$) and venous oxygen concentration ($CvO_2$) (normal is 4.5 to 5.5%) increase as cardiac output decreases.
   4. Urine output decreases as cardiac output decreases.
   5. Peripheral pulses: Thready to loss of peripheral pulses with decreased cardiac output.
   6. Skin perfusion: Increased capillary refill time, decreased temperature, and loss of color.
   7. CNS perfusion: Confusion and/or lack of appropriate answers to time, place, and person indicate poor perfusion from decreased cardiac output.

D. Determinants of cardiac output
   1. CO is determined by stroke volume times heart rate: 70 mL of blood × 80 beats/min = 5.6 L/min.
   2. Stroke volume is determined by preload, afterload, and contractility.
   3. Preload
      a. Preload is the filling pressure in the ventricles of the right and left ventricles.
      b. Preload is determined by blood volume, distribution of blood volume, atrial kick, and left ventricular function.
      c. Clinical indicators of preload include central venous pressure (CVP) of the right side of the heart and pulmonary capillary wedge pressure (PCWP) of the left side of the heart.
      d. Conditions altering preload include hypovolemia (burns, dehydration), congestive heart failure (CHF), renal failure, and altered vascular space (sepsis, anaphylaxis).
   4. Afterload
      a. Force that the ventricle muscle must contract against to eject blood into the arterial circulation
      b. Afterload is determined by vascular resistance, mass and viscosity of the blood, and compliance of the circulatory system.
      c. Conditions altering afterload include blood viscosity, hypoxemia, hypertension, and atherosclerosis. In general, conditions that alter vascular resistance will alter afterload. Since vascular resistance affects afterload, calculating PVR and SVR will give a clinical picture of afterload.
   5. Contractility
      a. Force of contraction by the myocardium

b. Contractility determinants include ventricular muscle mass, catecholamines, heart rate, metabolic state, and drugs such as (+) inotropic agents (digitalis dopamine) or (–) inotropic agents (beta blockers, antidysrhythmics).
c. Conditions that decrease contractility include myocardial infarction (MI), cardiomyopathy, ischemia, hypoxia, and acidosis.

6. Calculation of cardiac output and cardiac index
a. $$CO = \frac{\dot{V}O_2 \text{ (oxygen consumption)}}{CaO_2 - CvO_2 \times 10} = \text{L/min}$$
b. $$\text{Cardiac index} = \frac{\text{cardiac output}}{\text{body surface area (BSA in m}^2\text{)}} = \text{L/min/m}^2$$
7. Normal hemodynamic values (Table 7–5)

E. Central venous pressure
1. Indications.
a. Monitor right heart pressure.
b. Monitor fluid administration.
c. Monitor blood volume.
2. Increased CVP occurs with increased pressures resulting from chronic obstructive pulmonary disease (COPD) (cystic fibrosis), primary pulmonary hypertension, pulmonary embolism, and sepsis.
3. Decreased CVP results from hypovolemia (hemorrhage, dehydration) relative to the intravascular space.

F. Pulmonary artery catheter (PAC) (balloon-inflated, flow-directed catheter, or Swan-Ganz catheter).
1. Description of the PAC.
a. The PAC is a multilumen catheter (the triple-lumen catheter is common) that rests in the pulmonary artery and has the capability of measuring left heart pressures when the balloon at the end of the catheter is inflated.
b. Make-up of the triple-lumen PAC.
(1) A thermistor hub connects to a cardiac output computer to measure cardiac output.
(2) The distal lumen hub measures PAP and pulmonary capillary wedge pressure (PCWP); IV flush solution emits from end of catheter. A mixed venous blood sample is drawn from this lumen.
(3) The balloon inflation valve connects to the balloon at the distal end of the catheter to inflate the balloon to obtain wedge pressures (left ventricular end-diastolic pressure). A syringe attached to the hub inflates the balloon.
(4) The proximal lumen hub measures CVP and cardiac output (injected solution to measure cardiac output injected in this hub).
(5) The proximal lumen port rests in the right atrium.
(6) The balloon rests in pulmonary artery.
(7) Thermistor detects blood temperature changes to calculate cardiac output rests in pulmonary artery.
(8) The distal lumen port allows flush solution to be emitted or blood to be drawn for shunt calculation.

TABLE 7–5. ***Normal Hemodynamic Values***

| | **Newborn (up to 30 days of age)** | **Infant (up to 1 y of age)** | **Child (>1 y of age)** |
|---|---|---|---|
| MAP (mm Hg) | 62–76 | 67–79 | 1–8 yr 67–85<br>> 8 yr 81–96 |
| PVR: | | | |
| dyn/s/cm$^{-5}$ | | 2000–3200 | 40–320 |
| PVRI: | | | |
| dyn/s/cm$^{-5}$/m$^2$ | | 560–1200 | 80–240 |
| SVR: | | | |
| dyn/s/cm$^{-5}$ | | 2800–4000 | 1200–2000 |
| SVRI: | 0.9 | | |
| dyn/s/cm$^{-5}$/m$^2$ | | 800–1200 | 1200–2400 |
| CO (L/min) | | 1.2 | 1–8 yr 1.5–3.6<br>> 8 yr 3.4–6.0<br>(Reduces to 100 mL/kg/min) |

2. Indications for PAC
   a. Monitor left heart.
   b. Adult respiratory distress syndrome (ARDS)
   c. Sepsis
3. Direct data obtained from a PAC
   a. Cardiac output
   b. Mixed venous oxygen ($PvO_2$)
   c. Pulmonary artery pressure
   d. Central venous pressure
   e. PCWP or pulmonary artery occluding pressure (PAOP)
   f. Mixed venous oxygen saturation ($SvO_2$ contained in special PAC)
4. Insertion of the PAC
   a. The PAC is commonly inserted into the internal jugular or subclavian vein.
   b. As the catheter is inserted and advanced into the right atrium, the balloon at the end of the catheter is inflated, which assists in the advancement of the catheter.
5. Fluid-filled monitoring equipment for PAC pressures
   a. The equipment required for a PAC is similar to the setup for a peripheral arterial catheter, except for the catheter.
6. Obtaining PCWP with the PAC
   a. Once the catheter is wedged (balloon inflated), pressures from the left heart are obtained.
   b. The balloon obstructs blood flow to the tip of the catheter. Pressure developed in the left atrium and left ventricle transmits back to the catheter tip.
7. Confirmation of a wedged PAC
   a. The pulmonary artery waveform changes into a pulmonary wedge waveform. When the balloon is deflated, the pulmonary artery waveform reappears.
   b. If blood is withdrawn from the distal lumen with the balloon inflated, the sample will have a slightly higher $PaO_2$ and will be fully saturated as compared to an arterial sample drawn from another site in the body.
8. Waveforms from a PAC from the right atrium to PCWP (Fig. 7–1)
9. Normal pediatric hemodynamic values (Table 7–6)
10. Mixed venous sample to determine shunting
   a. Blood is slowly withdrawn from the distal lumen of the PAC, while at the same time an arterialized sample is obtained. The two samples are then analyzed.
   b. Rapid aspiration may contaminate the mixed venous sample. A true mixed venous sample has a $CO_2$ equal to, or lower than, a simultaneously obtained arterial blood sample.
   c. Percent shunt equation

$$\% = \frac{(PAO_2 - PaO_2)\ (0.003)}{(PAO_2 - PaO_2)\ (0.003) + a\text{-}vDO_2} \times 100$$

11. Troubleshooting arterial lines (Table 7–7)

G. Respiratory effects on hemodynamic pressures
   1. During normal spontaneous inspiration, a negative intrapleural pressure

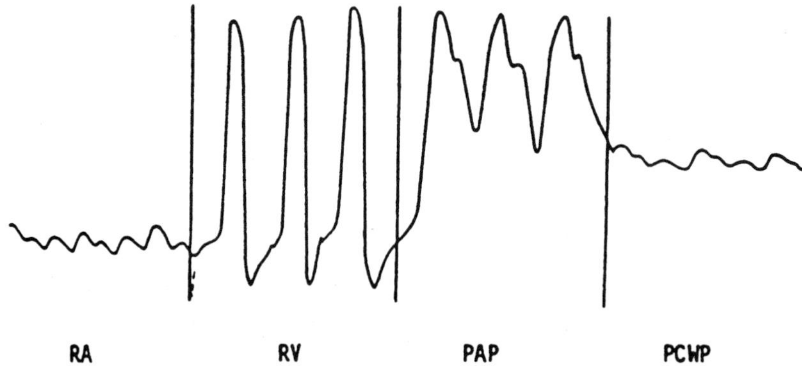


**FIGURE 7–1** Hemodynamic waveform obtained from insertion of a pulmonary artery catheter from the right atrium (RA) into the right ventricle (RV) into the pulmonary artery (PA). The pulmonary capillary wedge pressure (PCWP) is seen when the catheter balloon is inflated and the catheter wedges into the capillary.

TABLE 7–6. ***Normal Pediatric Hemodynamic Values***

| Value | Abbreviation | Normal Value | How Measured or Obtained |
|---|---|---|---|
| Central venous pressure | CVP | 0–3 mm Hg | Central venous triple-lumen catheter located in superior vena cava |
| Right ventricular pressure | RVP | 30/3 | Pulmonary artery catheter |
| Pulmonary artery pressure | PAP | 30/10 mPAP = 16 | Pulmonary artery catheter |
| Left atrial pressure | LAP | 4–12 with a mean pressure of 8 | Pulmonary artery catheter with balloon inflated during ventricular systole |
| Left ventricular pressure | LVP | 100/4–12 | Systolic pressure—Obtained from arterial line or blood pressure cuff<br>Diastolic pressure—PCWP<br>PAC with the balloon inflated during ventricular diastole |
| Pulmonary capillary wedge pressure | PCWP | 4–12 mm Hg | Pulmonary artery catheter with the balloon inflated in the wedged position |
| Mixed venous pressure | $PvO_2$ | 40 mm Hg | Blood from pulmonary artery |
| Atrial-venous oxygen content difference | $CaO_2$–$CvO_2$(a-$vDO_2$) | 3.5–5.5 vol % | Contents from arterial and venous blood obtained from arterial stick or arterial line and pulmonary blood |
| Stroke volume | SV | 10–85 mL | Cardiac output ÷ heart rate |

causes a fall in right atrial, right ventricular, pulmonary artery, pulmonary artery wedge, and left atrial pressure. Right ventricular preload and pulmonary arterial outflow increases. The elasticity and compliance of the pulmonary vasculature pools blood, reducing left ventricular filling. This results in a decreased stroke volume.

2. During normal spontaneous expiration, pulmonary venous return increases as intrapleural pressure begins returning to normal. This increases left ventricular filling and stroke volume.
3. During inspiration from mechanical ventilation, right atrial pressure increases. Right atrial preload decreases (venous return). PAP is increased because of increased PVR from increased airway pressure, squeezing vessels. Pulmonary blood flow and cardiac output fall. PCWP and LAP are elevated and diastolic filling of the left ventricle is decreased.
4. During expiration, intrathoracic pressures decrease. Right atrial pressure decreases and preload increases. PAP decreases and pulmonary blood flow and cardiac output increases. Because of these changes, hemodynamic pressures are obtained at end-expiration.

H. $SvO_2$ monitoring.

1. $SvO_2$ is the saturation of the mixed venous blood. The $SvO_2$ monitoring device is incorporated into the PAC and uses reflective spectrophotometry through fiber optics to obtain the saturation.
2. The normal $SvO_2$ is 60 to 80%. A change of 5% or less is not clinically significant and does not require intervention. A change in $SvO_2$ greater than 10% is significant and requires intervention.
3. Causes of fluctuations in $SvO_2$ (Tables 7–8 and 7–9)

## IV. Noninvasive monitoring.

A. Noninvasive blood pressure measurement

1. Routine blood pressure measurement is accomplished by using a cuff on an arm or leg. There is no clinical significant difference in blood pressure when either of these sites is used for the newborn.
2. The most widely used method for measuring blood pressure is the oscillometric technique. Disadvantages to this method are that spontaneous movement by the infant, respiratory artifact, and cardiac dysrhythmia can cause inaccurate readings.
   a. The cuff is inflated to above systolic pressure. Oscillatory pressure changes are noted at this level. As the cuff pressure is released, oscillatory pressure

TABLE 7–7. ***Troubleshooting the Arterial and Pulmonary Artery Catheter***

| Problem | Cause | Action |
|---|---|---|
| No waveform seen on monitor. | Transducer not open to catheter. | Check position of stopcock. |
| | Catheter clotted. | Aspirate blood clot. |
| Damped waveform on monitor (systolic pressure decreases, diastolic pressure increases). | Air bubbles in setup. | Remove bubbles. Use fast-flush device to purge system. |
| | Blood clot in catheter. | Aspirate clot. |
| | PAC—Forward migration of catheter into the pulmonary artery. | Reposition catheter and secure. |
| | PAL—Catheter lodged against the artery. | Manipulate catheter until appropriate waveform is seen. |
| | Leak in setup. | Secure all connections. |
| | Pressure bag not inflated to 300 mm Hg. | Inflate bag to 300 mm Hg. |
| False low measurement. | Transducer level too high. | Reposition transducer vent port at phlebostatic axis (4th intercostal space sternal border). |
| False high measurement. | Transducer level too low. | Reposition transducer vent port at phlebostatic axis (4th intercostal space sternal border). |
| Active bleedback from the patient to the transducer. | Pressure bag less than 300 mm Hg (not used in neonate). | Inflate bag to 300 mm Hg. |
| | Leak in system | Secure all connections. |
| PAC—Cannot obtain a wedge (PCWP) reading. | Balloon ruptured. | Use pulmonary end-diastolic value to approximate wedge pressure. |
| | Catheter not advanced enough for balloon to wedge. | Inflate balloon and advance catheter until a wedge pressure is seen. |
| Arterial—Hematoma after withdrawal of the catheter. | Bleeding at puncture site. | Hold puncture site for 5 min or until bleeding stops. |
| Micro drip chamber has continuous flow of fluid. | Fast-flush device broken. | Replace fast-flush device. |
| PCWP waveform appears on monitor with balloon deflated. | Forward migration of catheter. | Pull catheter back until a PAP waveform is seen. |
| Right ventricular waveform appears on monitor. | Catheter has migrated back into right ventricle. | Observe for ventricular dysrhythmia. Advance catheter to PAP if sterile. Pull back to RA if catheter is contaminated. |

increases until a mean arterial pressure is reached and then falls below the diastolic pressure.

3. The Doppler ultrasound method is another noninvasive method of measuring blood pressure, but the technique requires precise placement of the cuff and transducer. The Doppler transducer is placed under the cuff or distal to the occluding cuff over the artery to be occluded. Vessel wall vibration from the occluded vessel is transmitted to the transducer. As cuff pressure is reduced, less vibration occurs. The doppler ultrasound blood pressure method gives clinically acceptable systolic and diastolic pressures.

B. Transcutaneous oxygen ($PtcO_2$) and carbon dioxide ($PtcCO_2$) monitoring
   1. The transcutaneous method measures gases as diffusion occurs through the skin. A heated electrode placed on the surface of the skin measures the gases.
   2. $PtcO_2$ uses the Clark electrode and the $PtcCO_2$ uses the Severinghaus electrode.
   3. Transcutaneous monitoring is used as a trend monitoring device.
   4. The transcutaneous electrode is heated, which hyperperfuses the dermis layer of the skin.
      a. The transcutaneous oxygen electrode increases the capillary $PO_2$ by offsetting the drop in oxygen from consumption by tissues and diffusion barrier.
      b. The transcutaneous carbon dioxide electrode heat raises the capillary $PCO_2$. Further increases in $PCO_2$ occur because of a local increase in production of carbon dioxide, resulting in the transcutaneous $CO_2$ being greater than the arterial $CO_2$. Correction factors are used by the manufacturer so that both values approximate each other.
      c. Electrode temperature is in a recommended range of 43 to 45°C. Because of the thinness of their skin, micropremies (weighing less than 1000 gm)

TABLE 7–8. ***Causes of Increased $SvO_2$***

| Causes of Increased $SvO_2$ | | |
|---|---|---|
| ↑ Oxygen supply | ↑ Cardiac output | Septic shock, Inotropic agents |
| | ↑ $SaO_2$ | Hyperoxia, ↑ $FiO_2$ |
| | ↑ Hemoglobin | Polycythemia |
| ↓ Oxygen demand | ↓ $\dot{V}O_2$ | Hypothermia, paralysis, anesthesia |
| Catheter not able to "see" blood | | Wedged into the pulmonary capillary, catheter tip facing wall of vessel |

and premature infants may require the electrode temperature to be set at the lower end of this scale and/or changed more frequently. Erythema, a red, circular area caused by the heated electrode's contact with the skin, is normal and fades over time. Blistering requires more frequent electrode site changes (from every 3 h to every 2 h) or decreases in electrode temperature. Care must be taken not to decrease the electrode temperature below manufacturer specifications because this will affect the accuracy of the device.

5. Placement of the electrodes
   a. With a newborn or a pediatric patient, the electrode is placed on a flat portion of the skin that also has good perfusion. An electrolyte solution, placed on the electrode, is a medium for the diffusion of gases from the skin to the electrode. The proper electrolyte solution is important for accurate transcutaneous values.
   b. For newborn infants and children, the chest, thigh, and abdomen are good locations. For the newborn, the upper right chest and the area over the liver are used for determining ductal shunting when compared to a location with perfusion from the postductal site (see Chapter 5). Also fetal scalp placement provides monitoring during labor.
6. As infants and children grow, changes in skin thickness, texture, disease, and capillaries alter the relationship between the $PtcO_2$ and the $PaO_2$ (ratio decreases) and the $PtcCO_2$–$PaCO_2$ (ratio increases). In general, blood gases are done periodically to correlate the transcutaneous values with the arterial values.
7. Transcutaneous monitoring requires calibration of the oxygen and carbon dioxide electrodes. The carbon dioxide calibration requires two different percentages of carbon dioxide gas. The oxygen calibration uses room air.
8. Following individual use of an electrode, it should be disinfected according to manufacturer's specifications. The monitor is cleansed following individual patient use.
9. Troubleshooting (Table 7–10)

C. Pulse oximetry ($SpO_2$)
   1. Indications
      a. Monitoring adequacy of arterial oxyhemoglobin saturation
      b. Quantify the response of arterial oxyhemoglobin saturation to a therapeutic procedure.
      c. Comply with the regulations and recommendations of authoritative groups.
   2. Contraindications
      a. The need to measure pH, $PaCO_2$, total hemoglobin, and abnormal hemoglobin
   3. Hazards and complications

TABLE 7–9. ***Causes of Decreased $SvO_2$***

| Causes of Decreased $SvO_2$ | | |
|---|---|---|
| ↓ Oxygen supply | ↓ Cardiac output | Heart failure, ↑ PEEP, dysrhythmia |
| | ↓ $SaO_2$ | Respiratory failure, ventilator disconnect, suctioning |
| | ↓ hemoglobin | Anemia, hemorrhage |
| ↑ Oxygen demand | ↑ $\dot{V}O_2$ | Hyperthermia, shivering, seizures |
| | | ↑ Work of breathing, fever, activity, sepsis |

TABLE 7–10. ***Troubleshooting $PtcO_2$ and $PtcCO_2$ Transcutaneous Monitors***

| Problem | Cause | Remedy |
|---|---|---|
| High $PtcO_2$/low $PtcCO_2$ does not correlate with $PaO_2$/$PaCO_2$ condition of patient. | Air leak between skin and electrode. | Press electrode firmly against skin. Reapply electrode. If necessary, recalibrate. |
| | Incorrect calibration. | Recalibrate. |
| | Air bubbles under membrane. | Change membranes and electrolyte solution and reapply. |
| $PtcO_2$/$PtcCO_2$ does not correlate with $PaCO_2$/$PaO_2$ condition of patient. | Poor perfusion of skin site. | Evaluate heating power. |
| | Unsuitable skin site for diffusion. | Reapply electrode to more suitable site |
| | Membrane needs cleaning. | Change membrane and electrolyte solution and reapply. |
| | Incorrect calibration. | Recalibrate away from oxygen source. |
| | | Check gas tanks for proper gas concentration for $PtcCO_2$. |
| Electrode will not stabilize at calibration values; drifting. | Not enough warm-up time. | Allow greater warmup time. |
| | Electrode needs cleaning. | Change membrane and electrolyte solution and reapply. |
| Blistering or burns are noticed when changing electrode site. | Electrode temperature is too high. | Reduce temperature (premature infant). Check manufacturer's guidelines. |
| | Electrode is left on site too long. | Change site more often. |

a. Tissue injury at the site of measurement from misuse of the probe, such as pressure sores, or burns from incompatible sensors

4. Alteration in results and device limitations
   a. Motion artifact
   b. Low perfusion states
   c. COHb and methemoglobin presence
   d. Intravascular dyes
   e. Exposure of probe to ambient light (bilirubin lights)
   f. Skin pigmentation
   g. Nail coverings and polish
   h. Low saturation states (less than 83%)
   i. Hyperoxemia level undetermined.
5. To validate, the pulse oximeter and arterial oxyhemoglobin saturation should be performed with the initial setup, and then periodically.
6. For consistency of care, select an appropriate probe site; set high and low alarms appropriately; apply and adjust response time and electrocardiographic coupling; and assure that the device is detecting an adequate pulse by observing the amplitude of the pulse waveform.
7. In the chart, document $SpO_2$ values and the conditions under which these values were recorded, including the following:
   a. Date, time, and pulse oximeter reading
   b. Activity and position
   c. Inspired oxygen concentration, device, and liter flow
   d. Probe type and placement site
   e. Stability of readings
   f. Results of determining arterial blood gas values and pulse oximetry values simultaneously. Report any disparity between these two values and explore possible causes. If there is any disparity, suggest altering the probe site or replacing the probe. If the disparity is not remedied, obtain arterial blood gas values and do not report the saturation value. Document the corrective action.
   g. Clinical appearance of patient
   h. Heart rate and pulse oximeter agreement determined by palpation and heart monitor.
8. Needs assessment
   a. Measurement of $SaO_2$ is not possible or available.
   b. Appropriate for prolonged monitoring during procedures or continuous monitoring

c. Appropriate when acid-base assessment is not required
9. Outcome assessment
a. The $SpO_2$ reflects the patient's condition (validate ordering a test).
b. Documentation of intervention or lack of intervention results; clinical decisions based on $SpO_2$ value
10. The frequency of measurement is based on the clinical status of the patient. Invasive procedures require continuous monitoring to detect desaturation. Periodic or "spot" evaluation may be used in stable patients to wean them from oxygen.
11. Disposable probes should be discarded following individual patient use. The monitor is cleaned following individual use.

D. Capnography and capnometry
1. Capnography is the continuous analysis and recording of carbon dioxide at the patient's airway. Capnometry is analysis without a continuous written record or waveform.
2. Normal end-tidal carbon dioxide ($PetCO_2$) is 4.5 to 5.5%, which is equivalent to a $PaCO_2$ of 35 to 45 mm Hg.
3. Measured by an analyzer using a mainstream or sidestream device located between the endotracheal tube (ETT) and the wye adaptor of the patient's ventilator circuit
4. Indications
a. Evaluation of $PetCO_2$
b. Monitoring severity of pulmonary disease; response to therapy to improve ratio of dead space to tidal volume (VD/VT); matching of ventilation to perfusion and therapy to increase coronary artery blood flow
c. Determination of tracheal versus esophageal intubation (reduced or absent cardiac output may negate its use for this purpose)
d. Determine efficiency of mechanical ventilator support by comparing the $PaCO_2$ and $PetCO_2$ difference.
e. Monitoring coronary artery blood flow adequacy
f. Monitoring the administration of $CO_2$ when it is used as a therapeutic gas
g. Evaluate waveform of the ventilator-patient interface to determine abnormalities (see Clinical Conditions Altering Carbon Dioxide Waveform later in this section).
5. Normal carbon dioxide waveform (Fig. 7–2)
6. Difference between $PetCO_2$ and $PaCO_2$
a. Under normal conditions and where $PaCO_2$ is corrected for body temperature, the difference in this gradient is less than 5 mm Hg.
b. Dead-space ventilation increases the $PetCO_2$–$PaCO_2$ difference. Dead-space ventilation conditions include the following:
(1) Reduced blood flow in pulmonary circulation
(2) Pulmonary thromboemboli
(3) Patient position—lateral decubitus
(4) High tidal volume

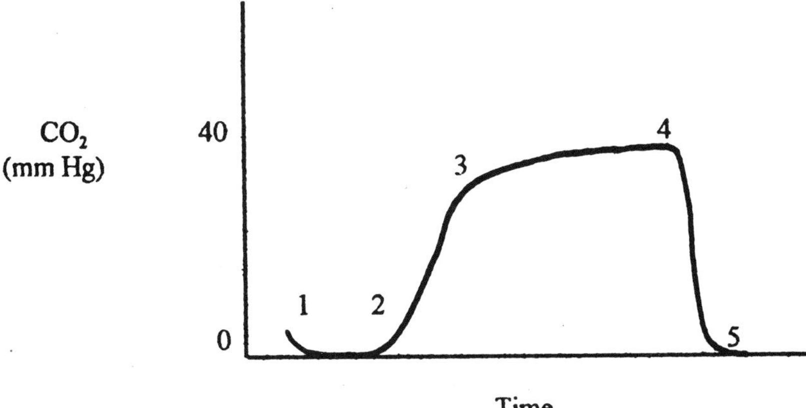


**FIGURE 7–2** From 1 to 2 is baseline and represents gas that has minimal dead-space (low $CO_2$); from 2 to 3 represents more alveolar gas entrained, thus increasing $PetCO_2$, 3 to 4 represents mostly alveolar gas—this line will level out or plateau, representing $CO_2$ in the alveoli; 4 represents $PetCO_2$ and is the point just before inspiration occurs; 4 to 5 represents inspiration and reduction of $CO_2$ in inspiratory gas.

c. Another problem that alters the $PetCO_2$–$PaCO_2$ difference is shunting. Shunting results in a reduced $PaCO_2$–$PetCO_2$ difference. Shunt conditions include the following:
   (1) Atelectasis
   (2) Mucus plugging
   (3) Bronchial intubation
d. Periodic arterial blood gas evaluation is necessary to assess ventilatory adequacy.

7. Causes of increased $PetCO_2$
   a. Increased production of $CO_2$ and delivery to lungs caused by the following:
      (1) Fever
      (2) Sepsis
      (3) Seizures
   b. Decreased alveolar ventilation caused by the following:
      (1) Hypoventilation
      (2) Muscular paralysis
      (3) Overdose (respiratory center depression)
      (4) Chronic lung disease as a result of asthma or cystic fibrosis
8. Causes of decreased $PetCO_2$
   a. Decreased production of $CO_2$ and delivery to the lungs caused by the following:
      (1) Hypothermia
      (2) Hemorrhage
      (3) Pulmonary hypoperfusion
      (4) Thromboembolism
   b. Increased alveolar ventilation
   c. Equipment-related problems, such as the following:
      (1) Patient disconnected from ventilator
      (2) Esophageal intubation
      (3) Airway obstruction
      (4) Leak around the endotracheal tube cuff
      (5) Water in sample line in side-stream sampling device
      (6) Water obstructing cuvette or light sensor in mainstream sampling device
9. Specific situations in which capnography and capnometry are used
   a. Esophageal intubation
      (1) Although clinical criteria are useful (such as breath sounds, bilateral chest rise, no gastric distension, and so on), they still may not be adequate to determine improper tube placement in the esophagus.
      (2) In most people, esophageal $CO_2$ falls to zero after several insufflations. If the patient was mask ventilated, it may take longer because of some gastric insufflation. However, the end-tidal $CO_2$ should fall to zero within a minute.
   b. Pulmonary emboli (PE)
      (1) Reduction in end-tidal $CO_2$ caused by blood flow obstruction. Minute volume increases in these patients to maintain appropriate V/Q balance in the nonobstructed segments of the lung.
      (2) The $PaCO_2$–$PetCO_2$ gradient widens more than 5 mmHg.
      (3) These patients form a normal alveolar plateau; with the performance of a maximal expiratory maneuver, the $PaCO_2$–$PetCO_2$ gradient does not decrease. In other diseases such as emphysema, the gradient decreases following a maximal expiratory maneuver. This differentiates perfusion inequality from ventilation inequality.
   c. Cardiac arrest
      (1) Appropriate chest compression depth can be determined by measuring end-tidal $CO_2$.
      (2) End-tidal $CO_2$ will increase with the return of circulation from the appropriate depth of compressions.
      (3) The greater the $PetCO_2$, the greater the success of resuscitation.
      (4) Following successful resuscitation, the $PetCO_2$ may be greater than at prearrest levels. This occurs because during cardiac arrest with compressions, the $CO_2$ removal is impaired and the $PvCO_2$ increases, causing respiratory acidosis. With ventilatory support, the small amount of $PaCO_2$ present during the arrest will be reduced, causing respiratory alkalosis.
      (5) When spontaneous circulation returns, large quantities of $CO_2$ are presented to the lungs from the tissue. Given the same level of venti-

TABLE 7–11. *Capnograph Alterations*

| Waveform | Problem | Indication/ Correction |
|---|---|---|
| 1. 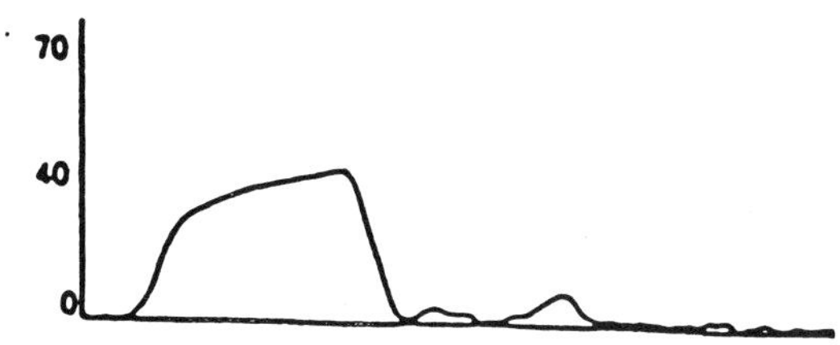 | Loss of $CO_2$ waveform and baseline to zero. | |
| | Endotracheal tube in esophagus. | Reintubate patient. |
| | Cardiac arrest. | Initiate CPR. |
| | Airway is disconnected. | Reconnect patient. |
| | Airway is completely obstructed. | Suction airway, extubate and reintubate patient. |
| | Sidestream analyzing port obstructed. | Free port of obstruction or replace sidestream device. |
| 2. 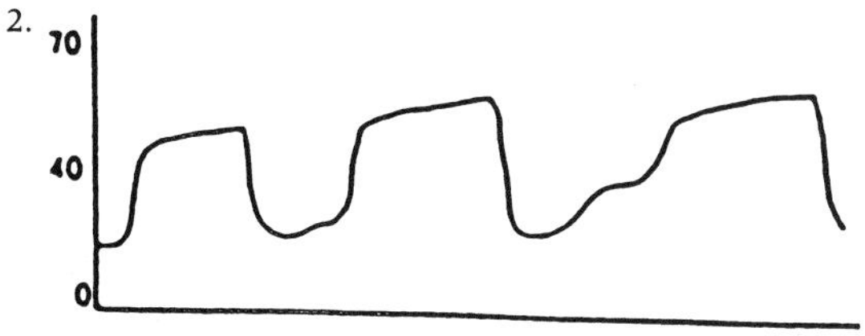 | Baseline rise in waveform. | |
| | Patient rebreathing $CO_2$. | Adjust minute ventilation on ventilator (tidal volume, frequency), place patient on assisted ventilation (remove from SIMV, PSV, CPAP). |
| | Mechanical dead space is added to the patient circuit between the ETT and wye adaptor. | Remove mechanical dead space. |
| 3. 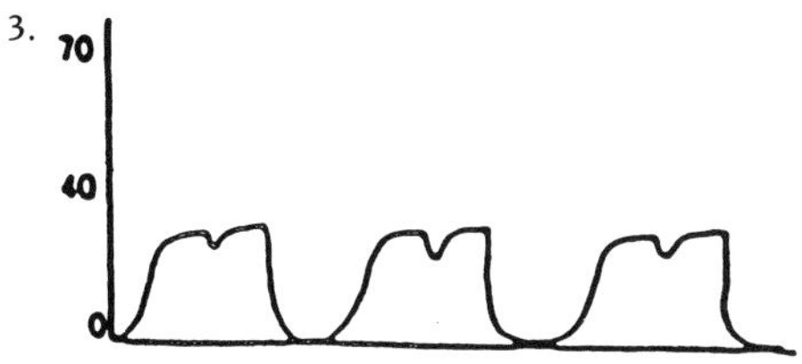 | "Curare cleft," indicating reversal of neuromuscular blocking agent. | Allow agent to reverse. Administer more neuromuscular blocking agent. |
| 4. 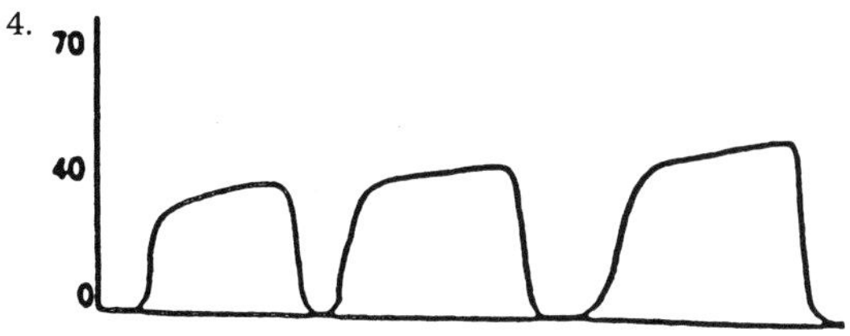 | Rise in the end-tidal point. | |
| | Hyperthermia. | Correct or remove elements that are causing the patient to be hyperthermic (blankets, excessive isolette temperature, procedure lights); increase work of breathing. Check for infection—antibiotics. |
| | Hypoventilation. | Increase minute ventilation. |

lation, the $PetCO_2$ begins to rise and transiently increases beyond pre-arrest values.

10. Hazards and complications
    a. The mainstream analyzer may add too much dead space to the breathing circuit.

b. Excessive weight placed on a small endotracheal tube may kink or displace the endotracheal tube.

11. Alteration in composition of the respiratory gas may alter the capnogram.
    a. High concentrations of both oxygen and nitrous oxide may alter the capnograph. Calibration of the device requires a correction factor in this situation.
    b. The presence of helium will increase the $CO_2$ values in proportion to the helium concentration.
    c. The device's response capabilities may be altered by high breathing frequency.
    d. Freon, a propellant in metered-dose inhaler (MDI) canisters, has been shown to artificially increase $CO_2$ values.
    e. Unreliable results occur if the sampling tube or chamber is obstructed with secretions or condensation, if the sampling tube is too long, or if the sampling rate is too high.
12. Capnograph alterations (Table 7–11)
13. Monitor the following when using capnography:
    a. Tidal volume
    b. Respiratory rate
    c. PEEP
    d. Inspiratory vs expiratory ratio
    e. PIP
    f. Concentration of respiratory gases
    g. Hemodynamic variables, including pulmonary and systemic blood pressure; cardiac output; and shunt, ventilation, and perfusion inequalities
    h. Monitoring frequency depends on the condition of the patient, the therapy being administered, and the information required. During intubation, capnometry should be available.
14. Because of the location in the airway, the mainstream or side-port sensor should be subjected to high-level disinfection. The monitor should be cleaned following individual use.

## V. Pediatric advanced life support

A. Electrocardiogram
1. Chest leads are attached to the infant and are used to monitor the heart.
2. Generally electrodes are placed on the chest (above the nipple area) or shoulder with the ground placed on the abdomen or thigh. Forming a triangle, these three electrodes are labeled leads I, II, and III.
    a. Lead I measures electrical activity from the right side of the chest to the left side of the chest.
    b. Lead II measures electrical activity from the right side of the chest to the thigh or abdomen.
    c. Lead III measures electrical activity from the left side of the chest to the thigh or abdomen.
3. When electrical activity flows from negative pole to positive pole, it causes an upward deflection of the ECG tracing. Lead II is commonly used because it shows a clear P wave and is parallel to the electrical activity of the heart.
4. Precordial leads are used to differentiate right-sided and left-sided heart conditions. On a 12-lead ECG, 6 chest leads and 6 leg leads are used.
    a. Chest leads include $V_1$, $V_2$, $V_3$, $V_4$, $V_5$, and $V_6$.
    b. Limb leads include I, II, III, AVR (augmented vector right), AVL (augmented vector left), and AVF (augmented vector foot).
5. By placing these leads a certain way, the technician can inspect each side of the heart and the inferior heart
    a. Leads $V_1$ and AVR measure activity on the right side of the heart
    b. Leads $V_2$, $V_3$, and $V_4$ measure the transition between the right and left side of the heart
    c. Leads $V_5$, $V_6$, I, and AVL measure activity on the left side of the heart
    d. Leads II, III, and AVF measure activity at the inferior heart
6. Looking at the different leads can determine the area where the heart problem is located. If an abnormal tracing shows up on leads V1 and AVR, this would indicate a problem on the right side of the heart.

B. Drug administration for advanced life support (Table 7–12)

C. If peripheral access cannot be established, then the following drugs can be administered through the endotracheal tube:
1. Narcan
2. Atropine
3. Epinephrine

TABLE 7–12. ***Resuscitative Medications, Mechanism of Action, and Indications for Use***

| Medications | Mechanism of Action | Indication(s) |
|---|---|---|
| Epinephrine | Increases SVR, BP, heart rate, myocardial contraction, coronary and cerebral blood flow. | Asystole, brady arrhythmias associated with pulselessness. |
| Atropine | Parasympatholytic, vagolytic action. | Bradycardia with hypotension, asystole (infants <6 months old). Treat vagally induced bradycardia from intubation. |
| Lidocaine | Suppresses ventricular dysrhythmia. | Suppresses ventricular tachycardia, ventricular fibrillation. |
| Bretylium | Adrenergic and myocardial effects, antidysrhythmic drug, reduces the potential of ventricular fibrillation. | Ventricular tachycardia and ventricular fibrillation. Used when lidocaine and countershock fail to convert ventricular fibrillation. |
| Sodium bicarbonate | Buffer H+ ions converting them to $CO_2$. Buffering acid pH. | Documented metabolic acidosis. Generally used after defibrillation, chest compressions, ETT, 100% oxygen, lidocaine, epinephrine. Patient must be ventilated when bicarbonate is given. |
| Dopamine | Stimulates release of norepinephrine, vasodilation of renal, cerebral arteries at low dosages. Increased dosages stimulate beta-adrenergic receptors of the heart. | Hypotension in the absence of hypovolemia (oliguria, poor tissue perfusion, mental status change) and a stable heart rate or heart rate has been restored. |
| Dobutamine | (+) Inotropic effect, contractility little effect on peripheral vascular resistance. Decreases PCWP in patients with cardiogenic shock. | Hypotension and/or poor in the postresuscitative phase. May not be as effective as dopamine. |
| Isoproterenol | Increases heart rate, conduction, and contractility. Systemic vasodilation, increases cardiac output if normovolemic. | Bradycardia caused by heart block that is resistant to atropine. Isoproterenol increases cardiac output in rate-dependent infants <6 months of age. |
| Glucose | To restore depleted glucose and reverse hypoglycemia. Helps restore myocardial contractility. | Hypoglycemia during cardiac arrest. |
| Furosemide (Lasix) | Diuretic (inhibits reabsorption of Na and $Cl^-$ in ascending loop of Henle). | Reduce PCWP caused by left heart dysfunction. |

4. Lidocaine

D. Dysrhythmias
1. Bradycardia
   a. Bradycardia in children and adolescents is defined as a rate of less than 60 beats/min.
   b. Causes include hypoxemia, hypotension, and acidosis.
   c. Treatment (with low cardiac output) includes oxygen, chest compressions, atropine, and epinephrine.
2. Sinus tachycardia
   a. Sinus tachycardia is dependent on age (see Chapter 8).
   b. The cause of sinus tachycardia may be fear, anxiety, or loss of blood.
   c. Treatment includes identifying the underlying cause and then treating it.
3. Ventricular tachycardia
   a. The cause of ventricular tachycardia may be underlying heart disease, hypoxia, electrolyte imbalance, or acidosis.
   b. The treatment includes cardioversion, if the patient is unstable. Cardiovert initially with 0.5 to 1 joules(J)/kg. For repeated cardioversion, use 2 J/kg. Oxygen and lidocaine may be given before cardioversion. Bretylium may be given if lidocaine is unsuccessful.
4. Ventricular fibrillation
   a. The causes of ventricular fibrillation are the same as for ventricular tachycardia.
   b. Treatment includes beginning or continuing cardiopulmonary resuscitation (CPR) and defibrillating as soon as possible. Begin defibrillation with 2 J/kg. For repeated defibrillation, use 4 J/kg two more times. If the patient is still in defibrillation, check oxygen, ventilation, and presence of acidosis.

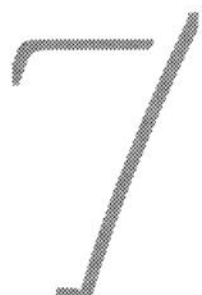

# REVIEW QUESTIONS

1. Fill in the table concerning causes of acid–base imbalance.

| | Causes |
|---|---|
| Respiratory acidosis | |
| Respiratory alkalosis | |
| Metabolic acidosis | |
| Metabolic alkalosis | |

2. List factors that affect the accuracy of a CBG.

   a.

   b.

3. Describe the location on the foot where a CBG can be obtained.

4. List three contraindications for performing a percutaneous arterial blood gas

   a.

   b.

   c.

5. Describe what action is taken if the modified Allen's test shows reduced collateral flow in the right hand.

6. What changes in the $PaCO_2$ and $PaO_2$ occur when there are air bubbles in the sample obtained with a CBG?

7. After obtaining a PAL, the blood pressure waveform does not reappear on the screen. What could be the problem?

8. What is the low- and high-position location for an umbilical artery catheter?

9. On radiograph, how is the umbilical artery catheter differentiated from the umbilical venous catheter?

10. What are the normal venous and arterial cord blood gases?

| | **Arterial** | **Venous** |
|---|---|---|
| pH | | |
| $PaCO_2$ | | |
| $PaO_2$ | | |

11. The following hemodynamic data have been obtained:

| | |
|---|---|
| Blood pressure: 120/90 | CVP, 8 mm Hg |
| mean PAP: 16 mm Hg | PCWP, 8 mm Hg |
| $CaO_2$–$CvO_2$: 5 vol% | oxygen consumption, 250 mL/min |
| Body surface area: 1.2 $m^2$ | |

Given this information, determine the following:

a. Pulmonary vascular resistance

b. Systemic vascular resistance

c. Cardiac output

d. Cardiac index

e. Mean arterial pressure

12. List two indications for insertion of a central venous catheter.

a.

b.

13. What is the difference between a pulmonary artery catheter and a central venous catheter?

14. In the accompanying table, fill in the normal values and how each value is measured.

| Value | Abbreviation | Normal value | How measured or obtained |
|---|---|---|---|
| Central venous pressure | CVP | | |
| Right ventricular pressure | RVP | | |
| Pulmonary artery pressure | PAP | | |
| Left atrial pressure | LAP | | |
| Left Ventricular Pressure | LVP | | |
| Pulmonary Capillary Wedge Pressure | PCWP | | |
| Mixed Venous | $PvO_2$ | | |
| Arterial-Venous Oxygen Content Difference | $CaO_2$-$CvO_2$(a-$vDO_2$) | | |

15. In the accompanying table, fill in the causes and actions for troubleshooting a peripheral arterial line and a pulmonary artery catheter.

| Problem | Cause | Action |
|---|---|---|
| No waveform seen on monitor. | | |
| Damped waveform on monitor (systolic pressure decreases, diastolic pressure increases). | | |
| False low measurement. | | |
| Active bleedback from the patient to the transducer. | | |
| **PAC**—Cannot obtain a wedge (PCWP) reading. | | |
| **Arterial**—Hematoma after withdrawal of the catheter. | | |

16. What is the normal $SvO_2$?

17. Answer the following questions with either TRUE or FALSE:

   a. Hypothermia, paralysis, and anesthesia may cause an increased $SvO_2$.

   b. Increased cardiac output reduces oxygen supply to the tissue, thus decreasing $SvO_2$.

   c. Hyperthermia, shivering, and seizures increases $VO_2$ and decrease $SvO_2$.

   d. Increasing PEEP can reduce cardiac output and decrease $SvO_2$ by reducing oxygen supply to the tissues.

18. A $PtcO_2$ has just been calibrated and the electrode temperature is set at 37°C. An arterial blood gas has been returned and shows a $PaO_2$ of 80 mm Hg, but the $PtcO_2$ value is 52 mm Hg. What is the problem? What should be done?

19. A newborn with a $PtcCO_2$ monitor in place has a value of 46 mm Hg. Over the next few minutes, it is noticed that this value is dropping without any change in patient status. What is the problem? What should be done?

20. If blistering is found on the skin after removal of a transcutaneous electrode, what should be done about preventing further blistering?

21. What are two dead-space conditions that would cause an increase in $PetCO_2$?

   a.

   b.

22. Draw a normal capnographic tracing and label the end-tidal $CO_2$ point. How would the capnographic tracing appear if the following problem occurred?

   a. Endotracheal tube in the esophagus

   b. Patient rebreathing carbon dioxide

   c. Hypoventilation

23. Give an indication for use with the following drugs:
    a. Atropine
    b. Lidocaine
    c. Sodium bicarbonate
    d. Dopamine

24. List four drugs that can be administered down the endotracheal tube when peripheral access cannot be established.
    a.
    b.
    c.
    d.

25. Give the recommended treatment for each of the following dysrhythmias:
    a. Ventricular fibrillation.
    b. Ventricular tachycardia.
    c. Bradycardia.
    d. Sinus tachycardia.

## BIBLIOGRAPHY


American Association for Respiratory Care. (1991). Clinical practice guideline: Pulse oximetry. *Respiratory Care* 36:1406.

American Association for Respiratory Care. (1995). Clinical practice guideline: Capnography/capnometry during mechanical ventilation. *Respiratory Care* 40:1321.

American Association for Respiratory Care. (1994). Clinical practice guideline: Capillary blood gas sampling for neonatal and pediatric patients. *Respiratory Care* 39:1180.

American Association for Respiratory Care. (1992). Clinical practice guideline: Sampling for arterial blood gas analysis. *Respiratory Care* 37:913.

American Association for Respiratory Care. (1993). Clinical practice guideline: In vitro pH and blood gas analysis and hemoximetry. *Respiratory Care* 38:505.

American Heart Association. (1988). *Textbook of Pediatric Advanced Life Support*. Dallas: American Heart Association.

Beachey, W., and Scanlan, C. L. (1995). Acid-base balance and the regulation of respiration. In Scanlan, C. L., Spearman, C., and Sheldon, R, L. (Eds.). *Egan's Fundamentals of Respiratory Care*, ed 6. St. Louis: Mosby–Year Book.

Blowers, M. G., and Sims, R. S. (1988). *How to Read an ECG*, 4 ed. Albany: Delmar Publishers.

Christian, S. S., and Brady, K. (1991). Cord blood acid-base values in breach presenting infants born vaginally. *Obstetrics and Gynecology* 75:778.

Clinical Information and Technology Series. (1995). *Neonatal Intensive Care*. Redmond: SpaceLabs Medical.

Courtney, S., et al. (1990). Capillary blood gases in the neonate: A reassessment and review of the literature. *AJDC* 144:168.

Creasy, R., and Resnik, R. (1990). *Maternal-Fetal Medicine, Child, Adolescent*, ed 2. Philadelphia: Lea & Febiger.

Daily, E., and Schroeder, J. (1990). *Techniques in Bedside Hemodynamic Monitoring*, ed 4. St. Louis: Mosby.

Dickinson, J., et al. (1992). The effect of preterm birth on umbilical cord blood gases. *Obstetrics and Gynecology* 79:959.

Duerbeck, N., et al. (1992). A practical approach to umbilical artery pH and blood gas determinations. *Obstetrics and Gynecology* 79:959.

Gomella, T., and Cunningham, M. (1994). *Neonatology Basic Management: On Call Problems, Diseases, Drugs*, ed 3. Norwalk, Connecticut: Appleton & Lange.

Hazinski, M. F. Pediatric evaluation and considerations. In Daravic, G. (Ed.). (1995). *Hemodynamic Monitoring: Invasive and Noninvasive Clinical Application*, ed 2. Philadelphia: J. B. Lippincott.

Hess, D. (1993). Capnography: Technical aspects and clinical applications. In Kacmarek, R., Hess, D., and Stoller, J. (Eds.) *Monitoring in Respiratory Care*. St. Louis: Mosby–Year Book.

Johnson, N., et al. (1990). The effect of meconium on neonatal and fetal reflectance pulse oximetry. *Journal of Perinatal Medicine* 18:351.

Koff, P., and Hess, D. (1993). Transcutaneous oxygen and carbon dioxide measurements. In Kacmarek, R., Hess, D., and Stoller, J. (Eds.). *Monitoring in Respiratory Care*. St. Louis: Mosby–Year Book.

Kacmarek, R., Mack, C., and Dimas, S. (1990). *The Essentials of Respiratory Care*, ed 3. Chicago: Yearbook Medical Publishers.

Murenstein, G, and Gardner, S. (1994). *Handbook of Neonatal Intensive Care*, ed 3. St. Louis: Mosby.

McCarthy, K., et al. (1993). Pulse oximetry. In Kacmarek, R., Hess, D., and Stoller, J. (Eds). *Monitoring in Respiratory Care*. St. Louis: Mosby–Year Book.

McNamara, H., et al. (1992). Do fetal pulse oximetry readings at delivery correlate with low blood oximetry and acidemia? *British Journal of Obstetrics and Gynaecology* 99:735.

Norman, D., et al. (1992). A practical approach to umbilical artery pH and blood gas determinations. *Obstetrics and Gynecology* 79 959.

Sail, A., Dutta, A. K., and Sonna, M. S. (1992). Reliability of capillary blood gas estimation in neonates. *Indian Journal of Pediatrics* 29:567.

Scarpelli, E.(1990). *Pulmonary Physiology: Fetus, Newborn, Child, Adolescent,* ed 2. Philadelphia: Lea & Febiger.

Shapiro, B., Harrison, R., and Walton, J. (1990). *Clinical Application of Blood Gases,* ed 5. Chicago: Year Book Medical Publishers.

Veyckemans, F., et al. (1989). Hyperbilirubinemia does not interfere with hemoglobin saturation measured by pulse oximetry. *Anesthesiology* 70:118.

Welch, J. P., DeCesare, R., and Hess, D. (1990). Pulse oximetry: Instrumentation and clinical applications. *Respiratory Care* 35:584.

Zijlkra, W. G., Buursma, A., and Meeuwsen vander Roest, W. P. (1991). Absorption spectra of human fetal and adult hemoglobin, de-oxy hemoglobin, carboxyhemoglobin, and methemoglobin. *Clinical Chemistry* 37:1633.

Zubrow, A. B., et al. (1990). Pulse oximetry in sick premature infants and the effects of phototherapy and radiant warmers on the oxygen saturation readout. *American Journal of Perinatalogy* 7:75.

# Pediatric Assessment

**I. Introduction**

A. Acute illness (sudden, rapid onset) may be caused by a motor vehicle accident, asthma attack, pneumonia, and/or upper airway obstruction. Chronic illness (long-term, recurrent) may be caused by infection, congenital anomalies, heart disease, or neoplastic processes.

B. History from birth to present

1. A neonatal history of long-term ventilation and BPD may predispose children to disease or intensify the effects of disease.
2. Prenatal care and testing are of greatest use in newborn assessment but are also of use in identifying congenital anomalies and assessing care of the child in later years.
3. Immunization history is important in the pediatric population to rule out such problems as measles, mumps, and rubella and to isolate children exposed to these diseases to avoid infecting other patients and staff.
4. Family illness, especially a history of allergies, asthma, and cystic fibrosis, may predispose children to disease.

**II. Age and physical changes from infancy to adolescence (Table 8–1)**

**III. Preparing for the physical exam**

A. Different age groups present distinct problems for the practitioner. Most children feel more comfortable and allow the practitioner to conduct an examination or give treatments in the presence of parents, siblings, or other family members.

B. Soliciting help from the family and allowing time for the practitioner to get acquainted with the child make the physical exam a good experience. Table 8–2 gives suggestions pertaining to treatment and physical examination according to the age of the child.

**IV. Interviewing**

A. By interviewing the patient or parent, the clinician can learn the patient's problems and can collect and evaluate pertinent clinical information.

B. The clinician first needs to gain the patient's trust and respect.

1. Introduce yourself and describe the purpose of your visit.

TABLE 8–1. ***Age and Physical Changes from Infancy to Adolescence***

| Description | Age | Physical Changes |
|---|---|---|
| Infant | 30 days to 1 year | By the end of 6 months, weight doubles. |
| Toddler | 1 year to 3 years of age | Yearly gain of 4.5 to 6.5 lb. By end of the third year, the toddler achieves one-half of eventual adult height. |
| Early childhood (preschool age) | 3 years to 6 years of age | Yearly height gain averages 2.5 to 3.2 in. |
| Middle childhood (school age) | 6 years to 12 years of age | Birth length triples by 12 years of age. |
| Adolescence | 13 years to 18 years of age | Marked physical changes. Greatest physical changes between 10 and 14 years of age. |

TABLE 8–2. ***Suggestions for Preparing the Child for Physical Examination and Treatment***

| Age of the Child | Suggestions |
|---|---|
| Infant: Up to 1 year of age | Allow infant to sit in parent's lap. Keep the parent in view of the infant while performing the examination. Respond to crying by gentle touching, rocking, or patting. |
| Toddler: 1–3 years of age | Describe several times what is about to happen. Communicate in short, concrete terms. Allow toddler to sit in parent's lap, on examining table next to parent, or in a chair close to parent. Allow the parent to give the treatment if the toddler is uncooperative. Approach the child and perform assessments that do not require the child to become fearful. Initially, just observe, then check pulse, auscultation, and pulse oximetry. Once confidence has been established, administration of oxygen devices and treatment can follow. |
| Early childhood: 3–6 years of age | Use visual aids to demonstrate procedure. Allow the child to handle instruments and perform the procedure on himself or herself (stethoscope). The child may react in a way that represents what the previous hospital experience was like. |
| Middle childhood: 6–12 years of age | Offer parents the option to remain in the room during the examination and treatment. Explain in more sophisticated terms but keep it simple. Patient may already be receiving these treatments. Remain in the room to evaluate the treatment. Child may be able to self-administer some of the treatment. |
| Adolescence: 13–18 years of age | Adolescent takes own treatment. At this age, privacy and confidentiality are important. Attitude may be less than desirable. Keep the explanation of procedures simple. |

2. The patient should be comfortable, and there should be privacy and few interruptions.
3. Start off the interview with casual talk to get acquainted and develop relaxation.
4. Use lay terms that the patient and family understand.

C. Record patient data by taking the patient's past medical history. Note pertinent facts such as the following:
1. Chief complaint
   a. Cough
   b. Fever
   c. Shortness of breath
   d. Difficulty breathing
   e. Wheezing
   f. Difficulty with activities of daily living (ADLs) (child becomes fatigued easily, cannot keep up with peers, becomes breathless)
2. Symptoms associated with the chief complaint
   a. Time of onset
   b. Severity
   c. Duration
3. Circumstances leading up to the chief complaint. Also look at events that occurred before the patient started having these problems.

D. Observe the patient.
1. Check the patient's level of consciousness by evaluating verbal responses.
2. Verbal responses are the most reliable indicator of cerebral function. Recognize normal and abnormal responses (Table 8–3).
3. Often anxiety can influence the patient's condition and change findings. To determine anxiety, look for the following:
   a. Rigidity
   b. Restlessness
   c. Short attention span
   d. Inability to follow directions
   e. Asking numerous questions and shifting topic of conversation

E. Focus on data that pertain to the chief complaint.
1. Start focusing on symptoms that have been explained by the patient or family.
2. Ask open-ended questions that are simple to understand.
3. Maintain eye contact and give responses to the patient or family.
4. Do not pursue questions that may be embarrassing for the patient.

F. Conclude the interview by answering questions that are pertinent to the respiratory care plan.

TABLE 8–3. ***Normal and Abnormal Responses to Questioning during Physical Examination***

| Normal | Abnormal |
|---|---|
| Oriented to time, place, and person. Able to recognize family members. | Does not recognize family; disoriented, confused. |
| Speaks clearly. | Unable to understand, irritable, defensive (may be associated with the age group). Weak cry, moaning, whimpering. |
| Alert and active. | Weak, lethargic, lies in parent's lap. |
| Responds to verbal command. | Difficult to awaken, arouse, and focus. Gives no resistance during examination. |

**V. Developing a respiratory care plan**

A. An appropriate respiratory care plan requires a complete review of the patient's chart and accurate documentation of findings.
B. SOAP notes provide a plan of care.
C. SOAP notes:
   1. **S**ubjective: Information provided by the child or parent. Example: "David has been coughing all night and it sounds like a dog barking. He has been sick the last 3 to 4 days until this evening, when he got worse."
   2. **O**bjective: Findings obtained from physical assessment of the patient. For example:
      a. Two-year-old boy, awake, alert and oriented to time, place, and person. Respiratory rate is 44 breaths per minute (bpm), blood pressure is 136/88, color is pale with diaphoresis, pulse is 146 beats per minute. Loud stridor on inspiration and forceful cough with barking sound and no expectoration. Patient is restless, sitting in mother's lap. Excessive accessory muscle usage. Lateral neck radiograph shows hypopharyngeal swelling.
   3. **A**ssessment: Derived from the subjective and objective findings. In this example, the assessment would determine that the child has croup.
   4. **P**lan: Treatment for the child based on the subjective, objective, and assessment findings. Treatment includes the following:
      a. Education: Explain to parents and child what treatment will be provided, what equipment will be used, and how the equipment will be used during the child's hospital stay. Allow the parents to give treatments with the respiratory practitioner present.
      b. Provide a low concentration of oxygen with a croup or mist tent.
      c. Provide small-volume nebulizer treatment with 2.25% racemic epinephrine every 2 to 4 h while child is awake and as needed (PRN).
      d. Monitor oxygen saturation with pulse oximeter, keeping saturation above 90%.
      e. Monitor breath sounds.

**VI. Factors influencing respiratory infection**

A. Factors that influence respiratory infection include the following:
   1. Nature of the infectious agent.
   2. The size and frequency of the dose. The larger and more frequent the dose exposure, the more significant the infection.
   3. The age of the child. Nursery- and grade-school children are exposed more frequently to illnesses.
   4. The ability to resist invading organisms. School-age children have greater resistance than newborns and infants.
   5. Presence of general conditions such as the following:
      a. Malnutrition
      b. Anemia
      c. Fatigue
      d. Chilling of the body
      e. Immune deficiency
      f. Presence of disorders such as cystic fibrosis, congenital heart defects, and allergies

**VII. Most common signs and symptoms of respiratory infection**

A. Cough
B. Nasal blockage: The infant's small nares are blocked by swelling and secretions. Infants must breathe through the mouth, interrupting feeding to do so.

C. Fever: Even in mild infections, temperature may reach 103 to 105°F (39.5 to 40.5°C).
D. Febrile seizures: A sudden increase in temperature to 40°C may elicit seizures.
E. Vomiting: Common and frequent; may cause hypovolemia
F. Diarrhea from viral infection
G. Abdominal pain that may be indistinguishable from appendicitis. A tender abdomen is identified by a painful response to pressure on the abdomen.

**VIII. Respiratory physical examination of the infant and child**

A. Vital signs
   1. Respiratory rate
      a. An infant up to 1 year of age has a normal respiratory rate of 20 to 25 bpm.
      b. A child of 1 to 2 years of age has a normal respiratory rate below 20 bpm.
      c. From 12 to 18 years of age, the normal respiratory rate is 16 to 18 bpm.
   2. Tachypnea—rapid, shallow breathing that may be caused by metabolic acidosis, drug overdose, or respiratory distress. Respiratory problems may initially cause tachypnea, but with fatigue the patient's respiratory rate drops, an ominous sign of impending respiratory failure. A child who is fatigued has a drop in respiratory rate and develops "head bobbing" because fatigue causes poor muscle tone in the neck region.
   3. Pulse
      a. In infants from 1 month of age to children 2 years of age, the normal pulse rate is 100 to 160 (mean 130) beats per min.
      b. In children 2 to 10 years of age, the normal pulse rate is 60 to 140 (mean 80) beats per minute.
      c. In children over 10 years of age, the normal pulse rate is 50 to 100 (mean 75) beats per minute.
      d. Sinus tachycardia (excessively rapid pulse rate) is the heart's response to stimuli such as hypoxemia, stress, and fever.
      e. Sinus bradycardia (excessively slow pulse rate) in infants and children is a secondary response to untreated hypoxemia. Bradycardia in a distressed child is an ominous sign of cardiac arrest.
   4. Blood pressure
      a. In children over 2 years, the following equation is used to determine the upper limit for systolic pressure: $90 + (2 \times \text{age in years})$.
      b. The lower limit for systolic pressure is determined using the following equation: $70 + (2 \times \text{age in years})$.
   5. Normal oral temperature
      a. In infants up to 1 year of age, the normal oral temperature is 37.5 to 37.7°C.
      b. In children from 1 to 5 years of age, the normal oral temperature is 37°C.
      c. In children from 5 to 12 years of age, the normal oral temperature is 36.6 to 37°C.

B. Inspection of the chest
   1. Orthopnea is the condition of being dyspneic while lying down. The degree of orthopnea may be described in terms of the number of pillows the patient requires to feel comfortable, such as "two-pillow orthopnea."
   2. Skin color
      a. Normal skin color is pink, tan, brown, or black, depending on the child' s ethnic background.
      b. A decrease in skin color may be caused by anemia or lack of blood flow to a specific region of the body. This is described as an ashen appearance or pallor.
      c. A yellowish discoloration, or jaundice, is the result of an increase in bilirubin level in the tissue. This may be present in children with hepatic disease.
      d. Redness of the skin resulting from capillary congestion, inflammation, or infection is called erythema.
      e. A bluish discoloration of the skin caused by increased amounts of reduced hemoglobin is called cyanosis.
   3. Skin texture
      a. Normal skin texture is smooth and slightly dry.
      b. Tissue turgor is the amount of elasticity in the skin. Assessment of skin turgor helps determine the level of hydration. When the skin is pulled up, poorly hydrated skin remains suspended, then eventually returns to normal.
      c. The presence of excessive fluid in the tissue is called edema. The severity of the edema is assessed by pressing a finger into the area of edema. If an

impression remains after removing the finger, edema is present. Pitting or peripheral edema occurs in dependent portions of the body such as the arms, hands, legs, ankles, and feet.

4. Jugular venous distention is the result of congestion of blood within the jugular veins. This may be caused by pressure within the thoracic cavity reducing venous return by obstructing the flow into the right atrium. Conditions such as obstructive pulmonary disease and heart failure cause reduced venous return and result in distended jugular veins.
5. Capillary refill assesses peripheral circulation. Capillary refill should occur within 1 to 3 s after occluding of a vessel. Reduced capillary refill may be caused by poor cardiac output or vasoconstriction.
6. Clubbing of the digits is an enlargement of the fingers and/or toes. The condition is suggestive of cardiopulmonary disease, gastrointestinal (GI) disease, and renal disease.
7. Sputum
   a. Infants and children may not expectorate sputum until they get older; therefore it may be impossible to inspect it for color, consistency, amount, and odor.
   b. Older children should be instructed to expectorate sputum and save it for assessment. The gross appearance of sputum can indicate an underlying condition in the lungs.
      (1) Mucoid sputum is white in color, viscous, and present in conditions such as asthma and bronchitis.
      (2) Yellow sputum indicates infection and is made up of white blood cells. This sputum may have an unpleasant taste and odor.
      (3) Green sputum contains pus and enzymes that discolor and add odor to the sputum. Gram-negative infection causes this type of sputum; green sputum is also present with cystic fibrosis.
      (4) Hemoptysis is expectoration of bright red blood arising from hemorrhage from the trachea, bronchi, or larynx. This is different from hematemesis, which is vomiting dark, frothy, and often clotted blood.
8. Coughing (Table 8–4)
9. Breathing Patterns (Table 8–5)
   a. In children under 7 years of age, normal respirations are diaphragmatic, with the abdomen rising with inspiration.
   b. In later years, breathing becomes more thoracic. Abdomen and chest rise together.
   c. In older children with respiratory disorders or injury to the chest, breathing is abdominal, with labored breathing causing the abdomen to push out abruptly.
10. Chest configuration
    a. Scoliosis
       (1) Scoliosis is a lateral deviation in the normally straight vertical line of the spine. It occurs in both sexes, but girls are more likely to have severe curvature.
       (2) Signs of scoliosis include one shoulder being higher than the other, tilting of the hips with one hip more prominent, and a prominence of the posterior chest or the shoulder when the child bends over.
       (3) Scoliosis is a restrictive disorder causing one lung to be affected by the lateral curvature. This lung has a greater tendency to develop pneumonia. Lung volumes are reduced in the affected lung.

TABLE 8–4. ***Causes, Descriptions, and Types of Coughing***

| Causes | Description | Types |
|---|---|---|
| Inflammation from pneumonia | Acute, short in duration | Barking from croup |
| Obstruction from aspiration due to acid content | Paroxysmal, which is periodic forceful and prolonged | Brassy from laryngitis |
| Bronchial abnormalities from chemical, smoke inhalation | Effective, mucus-producing | Stridor from inflammation and laryngospasm |
| High temperature causing inflammation and burning of the lung mucosa | Dry, nonproductive | Wheezing from bronchospasm |

TABLE 8–5. ***Breathing Patterns in Children***

| Breathing Pattern | Description | Cause |
|---|---|---|
| Eupnea | Normal respiratory rate, depth, and rhythm | Normal breathing pattern |
| Apnea | Cessation of breathing | Cardiac arrest, respiratory arrest |
| Cheyne-Stokes | Gradually increasing, then decreasing rate and depth in a cycle lasting from 30–180 s with periods of apnea | Central nervous system disease, congestive heart failure |
| Biot's | Increased respiratory rate and depth with irregular periods of apnea | Increased intracranial pressure |
| Kussmaul's | Increased respiratory rate and depth | Metabolic acidosis |
| Apneustic | Prolonged inhalation | Brain damage |
| Paradoxical | Chest wall movement, in which the wall moves in during inspiration and out during expiration | Chest trauma |

b. Kyphosis
   (1) Kyphosis is an abnormal convexity in the curvature of the thoracic spine as viewed from the side. Causes may include injury, congenital disorder, or disease. Symptoms may include back pain and increasing immobility.
   (2) Kyphosis is a restrictive disorder that affects both lungs. Lung volumes are reduced significantly because of compression of both lungs.

c. Kyphoscoliosis
   (1) Kyphoscoliosis is a combination of the curvature defects of both scoliosis and kyphosis.
   (2) Kyphoscoliosis is a restrictive disorder in which both lateral and convex curvature cause reduced lung volume and capacity.

d. Barrel chest
   (1) With a barrel chest, there is an increase in the anterior-posterior (AP) diameter that is caused by air trapping. As a result, the patient's chest appears to be inflated. Also, the slope of the ribs loses its normal 45-degree angle and becomes horizontal in relation to the spine.
   (2) As a result of air trapping, flow rates on exhalation are reduced, whereas lung capacity is increased above normal. Diseases such as cystic fibrosis cause barrel chest.

e. Pectus carinatum
   (1) Pectus carinatum (also called "pigeon breast") is a malformation of the chest wall in which the sternum is abnormally prominent.
   (2) Severe malformation causes dyspnea, reduced ability to perform ADLs, and exercise intolerance.

f. Pectus excavatum
   (1) Pectus excavatum is a restrictive formation of the chest wall characterized by a pronounced funnel-shaped depression. This is caused by a shortening of the central portion of the diaphragm, which pulls the sternum backward during inhalation.
   (2) Severe cases cause a reduction in the ability to perform ADLs, exercise intolerance, and dyspnea.

C. Percussion of the chest
   1. Percussion of the chest aids in determining densities and alteration of the densities of underlying structures.
   2. Percussion is performed by placing the third finger of the left hand on the surface of the chest and tapping the chest with the third finger of the right hand. The sounds emitted are determined by the ratio of air-containing tissue to solid tissue.
   3. In general, a low-pitched (resonant) sound is produced as a result of an increased amount of solid tissue. Specific sounds emitted according to pathology include the following:
      a. Dull to flat note—atelectasis, consolidation, or pleural effusion
      b. Hyperresonant—pneumothorax
      c. Tympany—air-filled organ such as the stomach
      d. Resonant—air-filled lung

D. Auscultation of the chest
   1. Normal breath sounds (Table 8–6)
   2. Abnormal breath sounds (Table 8–7)

TABLE 8–6. ***Findings of Normal Breath Sounds***

| | Vesicular | Bronchial | Bronchovesicular |
|---|---|---|---|
| Description | Low-pitched and soft on inspiration | High-pitched, loud, harsh, hollow on inspiration or expiration | Medium-pitched, muffled on inspiration and expiration |
| Position in the respiratory cycle | More prominent during inspiration than expiration | Less prominent during inspiration than during expiration | Equally heard during inspiration and expiration |
| Typical respiratory cycle | Inspiration is longer than expiration with no pause in between them | Inspiration is shorter than expiration with a pause in between them | Inspirations equal with no pause in between them |
| Normal findings | Over peripheral lung fields | Over the main-stem bronchus | Over large airways, either side of sternal angle and between scapula |
| Abnormal findings | Decreased sounds over peripheral lung fields | Bronchial sounds over peripheral lung fields | Sounds heard over peripheral lung field |

E. Palpation of the chest
   1. Palpation helps the examiner evaluate underlying lung structure and function by placing the hand on the chest wall. Palpation assesses the skin and subcutaneous tissues of the lung, estimates thoracic expansion, and evaluates vocal fremitus.
   2. Symmetrical chest movement occurs as sides of the chest move at the same time and with equal expansion. Assessment of chest movement is done by placing the hands on opposite sides of the chest, such as the apices, middle, and lower areas, anteriorly and posteriorly. During inspiration, the hands should separate equally and return to the original placement at end-exhalation. Diseases that can cause bilateral chest reduction include neuromuscular disease and cystic fibrosis.
   3. Asymmetrical chest movement is a dissimilarity in the expansion of the chest. One lung or both lungs may be affected, with reduced lung volume from lobar atelectasis, pleural effusion, or pneumothorax.
   4. Tactile fremitus is vibration caused by sound transmission passing through the chest wall. The hand is placed on the chest wall to detect fremitus. A

TABLE 8–7. ***Abnormal Breath Sounds***

| Breath Sound | Description | Position in Respiratory Cycle | Cause | Disease |
|---|---|---|---|---|
| Wheeze | High-pitched, continuous. Loud wheezing indicates airflow is occurring. Soft wheezing may occur with fatigue. | Heard predominantly during inspiration, but also on expiration | Narrowed airways. | Asthma, foreign body. |
| Crackle | High-pitched. | Occurs at end of inspiration | Fluid in alveoli. | Pneumonia, CHF. |
| Rhonchi | Low-pitched, loud, rattling. | Occurs at the beginning of inspiration and during expiration. Sounds may clear with coughing. | Excessive sputum in bronchi. | Pneumonia |
| Pleural Friction Rub | Low-pitched, coarse, grinding or crunching. | Loudest on inspiration, and sounds do not clear with coughing. | Pleura rubbing together. | Pleurisy, tuberculosis. |
| Stridor | High-pitched, heard in upper airway. | Heard during inspiration. | Narrowing of the larynx, trachea. | After extubation, upper respiratory tract infection (croup). |

cause of tactile fremitus is pneumonia. A decreased unilateral tactile fremitus may be caused by pneumothorax, pleural effusion, bronchial obstruction from a mucus plug, or a foreign object. Bilateral decreased tactile fremitus may be caused by obesity. Other types of fremitus include the following:
   a. Vocal fremitus is the vibration created by the vocal cords during speaking. This may be minimal in small children with high-pitched voices.
   b. Pleural rub fremitus is a grating sensation felt on the chest wall that is caused by a rubbing of pleural surfaces as a result of pleuritis.
   c. Rhonchal fremitus is vibration produced by air passing over loosely adhered secretions in the bronchus.
5. Crepitus, or subcutaneous emphysema, found in the loose tissue in the apical area of the thorax, is caused by tiny air bubbles released from the lungs during a tracheostomy or with a pneumothorax.

F. Using the four fundamental techniques of respiratory assessment provides the clinician with a way of diagnosing lung problems (Table 8–8).

**IX. Evaluation of the pediatric patient with respiratory stress**

A. Common pediatric disorders in children from 1 month to 2 years of age
   1. Upper airway obstruction
   2. Asthma
   3. Foreign body aspiration
   4. Cystic fibrosis
   5. Poisoning
   6. Bronchiolitis

B. Common pediatric disorders in children over 2 years of age
   1. Asthma
   2. Poisoning
   3. Drowning
   4. Burns
   5. Septicemia
   6. Trauma
   7. Bronchopneumonia
   8. Croup and epiglottitis

C. Once the history has been taken, focus on the primary complaint and look for severity of clinical signs (Table 8–9).

D. Monitoring pulmonary functions alerts the clinician to respiratory distress and failure.
   1. Pulmonary functions
      a. Respiratory rate is increased.
      b. Vital capacity is below 10 mL/kg (normal is 40 to 60 mL/kg).
      c. Tidal volume is subjective, but normal value is 5 to 8 mL/kg.
      d. Normal minute ventilation is 5 to 8 mL/kg times the respiratory rate.
      e. Alveolar-arterial oxygen difference (A-a$DO_2$) is increased (normal is less than 15 mm Hg on room air).
      f. Arterial blood gas values (ABGs) (Table 8–10).
      g. Watch for rapid, shallow breathing. Changes in oxygenation occur as the child hypoventilates.

TABLE 8–8. ***Clinical Diagnosis of Pulmonary Problems***

| Pathology | Inspection | Palpation | Percussion | Auscultation |
|---|---|---|---|---|
| Pneumothorax | Dyspnea, less motion on affected side, deviation of trachea away from affected side (tension pneumothorax) | Decreased fremitus | Hyperresonant | Diminished, absent breath sounds over affected side |
| Consolidation | Dyspnea, less motion on affected side | Decreased fremitus | Dullness | Decreased to absent breath sounds |
| Atelectasis | Dyspnea, less motion and decreased volume on affected side | Decreased fremitus | Dullness | Absent breath sounds |
| Pleural effusion | Dsypnea | Decreased fremitus | Flatness | Decreased or absent breath sounds over affected area |

TABLE 8–9. ***Severity of Clinical Signs Associated with Respiratory Failure***

| Clinical Sign | Mild Symptoms | Moderate Symptoms | Severe Symptoms |
|---|---|---|---|
| Respiratory effort | Increased effort with minimal retractions | Greater retractions, nasal flaring, mouth open | Head bobbing, mouth open, severe retractions, grunting, tracheal tug |
| Color | Pink | Pale, flushed, cyanosis on room air | Cyanosis on increased $FIO_2$ |
| Activity | Normal | Lethargic | Delirium, coma |
| Temperature | 97–101°F | 101–104°F | >104°F |
| CNS status | Normal to drowsy, headache, irritable | Restless, irritable, stupor | Convulsions, coma, unable to recognize parents |
| Breath sounds | Equal, bilateral | Unequal, diminished | Absent, silent chest |
| Blood pressure | Normal | Hypertension | Hypotension |
| Heart rate | Within normal range | Tachycardia | Bradycardia |
| Response (talking, smiling) | Alert, smiling, complete sentences | Broken sentences, phrases | Halting speech, not talking or smiling |
| Hydration | Moist skin, mucous membranes | Slightly dry mouth, cool extremities, reduced peripheral perfusion | Dry skin and mucous membranes, cold extremities, poor peripheral perfusion |
| Quality of cry | Not crying, crying with normal tone | Sobbing, whining | Moaning, weak cry, high-pitched |

h. Dead-space to tidal-volume ratio ($V_D/V_t$). Normal is 30%. As respiratory rate increases and tidal volume decreases, dead space increases.

## X. Common radiograph positions for infants and children

A. Posterior-anterior (PA) position
1. Patient stands upright and the chest is placed against the film. The shoulders are rotated forward, touching the film so as not to obscure a portion of the lung field.
2. Advantages of this type of film include the following:
   a. Better sharpness
   b. A reduction in the magnification of the heart
   c. More lung is viewed; the diaphragm is lower.

B. Anterior-posterior (AP) position
1. Common radiograph position for bedridden patients
2. Radiographic film is placed behind the back of the patient and the x-ray is taken approximately 36 to 40 in from the chest of the patient.
3. The technique may have some distortion (patient turned in bed), coarseness, and less resolution. The heart may appear larger.

C. Lateral position
1. Patient's side is placed against film with the arm raised over the head. This helps prevent obscuring of the thorax and allows the diaphragmatic dome and descending aorta to be seen, as well as the depth of the thorax.
2. The side of the chest that is suspected of having problems should be placed against the film.

D. Oblique position
1. This position is used to see around and behind overlying objects. A right or left oblique film refers to the position in which the shoulders are rotated in relation to the film plate. The chest is rotated 45°. This shifts the angle of the film in which the x-ray passes through the body.
2. In the right anterior oblique position, the patient's chest is against the film, whereas in the right posterior oblique position, the patient's back is against the film.

TABLE 8–10. ***Normal Arterial Blood Gas Values for the Infant and Child***

| | Infant Child |
|---|---|
| pH | 7.35–7.45 |
| $PaCO_2$ (mm Hg) | 35–45 |
| $PaO_2$ (mm Hg) | 80–100 |
| $HCO_3^-$ (mEq/L) | 20–28 |

E. Lordotic position
   1. This position is used to identify the upper lung fields that are obscured by the clavicles and first and second ribs. It is used to evaluate collapse in this area and to detect the presence of pleural fluid.
   2. The x-ray beam is shot at an upward angle into the chest.

F. Lateral decubitus position
   1. The patient lies on either side and the film plate is placed beneath the side to be evaluated.
   2. This position is used to determine the presence of pleural fluid.

G. Radiologic appearance of anatomic structures of the child (Table 8–11)

## XI. Common radiologic abnormalities in respiratory disease

A. Pneumothorax
   1. Shift of the mediastinum, radiolucent lung field, intercostal bulging, and no lung markings

B. Consolidation
   1. Minimal loss of volume; air bronchograms are present and densities may be seen late in the process.

C. Atelectasis
   1. Loss of volume, hemidiaphragms elevated on affected side, radiopaque lung field, and possible shifting of the mediastinum to the affected side

D. Pleural effusion
   1. Blunting of costophrenic angles; diaphragm appears elevated because of fluid.

## XII. Laboratory values (Table 8–12)

## XIII. Laboratory examination

A. Sputum
   1. Expectoration of sputum into a collection cup from an effective cough. Ultrasonic nebulization, suctioning of the airway, and bronchoscopy are all methods used to obtain sputum.
   2. Many pathogenic organisms from the lungs, such as *Streptococcus pneumoniae, Mycoplasma tuberculosis, Klebsiella pneumoniae, Haemophilus influenzae,* and *Pneumocystis carinii,* can be identified.
   3. Four types of tests may be performed on sputum to detect abnormal organisms or cells.
      a. Gram's stain
         (1) This test differentiates gram-positive from gram-negative bacteria.

TABLE 8–11. ***Radiologic Appearance of Anatomic Structures of the Child***

| Anatomy | Location and Appearance of Anatomy | Abnormal Appearance | Causes |
|---|---|---|---|
| Trachea | Midline, translucent and tubelike. | Shift to left or right of midline. | Tension pneumothorax, tumor, severe atelectasis. |
| Heart | Mediastinum, midline in chest. | Cardiothoracic ratio >50%. | Cor pulmonale, CHF, congenital heart disease. |
| Main-stem bronchus | May be visible 2.5 cm from hilum. Tubelike appearance with right bronchus angle less acute than the left. | Shifted away from affected side. | Tension pneumothorax. |
| | | Shifted toward affected side. | Severe atelectasis. |
| Bronchi | Normally not visible. | Visible bronchi called air bronchograms. | Atelectasis. |
| Diaphragm | Most inferior portion of both lung fields contour in shape with hemidiaphragms ending at the costophrenic angle. The right side is higher than the left. | Flattened diaphragm. | Hyperinflation from air trapping. |
| | | Obscured or blunted costophrenic angle. | Fluid in the base of the lung. |
| | | Elevated diaphragm. | Atelectasis. |

TABLE 8–12. ***Laboratory Values and Conditions***

| Measurement | Normal Value | Condition Altering Normal Value |
|---|---|---|
| Sodium | 135–140 mEq/L | Hypernatremia: Excessive water loss in excess of sodium (diabetes insipidus), prolonged hyperventilation. |
| | | Hyponatremia: Reduced sodium intake or excessive sodium loss from profuse sweating, GI suctioning, diarrhea, vomiting. |
| Potassium | 3.5–5.5 mEq/L | Hypokalemia: Reduced $K^+$ from diarrhea, vomiting, nonsupplemented IV, chronic diuretic use. |
| | | Hyperkalemia: Increased $K^+$ from renal failure, diuretics, burns. |
| Chloride | 99–105 mEq/L | Hypochloremia: Vomiting, diarrhea. |
| | | Hyperchloremia: Severe dehydration. |
| Calcium | 9.5–10.5 mg/dL | Hypocalcemia: Renal failure. |
| | | Hypercalcemia: Multiple fractures, adrenal insufficiency. |
| Bicarbonate | 21–28 mEq/L | Reduced bicarbonate: Acute metabolic acidosis, chronic respiratory alkalosis |
| | | Increased bicarbonate: Acute metabolic alkalosis, chronic respiratory acidosis |
| Magnesium | 1–2 mEq/L | Hypomagnesemia: Diarrhea, prolonged gastric aspiration, after mercurial diuretics |
| | | Hypermagnesemia: Following administration of magnesium sulfate in mothers before birth, renal failure |
| Hemoglobin<br>Hematocrit | 13–18 gm/dL<br>38–54% | Polycythemia: Increased levels of hemoglobin, increased hematocrit |
| | | Anemia: Reduced levels of hemoglobin, decreased hematocrit |
| Red blood cells | $4.2–6.2 \times 10^6/mm^3$ | Anemia, blood loss: Decreased red blood cells |
| | | Polycythemia: Increased red blood cells |
| White blood cells: | $4{,}500–10{,}000\ mm^3$ | Leukocytosis: Increased white blood count from infection |
| Eosinophils | 3.0% | Eosinophilia from allergic rhinitis, asthma |
| Lymphocytes | 20–45% | Lymphocytosis: Viral infection |
| Basophils | 0–1% | Basophilia: Myeloproliferative disorders |
| Neutrophils | 40–75% | Neutrophilia: Bacterial infection, inflammation |
| Monocytes | 2–10% | Monocytosis: Chronic infection |

(2) The test determines whether the specimen is from the lung (many white blood cells [WBCs], few epithelial cells) or from the oral cavity (few WBCs, many epithelial cells).

(3) The test provides early presumptive diagnosis of bacterial pneumonia.

(4) Gram staining may be performed on cerebrospinal fluid to test for meningitis or on urine to identify infection following catheterization and monitoring for colonization of microorganisms.

b. Acid-fast stain

(1) This test identifies organisms of the genus *Mycobacterium*.

(2) Acid-fast stain determines a presumptive diagnosis of tuberculosis.

c. Culture and sensitivity (C&S)

(1) C&S identifies and isolates microbes for positive identification and determination of their vulnerability to antibiotics.

(2) This test helps diagnose lower respiratory tract infection.

d. Cytologic examination

(1) This test is performed to identify cancer cells, malignant pulmonary lesions, granulomas, inflammation, and other benign conditions.

B. Other cultures

1. A nasopharyngeal culture or a nasal wash isolates respiratory syncytial virus, rhinoviruses, parainfluenza viruses, and adenoviruses that cause upper respiratory tract infection.
2. A blood culture identifies pathogens in bacteremia and septicemia. Within 72 h, blood culture can identify up to 90% of pathogens.
3. After catheterization, a urine culture is performed to identify urinary tract infection and to monitor for colonization of microbes.

## XIV. Hospital-acquired infections

A. Precautions against hospital-acquired infections

1. Hands must be washed after contact with a patient and after contamination with any bodily fluids or fluids that contain blood.

TABLE 8–13. ***Isolation Categories for Hospitalized Children***

| Isolation | Single Room | Mask | Glove | Gown |
|---|---|---|---|---|
| Strict | Yes | Yes | Yes | Yes |
| Respiratory | Yes | Yes | No | No |
| Contact | Yes | Yes (if close to patient) | Yes (if touching infected material) | Yes (if soiling possible) |
| Secretions | No | No | Yes (if soiling possible) | Yes (if soiling possible) |

(Adapted from Steele, R.W., p 362, 1994.)

2. Respiratory care procedures requiring direct contact with bodily fluids necessitate the use of gown, gloves, eye protection, and mask. These respiratory care procedures include the following:
   a. Intubation
   b. Suctioning the airway
   c. Arterial artery puncture
   d. Rinsing contaminated equipment
   e. Endoscopy
   f. Phlebotomy
   g. Tracheostomy
3. Blood spills must be cleaned up immediately with a diluted bleach mixture.
4. Universal precautions do not routinely require single rooms or masks.

B. Isolation for hospitalized children (Table 8–13)
C. Diseases requiring specific isolation (Table 8–14)

TABLE 8–14. ***Diseases Requiring Specific Isolation***

| Disease | Mask | Gown | Gloves |
|---|---|---|---|
| Bronchiolitis (respiratory syncytial virus) | No | Yes* | No |
| Bronchitis | No | Yes* | No |
| Croup | No | Yes* | No |
| Epiglottitis | Yes | No | No |
| Common cold | No | Yes* | No |
| Cytomegalovirus (pregnant personnel require counseling) | No | No | No |
| Chickenpox (varicella) | Yes (if not susceptible, mask is not necessary) | Yes | Yes |

*Yes, if soiling likely.
(Adapted from Steele, R.W., p 364, 1994.)

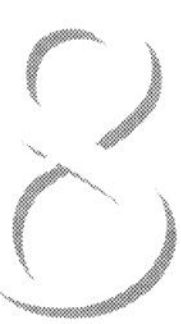

# REVIEW QUESTIONS

1. In the accompanying table, fill in the age and physical changes from infancy to adolescence.

| Description | Age | Physical Changes |
| --- | --- | --- |
| Infant | | |
| Toddler | | |
| Early childhood | | |
| Adolescence | | |

2. List suggestions that would be helpful when preparing to administer a respiratory treatment to the following age groups:
   a. Infants up to 1 year of age
   b. Toddlers up to 3 years of age
   c. Children 3 to 6 years of age
   d. Children 3 to 12 years of age

3. In the accompanying table, given the normal response from a child during physical exam questioning, fill in what would be an abnormal response.

| Normal Response | Abnormal Response |
| --- | --- |
| Speaks clearly | |
| Alert and active | |
| Able to recognize parents, siblings, other family members | |
| Responds to verbal command | |

4. What are SOAP notes?

5. List two common signs and symptoms of respiratory illness.
   a.
   b.

6. Fill in the normal vital signs for each of the following age groups:

   a. The normal respiratory rate for a child 1 year of age is __________.

   b. The normal pulse for a child 10 years of age is ________.

   c. The normal systolic range (high and low range) for blood pressure for a child 4 years of age is ________.

   d. The normal temperature for a child 5 years of age is ________.

7. Place a **T** for true or **F** for false with the following statements:

   a. _____ Orthopnea is a condition of being dyspneic while lying down.

   b. _____ Peripheral edema can be assessed by checking the temperature of the extremity.

   c. _____ Distended jugular veins indicate congestion of blood caused by right heart failure.

   d. _____ Hemoptysis is vomiting of blood that is dark, frothy, and often clotted.

   e. _____ A stridor associated with a cough is from bronchospasm caused by pneumonia.

   f. _____ The type of breathing pattern in which the chest wall moves in during inspiration and out during expiration is called paradoxical.

   g. _____ In children under 7 years of age, normal respirations are diaphragmatic and the abdomen rises with inspiration.

8. Describe the type of breathing problem (restrictive or obstructive) that occurs with the following chest abnormalities:

   a. Scoliosis

   b. Kyphosis

   c. Pectus carinatum

   d. Pectus excavatum

   e. Barrel chest

9. In the following list, match the findings in the lettered column with the conditions in the numbered column (all have to do with percussion and auscultation of the chest).

| | |
|---|---|
| a. _____ Hyperresonant | 1. Normal air-filled lung |
| b. _____ Low-pitched and soft on inspiration | 2. Crackles |
| c. _____ Normal findings heard over the main-stem bronchus | 3. Pleural effusion, atelectasis |
| d. _____ Resonant | 4. Pleural friction rub |
| e. _____ Dull to flat percussion rate | 5. Bronchial breath sounds |
| f. _____ High-pitched breath sound heard at the end of inspiration | 6. Vesicular breath sound |
| g. _____ Low-pitched, grinding breath sound loudest during inspiration | 7. Pneumothorax |

10. Describe the following findings from chest palpation:

    a. Vocal fremitus

    b. Pleural rub fremitus

    c. Rhonchal fremitus

11. Match the clinical sign with the severity of the clinical sign.

| | |
|---|---|
| a. _____ Head bobbing, mouth open, severe retractions | 1. Mild |
| b. _____ Hypertension | 2. Moderate |
| c. _____ Moist skin and mucous membranes | 3. Severe |
| d. _____ Absent and silent breath sounds | |
| e. _____ Restless, irritable, stupor | |
| f. _____ Lethargic | |

12. Match the following laboratory studies with their normal value or condition:

| | |
|---|---|
| a. _____ Bicarbonate | 1. 135 to 145 mEq/L |
| b. _____ Sodium | 2. 3.5 to 5.5 mEq/L |
| c. _____ Potassium | 3. Vomiting, diarrhea, nonsupplemented IV fluid |
| d. _____ White blood cells | 4. 4,500 to 10,000/$mm^3$ |
| e. _____ Allergic rhinitis, asthma | 5. Increased hemoglobin, red blood cells |
| f. _____ Lymphocytosis | 6. Eosinophilia |
| g. _____ Polycythemia | 7. Viral infection |
| h. _____ Hypokalemia | 8. 21 to 28 mEq/L |

13. Give a description as to why the following radiologic positions are used for infants and children:

    a. Anterior-posterior

    b. Posterior-anterior

    c. Lordotic

    d. Lateral

    e. Lateral decubitus

14. What is the indication for each of the following sputum examinations?

    a. Gram's stain

    b. Acid-fast stain

    c. Culture and sensitivity

    d. Cytologic examination

15. Determine if a mask, gown, or gloves are required by matching them to the disease (there may be more than one for each disease).

| | |
|---|---|
| a. _____ Respiratory syncytial virus | 1. Mask |
| b. _____ Croup | 2. Gown |
| c. _____ Epiglottitis | 3. Gloves |
| d. _____ Cytomegalovirus | |
| e. _____ Chickenpox | |

## BIBLIOGRAPHY


Burgess, W. R., and Cherniak, V. (1986). *Respiratory Therapy in Newborn, Infants and Children,* ed 2. New York: Thieme-Stratton.

Engle, J. (1993). *Pocket Guide: Pediatric Assessment,* ed 2. St. Louis: Mosby–Year Book.

Ferholt, J. D. L. (1980). *Clinical Assessment of Children: A Comprehensive Approach to Primary Pediatric Care.* Philadelphia: J. B. Lippincott Co.

Fishman, A. P. (1988). *Pulmonary Diseases and Disorders,* ed 2. New York: McGraw-Hill.

Gregory, G. A. (1981). *Respiratory Failure in the Child.* New York: Churchill Livingstone.

Graef, J.W., and Cone, T.E. (1980). *Manual of Pediatric Therapeutics,* ed 2. Boston: Little, Brown & Company.

Hazinski, M. F. (1992). *Nursing Care of the Critically Ill Child,* ed 2. St. Louis: Mosby–Year Book.

Hughes, J., and Griffith, J. (1984). *Synopsis of Pediatrics,* ed 6. St. Louis: Mosby.

*Illustrated Guide to Diagnostic Tests.* (1993). Springhouse, PA: Springhouse Corporation.{AU6}

MacDonald, K. F., Fahey, P. J., and Segal, M.S. (1987). *Respiratory Intensive Care.* Boston: Little, Brown & Company.

Morray, J. R. (1987). *Pediatric Intensive Care.* Norwalk, CT: Appleton & Lange.

Orlowski, J. (1988). *The Pediatric Clinics of North America: Intensive Care.* Philadelphia: W. B. Saunders Company.

Pascoe, D., and Grossman, M. (1984). *Quick Reference to Pediatric Emergencies,* ed 3. Philadelphia: J. B. Lippincott Co.

Robers, M. C. (1987). *Textbook of Pediatric Intensive Care,* Vol. 1. Baltimore: Williams & Wilkins.

Steele, R. W. (1994). *The Clinical Handbook of Pediatric Infectious Disease.* New York: Parthenon Publishing Group.

Wilkins, R., Sheldon, R., and Krider, S. J. (1990). *Clinical Assessment in Respiratory Care,* ed 2. St. Louis: Mosby.

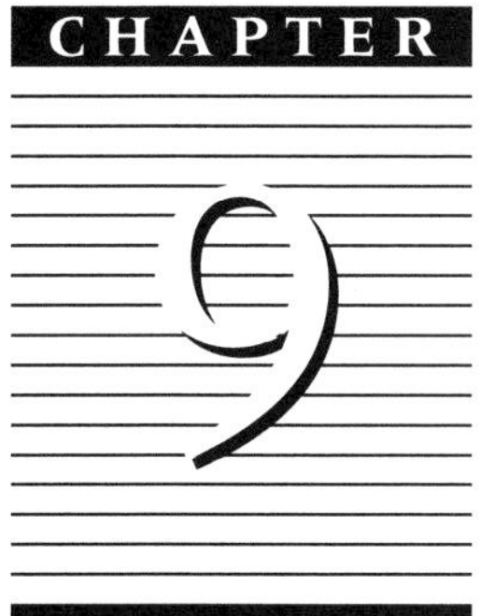

# Oxygen, Humidity, and Aerosol Therapy

**I. Indications for oxygen therapy**

A. Treat hypoxemia by increasing the alveolar $PaO_2$, thus increasing the pressure gradient for oxygen to diffuse into the bloodstream.
B. Treat the excessive work of breathing caused by hypoxemic stimulation of peripheral chemoreceptors. Increasing the arterial partial pressure of oxygen ($PaO_2$) reduces the stimulation of peripheral chemoreceptors.
C. Treat excessive myocardial work caused by an increased rate and force of contraction as a compensatory response to hypoxemia. Treating hypoxemia may reduce the stimulus to increased cardiac output.
D. Severe trauma
E. Short-term therapy (postanesthesia recovery)

**II. Precautions and possible complications of oxygen therapy**

A. Retinopathy of prematurity (ROP)
   1. Etiology
      a. Infants under 33 weeks of age who weigh less than 1500 gm have the greatest incidence of ROP.
      b. Very premature infants can develop ROP in the presence of very low concentrations of oxygen and in room air.
      c. Lengthy exposure to oxygen with $PaO_2$ above 80 mm Hg
      d. Exposure to fluorescent lights
   2. Factors contributing to ROP
      a. $PaO_2$ of blood supplying retina above 80 mm Hg
      b. Retinal vessel maturity
      c. Length of exposure to oxygen
      d. Increased $PaCO_2$
      e. Other risk factors include the following:
         (1) Exchange transfusion
         (2) Maternal hypertension
         (3) Heavy cigarette smoking by mother
         (4) Patent ductus arteriosus
   3. Pathophysiology
      a. Vascularization of the eye begins at approximately week 12.
      b. Newly formed capillaries are just under the inner surface of the retina. These capillaries receive blood from the central retinal arteries, which enter the eye along the optic nerve. These vessels begin to extend peripherally from the optic nerve toward the ora serrata.
      c. By 32 weeks' gestation, the nasal periphery of the eye is vascularized, and temporal vascularization is complete by term.
      d. Vascularization develops within the eye with a $PaO_2$ range of between 17 to 29 mm Hg.
      e. With hyperoxia:
         (1) Autoregulation causes arterioles to constrict and reduce blood flow.
         (2) Developing vessels may permanently constrict and become necrotic. This is referred to as vasobliteration.
         (3) Vasoactive substances are released from ischemic areas of the eye, resulting in rapid vascular growth and the formation of new vessels to oxygenate the eye. These vessels extend into the fluid portion of the

TABLE 9–1. ***Stages and Classification of ROP***

| Stages of ROP | Classification |
|---|---|
| 1 | A thin, white demarcation line is seen separating the avascular retina anteriorly from the vascularized retina posteriorly. |
| 2 | Proliferation of new vessels. Tortuous vessels are seen within the eye. |
| 3 | Scar tissue is formed from hemorrhaging of newly formed vessels. |
| 4 | Retina begins to become detached. |
| 5 | Retina is completely detached. |

eye (the vitreous humor) and hemorrhaging begins. This causes peripheral retinal clouding and scarring. With minor scarring behind the retina, vision may be normal if the causative factor is removed. No permanent injury results.

(4) Continual blood leakage into the eye behind the retina causes scar tissue formation. As this process continues, scar tissue formed from the hemorrhage shrinks and pulls on the retina, causing detachment, which results in blindness.

f. Stages and classification of ROP (Table 9–1)

4. Diagnosis
   a. ROP is diagnosed by ophthalmologic exam of the internal eye anatomy.
5. Treatment and prevention
   a. Directed toward maintaining $PaO_2$ levels at 50 to 70 mm Hg
   b. Reducing the time of exposure to high $FIO_2$ (over 0.50)
   c. Use oxygen blenders to provide specific $FIO_2$ during procedures (i.e., suctioning, apneic spell, endotracheal intubation) and avoid hyperoxygenation if possible.
   d. Ophthalmologic assessment is done on a consistent basis to assess the eye.
   e. Cover the eyes to protect them from fluorescent lights.
   f. Use laser surgery to treat glaucoma.

B. Oxygen toxicity
   1. Oxygen toxicity results from a series of reversible pathophysiologic inflammatory changes of lung tissue. An increase in free oxygen radicals depends on $PAO_2$. The greater the $PAO_2$, the greater the quantity of free radicals.
   2. Certain lung cells, such as alveolar types I, II, and III, are susceptible to hyperoxia. Pulmonary capillary endothelium is most susceptible. With continued exposure to a high concentration of oxygen, type I alveolar cells are destroyed and replaced with type II alveolar cells.
   3. Edema follows, with destruction and necrosis of endothelial cells. Hyaline membrane follows. Chronic changes in the lung, including thickening of the alveolar septa, develop.

C. Oxygen-induced alveolar hypoventilation
   1. Observed in patients with chronic carbon dioxide ($CO_2$) retention
   2. Increased $PaO_2$ eliminates the drive to breathe, causing hypoventilation.

D. Absorption atelectasis
   1. When a high fractional concentration of oxygen ($FIO_2$) is administered (above 0.50), nitrogen is washed out.
   2. Oxygen is removed from the alveoli faster than it can be replaced by normal ventilation, thus reducing alveoli size. When alveoli reach their critical volume, collapse and atelectasis occur.

E. Constriction or closure of ductus arteriosus
   1. Increased $PaO_2$ contributes to the constriction or closure of the ductus arteriosus.
   2. For infants with ductus-dependent heart lesions, this may be a concern.

## III. Oxygen delivery devices

A. Low-flow systems
   1. Low-flow systems, in which the fractional oxygen delivery varies with the patient's inspiratory flow, are classified as variable-performance oxygen delivery systems.
      a. A nasal cannula provides a variable that is dependent on the patient's inspiratory flow, tidal volume, and respiratory rate.
      b. A nasopharyngeal catheter is inserted into one naris to a depth equal to the distance from the ala nasi to the tragus of the ear. Proper distance is

determined by observing the tip of the catheter just below the uvula. The $FIO_2$ varies with the patient's inspiratory flow, tidal volume, and respiratory rate.

c. The tracheostomy oxygen adapter is a device that attaches either directly to a tracheostomy tube or to a heat-moisture exchanger (HME), which then attaches to a tracheostomy tube. The $FIO_2$ is variable and is provided to the patient by an oxygen supply tube and adapter attached to a tracheostomy. The patient inspires the blow-by gas source. These devices are intended for short-term periods such as during transportation or for increased patient mobility.

B. Reservoir systems
  1. A simple oxygen mask provides oxygen through a single oxygen connecting tube. Holes on each side of the mask allow exhaled $CO_2$ to escape and room air to entrain in the mask.
  2. Partial-rebreathing masks contain a reservoir at the base of the mask. The reservoir receives fresh gas plus the exhaled gas from the patient that is equal to the anatomic dead space. Exhaled gas plus fresh gas combine to achieve a variable $FIO_2$.
  3. A nonrebreathing mask is similar to the partial-rebreathing mask except it does not allow exhaled gas from the patient to enter the reservoir bag. One-way valves positioned at the opening of the reservoir prevent mixing of the gases. This device is designed to deliver a higher $FIO_2$ than the simple mask and partial-rebreathing mask.

C. High-flow systems
  1. An air-entrainment mask is used to attain a specific $FIO_2$. It uses a corrugated tube and jet orifice connected to an oxygen supply. The total flow is dependent on the oxygen flow rate, cross-sectional area of the entrainment ports, and diameter of the jet orifice. Aerosol can be added to the flow by a collar and can be adapted to fit a tracheostomy.
  2. An air-entrainment nebulizer is a gas-powered, large-volume nebulizer that contains an adjustable air-entrainment port. A specific oxygen concentration can be achieved with this device. A heating device may be attached to the nebulizer to achieve water vapor at body temperature. This device may be attached to a face tent, aerosol mask, tracheostomy collar, T-piece, or Briggs adapter.

D. Enclosure systems
  1. An oxygen hood is a transparent device that fits around the head of a newborn or small infant. Humidified oxygen is supplied to the hood by tubing attached to an air-entrainment device that provides a specific oxygen concentration. Larger units called tent houses or huts are used for infants who do not fit in the newborn-size hood. Very small infants may be placed inside a tent house to receive humidity.
  2. An oxygen tent is a device that uses an air-conditioning system to control the internal environment of the tent. Oxygen and humidification are provided in the tent. A transparent tent is placed around the patient and tucked into the mattress to provide an oxygen-enriched environment.
  3. Closed incubators are devices that provide a neutral thermal environment for newborn infants (see Chapter 4).

E. Indications for oxygen device use
  1. Documented hypoxemia
  2. Suspicion of hypoxia or suspicion of regional hypoxia where the hypoxia may respond to an increase in $PaO_2$

F. Contraindications
  1. Where there is a nasal cannula with nasal obstruction (choanal atresia, nasal polyps)
  2. Nasopharyngeal catheters are contraindicated with maxillofacial trauma or with basal skull fracture.
  3. Patients intubated for airway protection should probably be placed on continuous positive airway pressure (CPAP) rather than a T-piece to replace the loss of physiological end-expiratory pressure created by the endotracheal tube.

G. Physiological hazards, precautions, and possible complications
  1. Development of ROP (see Equipment-Related Hazards, Precautions, and Possible Complications later in this chapter). Preterm infants (under 37 weeks of age) receiving oxygen should not have a $PaO_2$ over 80 mm Hg.
  2. Reducing the respiratory drive in $CO_2$ retainers
  3. Apnea from cool oxygen directed over an infant's face
  4. Hypoxemia or hyperoxemia from incorrect oxygen device

H. Equipment-related hazards, precautions, and possible complications
   1. Nasal cannula
      a. Skin irritation from cannula material or material used to attach cannula
      b. Nasal irritation or improper sizing
      c. Displacement from nares can lead to loss of oxygen.
      d. Development of CPAP from tight-fitting cannula because of anatomy of nose, size of cannula, and gas flow. Excessive flows can irritate the nose.
      e. Low relative humidity from the cannula can dry mucus, obstructing the flow of oxygen into the nose.
   2. Nasopharyngeal catheter
      a. Nasal pharyngeal trauma during insertion
      b. Pain from excessive flow
      c. Skin irritation from device material or material used to secure device
      d. Gastric distention
   3. Masks
      a. Irritation from mask material or straps to hold mask on face
      b. Aspiration of vomitus when mask is in place
      c. Inadequate flow of oxygen, causing rebreathing of $CO_2$
   4. Air-entrainment devices
      a. High noise levels in incubators or hoods (suggest using entrainment port in the 100% setting powered by compressed air and blending in oxygen to achieve a specific oxygen concentration, or air-entrainment device set at 100% setting connected to a blender set at a specific $FIO_2$)
      b. Contamination
      c. Bronchoreactivity in patients with reactive airways when used with non-isotonic solutions
      d. Inadvertent extubation or decannulation of tracheostomy when used with a T-piece
      e. Nonheated device may produce cold stress in neonates.
      f. Excessive condensation in tube may cause inadvertent lavage when attached to an artificial airway.
      g. Overhydration in very small infants
   5. Hoods and transparent enclosure
      a. Cutaneous fungal infection from prolonged exposure to humidified oxygen
      b. Disconnection from device may cause hypoxia.
      c. Cold stress from improper temperature of gas
   6. Oxygen tent
      a. Electric shock or fire from battery-operated or electrical devices
      b. Electric shock from electrical discharge (static electricity) from the plastic tent
      c. Contamination of large nebulizer
      d. Buildup of heat from loss of cooling device
      e. Possible asphyxiation of infant lodged between plastic tent and mattress

I. Limitations of oxygen devices
   1. Nasal cannula
      a. Oxygen flow rate should be limited to 2 L/min in infants and newborns.
      b. Discrepancies in flow and oxygen concentrations between set and delivered values can occur in low-flow blenders at flows below the recommended range of the blender.
      c. The flow rate may differ in the same flowmeter at different flow settings and among different flowmeters.
      d. Easy to occlude
   2. Nasopharyngeal catheter
      a. The nasopharyngeal catheter is not commonly used because of the complexity of its care and its uncertain $FIO_2$.
      b. Catheter sizes less than 8 French are less effective in oxygen delivery. Use a flowmeter that delivers less than 3 L/min.
      c. Easy to occlude
   3. Masks
      a. Masks are not recommended for the precise concentration and delivery of oxygen.
      b. Masks are confining and interfere with feeding.
      c. Settings on air-entrainment devices with an $FIO_2$ of over 0.40 may not provide enough flow to meet the demand of the patient. Total flow output is determined by the $FIO_2$ setting and flow rate of oxygen (Table 9–2).
      d. Calculation of total flow from an entrainment device

TABLE 9–2. ***Specifics of Air-Entrainment Systems***

| $FIO_2$ | Flow Rate of Oxygen (L/min) | Entrainment Ratio (oxygen to air) | Total Flow to Patient (L/min) |
|---|---|---|---|
| 0.24 | 4 | 1:25 | 104 |
| 0.28 | 4 | 1:10 | 44 |
| 0.31 | 6 | 1:7 | 48 |
| 0.35 | 8 | 1:5 | 48 |
| 0.40 | 8 | 1:3 | 32 |
| 0.50 | 12 | 1:1.7 | 32 |

(1) What is the total flow coming from an air-entrainment device set at 40% with a flow rate of 10 L/min?

Total flow = oxygen flow rate × total entrainment ratio

Total flow = 10 L/min × (3 + 1 = 4) = 10 × 4 = 40 L/min

e. Calculation of flow using the "tic-tac-flow" method (if you cannot remember each ratio).
   (1) What is the total flow of an air-entrainment device set at 40% with an oxygen flow rate of 10 L/min?

| Air | | Oxygen |
|---|---|---|
| 20 | | 100 |
| | 40 | |
| 60 | ÷ | 20 |
| 3 | : | 1 |

   (2) Set up the tic-tac-flow box with air at 20% (rounded down) in the upper left hand box and oxygen in the upper right hand box. In the middle box, insert the $FIO_2$ at which the device is set (in this example, 40% is used).
   (3) Subtract 20 from 40 (ignore the negative sign) and subtract 100 from 40. This will equal 60 in the lower left-hand box and 20 in the lower right-hand box.
   (4) Next, dividing 60 by 20 is equal to 3, which is the number of parts of air entrained to give 40% oxygen (oxygen is always 1 part).
   (5) 3 parts of air to 1 part of oxygen is 4 total parts.
   (6) 4 total parts × 10 L/min = 40 L/min total flow coming from the system.

4. Air-entrainment nebulizers
   a. Temperature should be monitored to prevent cold stress. The temperature of the gas should be the same as that of the infant's environment.
   b. Condensation in tubing restricts air-entrainment and increases the delivered oxygen concentration.
5. Hoods and tents
   a. Measure the oxygen concentration as close to the mouth or nose as possible.
   b. The oxygen concentration that can be achieved in an oxygen tent is less than 0.40.
   c. The oxygen concentration in a hood varies between 0.21 to 1.0 and is more stable than a tent.
   d. High gas flows produce harmful noise levels.
6. Tracheostomy adapters using blow-by gas flow provide variable $FIO_2$.
7. The heat moisture exchanger must be monitored for excessive secretion buildup or for absorption of a large amount of water by the hygroscopic inserts.

J. Oxygen device assessment of need (Table 9–3)

TABLE 9–3. ***Oxygen Device Assessment of Need***

| Device | Needs Assessment |
|---|---|
| Nasal cannula | Provides low-level oxygen concentration. Infant can feed without interruption of oxygen delivery. Bubble humidifier may be used with a nasal cannula. Blenders and flowmeter with adjustable increments of 0.125 L/min are reliable for use with neonates. $FIO_2$ of 0.28 to 0.30 is delivered with a liter flow of 0.125 to 1 L/min. For older children 1–6 L/min is used to deliver $FIO_2$ of 0.24 to 0.44. |
| Nasopharyngeal catheter | Provides low-level oxygen concentration. Infant can feed without interruption of oxygen delivery. Increased mobility. |
| Simple oxygen mask | Used for delivery of supplemental oxygen in the range of 0.35–0.50 (depending on minute ventilation) at 6–10 L/min. Used for short periods during transport, procedures. |
| Partial rebreathing mask | Used for delivery of 0.40–0.60 oxygen concentration. Used for delivery of higher oxygen concentrations. |
| Non-rebreathing mask | Used to deliver oxygen concentrations of >0.60 or specific concentrations from a blender. |
| Air-entrainment mask | Used to deliver a predetermined oxygen concentration from 0.24 to 0.50. High oxygen concentration settings may not deliver high enough flow for larger infants and children. |
| Air-entrainment nebulizer | Used for high levels of humidity or aerosol. Used for patients with artificial airway, following extubation. Sterile water or normal saline solution used in nebulizer. |
| Hoods | Used for controlled $FIO_2$ in newborns and small infants. Useful with hyperoxia tests in spontaneously breathing infants. Flow should be >7 L/min to flush out $CO_2$. |
| Tents | Useful for larger infants and children requiring cool humidity and supplemental oxygen (<0.40). Infants with upper airway obstruction, such as laryngotracheobronchitis, artificial airways that cannot have other devices attached. Flow should be >7 L/min to flush out $CO_2$. |
| Tracheostomy oxygen adapters | Used to provide blow-by oxygen to patients with tracheostomy tube. Specific oxygen concentration may vary with patient's minute ventilation or if a reservoir tubing is not attached to the opposite end of the T-adapter. |

K. Monitoring
1. Oxygen tension and saturation by invasive and noninvasive monitoring of patient within an appropriate time (1 h of initiation of oxygen for a neonate) should be assessed.
   a. The acceptable oxygen blood level for a newborn is 50 to 70 mm Hg; for an infant, 60 to 80 mm Hg; and for a child, 80 to 100 mm Hg.
   b. When monitoring oxygen saturation by pulse oximetry, the high oxygen alarm should be set for less than 100% when the infant is on oxygen.
   c. All oxygen delivery systems should be checked once per shift, with a calibrated analyzer if possible.
2. Watch for signs and symptoms of hypoxemia.
   a. Early signs of moderate hypoxemia include tachycardia, tachypnea, and desaturation.
   b. With severe hypoxemia, there are signs and symptoms of bradycardia, apnea, and further desaturation. Other physical signs include increased inspiratory effort, lethargy, restlessness, irritability, and frog-leg appearance (infant or child on his or her back with legs in a froglike position as a result of lethargy).
3. The oxygen delivery device may not be appropriate for this level of hypoxemia, which requires changing to a new device that can deliver higher oxygen concentrations or higher flowrates.
   a. Determination of $FIO_2$ with any system combining flows:

$$FIO_2 = \frac{(FIO_2 \text{ of A device})\ (\text{Flow of A device}) + (FIO_2 \text{ of B device})\ (\text{Flow of B device})}{\text{Total flow of combined systems}}$$

$$FIO_2 = \frac{(0.30)\ (10\ \text{L/min}) + (0.50)\ (10\ \text{L/min})}{20\ \text{L/min}}$$

$$FIO_2 = \frac{0.3 + 0.5}{20} = \frac{0.8}{20} = 0.40$$

b. If hyperoxemia or a high oxygen saturation occurs, the oxygen concentration should be checked with a calibrated oxygen analyzer to ensure that the correct oxygen concentration is being delivered. If so, reduce the oxygen concentration to a lower value that will maintain an appropriate oxygen saturation.
c. Change the oxygen delivery device if the infant or child does not tolerate the device. Ensure that the same oxygen concentration is maintained with the new device.

L. Infection control
1. Nasal cannulas and masks do not require routine change.
2. Nasopharyngeal catheters should be changed every 24 h and inserted into the opposite naris if possible.
3. When connected to artificial airways, large-volume nebulizers require changing every 24 h. In nonintubated patients, replace the equipment on an as-needed basis.
4. Mist-tent nebulizers and head hoods are replaced on an as-needed basis.

## IV. Continuous positive airway pressure (CPAP)

A. CPAP provides a continuous positive pressure to the airways throughout the respiratory cycle of a spontaneously breathing patient.

B. CPAP may be applied through nasal prongs inserted into the nares (NCPAP), through an endotracheal tube (ETCPAP), or through a nasopharyngeal tube (NP-CPAP). Each has its advantages and disadvantages (Table 9–4). The device is attached to a continuous flow, humidified system. This may be a mechanical ventilator or a free-standing unit.

C. CPAP aids in maintaining lung volume by keeping inspiratory and expiratory pressures above ambient pressure. This results in an increase in functional residual capacity, an improvement in static compliance, and reduced airway resistance in patients with unstable pulmonary mechanics. An improvement in lung mechanics is evidenced by an increase in spontaneous tidal volume, stable minute ventilation, and a reduction in the work of breathing.

D. Indications for neonatal CPAP:
1. An increase in the work of breathing is identified on physical examination by a 30 to 40% increase in respiratory rate, substernal and suprasternal retractions, nasal flaring, and grunting.
2. An inability to maintain a $PaO_2$ above 50 mm Hg on an $FIO_2$ of 0.60 or less while maintaining a $PaCO_2$ of 50 mm Hg or less and a pH of 7.25 or higher.
3. Evidence of reduced lung volume and/or infiltrates on chest radiograph

TABLE 9–4. *Advantages and Disadvantages of CPAP Application*

| Device | Advantages | Disadvantages |
|---|---|---|
| Nasal prongs | Noninvasive.<br>Lightweight.<br>Easily removed to clean or replace and suction nose to maintain patency. | Easily dislodged.<br>Requires stabilization to face, nose, or head.<br>Nose and nasal septum may become damaged with long-term use or improperly fitting prongs.<br>Mucus plugging.<br>Level of noise from continuous flow device.<br>Requires intubation to mechanically ventilate.<br>Loss of CPAP when the infant cries. |
| Nasopharyngeal tube | More stable than prongs.<br>Optimal delivery pressure better than prongs.<br>Less frequent dislodgement as compared to prongs. | Mucus plugging.<br>Increased airway resistance.<br>Irritation and potential damage to nares, septum, and nasopharynx.<br>Requires stabilization to face and nose.<br>Level of noise from continuous flow device.<br>Requires intubation to mechanically ventilate. |
| Endotracheal tube | Optimal transmission of pressure provided by the tube directly into the lungs and less leak as compared to nasal prongs and nasopharyngeal tube.<br>Infant can be switched to mechanical ventilation. | High airway resistance.<br>Oral, tracheal, and vocal cord damage from intubation. |

4. Conditions responsive to CPAP present clinically as the following conditions:
   a. Respiratory distress syndrome
   b. Atelectasis
   c. Recent extubation
   d. Transient tachypnea of the newborn
   e. Pulmonary edema

E. Neonatal and pediatric contraindications
1. Anatomic abnormalities that would make NCPAP and NP-CPAP ineffective, such as choanal atresia, tracheoesophageal fistula, and cleft palate
2. Cardiovascular instability and impending arrest
3. Frequent apneic spells resulting in desaturation and/or bradycardia
4. An inability to maintain a $PaCO_2$ below 60 mm Hg and a pH greater than 7.25
5. Application to infants with diaphragmatic hernia, which may lead to gastric insufflation

F. Neonatal and pediatric hazards, complications, and potential problems with equipment
1. Mucus plugging causes a reduction in $FIO_2$ from entrainment of room air from other nare with NCPAP or NP-CPAP. If the infant desaturates (the $FIO_2$ delivery from the continuous-flow device has not been altered) remove the prongs or nasopharyngeal tube, provide flow-by oxygen with the resuscitation bag, and suction the nares. Inspect the prongs and nasopharyngeal tube for mucous obstruction and clear. After replacing device, monitor for increased oxygen saturation and auscultate.
2. Complete obstruction of NCPAP or NP-CPAP results in continued pressurization of CPAP system without activation of high and low airway pressure alarms.
3. Endotracheal tube or NP-CPAP tube kinking
4. With NCPAP and NP-CPAP, gastric insufflation may occur. Some ventilators provide a manual breath to be delivered, which also causes gastric insufflation. An open orogastric tube should be placed with infants on NCPAP or NP-CPAP.
5. Appropriate length for NP-CPAP is determined by measuring from the tragus of ear to tip of chin or nose.

G. Neonatal and pediatric hazards and complications associated with clinical conditions
1. Excessive pressure may cause overdistention, leading to pulmonary air leak syndrome (PALS) and increased work of breathing.
2. Hypercapnia
3. Increased pulmonary artery pressure, reduced cardiac output
4. Abdominal distention and reduced tidal volume
5. Nasal necrosis caused by inadequate humidification
6. Nasal irritation, septal distortion, tracheal stenosis
7. Hypotension

H. Neonatal application of NCPAP or NP-CPAP and assessment of outcome
1. Initiate CPAP at 4 to 5 cm $H_2O$. Increase levels gradually to 10 cm $H_2O$ to achieve the following:
   a. A $FIO_2$ less than or equal to 0.60 with $PaO_2$ levels above 50 mm Hg, acceptable noninvasive oxygen monitoring, and maintaining an acceptable minute ventilation as determined by a $PaCO_2$ of 50 to 60 mm Hg and a pH of 7.25 or higher
   b. A decrease in respiratory rate by 30 to 40% and a reduced severity of retractions, nasal flaring, and grunting
   c. Chest radiographic improvement of lung volumes and infiltrates
   d. Patient comfort improved
   e. Monitor for side effects at different CPAP levels (Table 9–5)
2. Optimal CPAP
   a. Optimal CPAP is defined by the disease state of the patient. The optimal CPAP for an infant with RDS differs from that for an infant being weaning from CPAP.
   b. In general, the optimal CPAP is the least amount of CPAP required to achieve the best $PaO_2$, oxygen saturation, lung compliance, pulmonary mechanics, cardiac output, and oxygen delivery.
   c. For infants with RDS and in whom oxygenation is a major problem, optimal CPAP is calculated by determining the oxygenation levels as measured by $PaO_2$, oxygen saturation, and oxygen delivery (arterial oxygen concentration [$CaO_2$] times cardiac output [CO]).

TABLE 9–5. ***Rationale for Use and Side Effects at Different CPAP Pressures***

| Levels of CPAP (cm $H_2O$) | Rationale for Use | Potential Side Effects |
|---|---|---|
| <4 | Used during weaning<br>Maintenance of lung volume in extremely low-birth-weight infants | Hypercapnia<br>Reduced lung volumes<br>Hypoxemia |
| 4–6 | Common level for RDS infants<br>Stabilizes lung volume and obstructed airway in low-birth-weight infants | Reduction in venous return in infants with normal compliance<br>Overdistention |
| 7–10 | Increased pressure requirement in infants with poor lung compliance and reduced FRC<br>Increased distribution of ventilation<br>Used in larger infants | PALS<br>Reduced compliance from overdistention<br>Increased work of breathing<br>Hypercapnia<br>Hypoxemia<br>Increased pulmonary vascular resistance, decreased cardiac output |
| >10 | In severe RDS infants with very low compliance and lung volumes<br>Prevents complete collapse of the lung | Same as for CPAP levels of 7 to 10 cm $H_2O$ |

d. For infants being weaned from CPAP and in whom oxygenation is not a problem, compliance, resistance, and lung volume determine the optimal CPAP level.

3. Monitor the patient every 2 h and document the following:
   a. CPAP settings
   b. Periodic sampling of arterial and capillary blood gas values
   c. Continuous noninvasive monitoring of oxygen
   d. Respiratory rate and heart rate
   e. Mean airway pressure; proximal airway pressure
   f. $FIO_2$
   g. Physical examination including chest appearance, color, evidence of retractions, and breath sounds
   h. Appearance of nose; taped skin; and stabilizing structure to head, mouth, and lips
   i. Changes in chest radiograph
4. If no improvement occurs or if the patient demonstrates agitation on application of NCPAP or NP-CPAP, consider ETCPAP. Mechanical ventilation is required when there is no improvement in the patient's condition and when there are increased episodes of apnea and/or bradycardia and desaturation.

I. Neonatal CPAP weaning
   1. Patient shows signs of clinical improvement (see Neonatal Application of NCAP or NP-CPAP and Assessment of Outcome earlier in this chapter).
   2. Reduce $FIO_2$ to under 0.40 in increments that are consistent with maintaining noninvasive monitoring of oxygen at acceptable levels (oxygen saturation above 90% with a transcutaneous oxygen pressure [$PtcO_2$] of 50 to 70 mm Hg). The $FIO_2$ may be reduced to 0.21 while maintaining CPAP.
   3. Reduce CPAP levels to 3 to 5 cm $H_2O$ in 1-cm $H_2O$ increments.
   4. Chest radiograph shows improvement.
   5. Remove CPAP when CPAP levels are at 5 cm $H_2O$ and under, and when the $FIO_2$ is less than 0.40.
   6. To maintain acceptable noninvasive oxygen values, insert a nasal cannula attached to a blender at the lowest $FIO_2$ level.
   7. Monitor for episodes of apnea and/or bradycardia. Before reapplying CPAP, consider a bumper bed and aminophylline or caffeine administration. If apnea and/or bradycardia persist and desaturation occurs, reapply CPAP.

J. Pediatric application of CPAP
   1. Indications for applying CPAP are the same for older infants and children as for neonates.
   2. Weaning the patient from mechanical ventilation is a common use of CPAP.
   3. Physical examination of older infants and children yields similar findings to that of the neonate for determining the need for CPAP.

4. Infants and older children may tolerate a higher level of CPAP. Initiate CPAP at 5 to 10 cm $H_2O$ and increase the CPAP level in increments of 2 to 3 cm $H_2O$ until an improvement in the overall condition is seen and the $PaO_2$ increases to 60 to 70 mm Hg. CPAP pressures above 10 cm $H_2O$ may be required for the extremely poor compliance, low-volume patient.
5. In addition to a CPAP above 20 cm $H_2O$, hypoxemia, hypercapnia, acidosis, increased retractions, respiratory rate, and desaturation may all indicate the need for mechanical ventilation.

K. Pediatric weaning from CPAP
1. Once the patient is stabilized, decrease oxygen to less than 50% in increments of 5 to 10%.
2. Decrease CPAP down in increments of 2 to 3 cm $H_2O$ until the pressure is 5 cm $H_2O$ or lower.
3. CPAP is removed when the pressure is 5 cm $H_2O$ or lower, the $FIO_2$ is below 0.40, and all pulmonary function, oxygenation, and cardiovascular assessments are acceptable.

L. Infection control
1. Following use, dispose of single-patient CPAP kits.
2. It is acceptable to change disposable CPAP circuits, humidifying devices, and continuous-feed water systems after 5 days.
3. The ventilator and CPAP unit should be wiped down periodically when soiled and when removed from the patient's room to prevent potentially communicable organisms from being transmitted to other patients.
4. Adhere strictly to sterile suctioning and handwashing procedures.

M. Nasal mask CPAP
1. Indication
   a. Used in the home for the treatment of obstructive sleep apnea in children over 3 years of age (because of the leak created by the flat, narrow nasal bridge that is present in infants under 3 years of age). Sleep apnea is diagnosed by polysomnography.
2. Contraindications
   a. Inability to maintain life-sustaining ventilation
   b. Barotrauma in patients with extensive bleb formation in the lung
   c. Hypotension
   d. Allergic reaction to mask material
3. Components of nasal CPAP
   a. Flow generator that raises the pressure slowly to the preset CPAP level
   b. Nasal mask
   c. Positive end-expiratory pressure (PEEP)—CPAP valve, which is an adjustable threshold valve with a pressure range from 2.5 to 20 cm $H_2O$
   d. One-way valve
   e. Patient circuit
   f. Low or disconnect CPAP alarm
   g. If oxygen is required, it will need to be blended into the device or the patient will need to use a nasal cannula.
4. The appropriate CPAP level is set according to one of the following choices:
   a. The lowest CPAP at which the apneic episodes cease (this may require pressures of up to 15 cm $H_2O$)
   b. The lowest level of CPAP that prevents arterial desaturation ($SpO_2$ less than 90%)
   c. Taking the patient's subjective response to different levels of CPAP into account, the level that achieves the least hypersomnolence and fewest headaches
5. Troubleshooting mask CPAP and patient complaints (Table 9–6)

**V. Bilevel positive airway pressure (BiPAP)**

A. BiPAP does not provide the total ventilatory requirements for the patient. The use of BiPAP may reduce the incidence of intubation. BiPAP reduces respiratory distress by reducing the work of breathing. BiPAP is administered by nasal mask or full mask.

B. Indications.
1. Alveolar hypoventilation
2. Ventilatory muscle fatigue or muscle dysfunction manifested by the following:
   a. Tachypnea
   b. Reduced tidal volume
   c. Hypercapnia
   d. Subjective complaints

TABLE 9–6. ***Troubleshooting Mask CPAP and Patient Complaints***

| Troubleshooting/Patient Complaint | Solution |
|---|---|
| Patient is unable to achieve desired CPAP. | Check for leaks in the circuit, around mask. Refit mask or obtain a proper fitting mask.<br>Check to assure blower device is working. Check and replace fuse if necessary.<br>Check filters and clean and replace as needed.<br>Check intake and outport for assured clear distance from wall.<br>Move device away from the wall.<br>Patient is mouth-breathing and needs to nose-breathe. |
| Patient complains of headache and hyper somnolence. | Optimal level of CPAP not achieved. Increase the CPAP level until headache and hyper somnolence are reduced or cease. |
| Snoring is still present. | Obstruction is still present. Increase the level of CPAP until snoring ceases. |
| Patient complains of dryness, epistaxis of the nose. | Add a humidifier. |
| Patient complains of conjunctivitis or eye irritation. | Check for proper fitting nasal mask. Change mask to proper fitting mask, if needed. |
| Irritation from nasal mask. | Assess nasal area where mask comes in contact with nose regularly. Note any redness, cracking, or bleeding. Clean mask regularly and replace if needed. |

3. Hypoxemia in spite of increasing $FIO_2$
4. Post-extubation difficulties (prevent reintubation)
5. Upper airway obstruction

C. Contraindications
1. Inability to maintain life-sustaining ventilation
2. Barotrauma (patient with extensive bleb formation in the lung)
3. Hypotension
4. Allergic reaction to mask material

D. Airway pressure
1. Two airway pressures that range from 4 to 20 cm $H_2O$ are available to the patient.
   a. Inspiratory positive airway pressure (IPAP), which is similar to pressure support, is given to the patient during inspiration to provide a pressure boost. This is directed toward reducing the patient's work of breathing and enhancing tidal volume to affect atelectasis.
   b. Expiratory positive airway pressure (EPAP), which is similar to CPAP, helps to maintain or increase functional residual capacity (FRC) in patients. EPAP is directed toward increasing the $PaO_2$ in patients who are hypoxemic in spite of an increased $FIO_2$.

E. Modes of operation
1. CPAP—for patients who are hypoxemic in spite of an increased $FIO_2$
   a. In this mode, EPAP is set.
2. Spontaneous—for individuals who have adequate respiratory rate. The patient determines his or her own respiratory rate, tidal volume, and flowrate.
   a. In this mode, IPAP and EPAP are adjusted. This helps to enhance inspiratory volume, reducing the work of breathing and also affecting $PaO_2$ in patients who are hypoxemic.
3. Spontaneous and controlled—for patients not maintaining adequate respiratory rate by having long periods of apnea
   a. In this mode, IPAP, EPAP, and breaths per minute (bpm) are set. The bpm functions to assist the patient who is not breathing in the given time as set on the bpm control. For example, if the bpm is set for 10/min, there is a 6-s cycle time. If the patient fails to take a breath in this time, an IPAP breath is delivered. If, however, the patient were to spontaneous breath in 5 s, the bpm is reset following exhalation. In this mode, it is similar to synchronized intermittent mandatory ventilation (SIMV), except that instead of a positive-pressure breath delivery occurring as with SIMV, a pressure support breath is initiated.

4. Controlled—for patients who do not synchronize with BiPAP. Generally, the patient is supported at a higher rate than his or her spontaneous rate until the patient's distress is relieved and the patient's spontaneous rate is reduced to a reasonable level.

F. Protocol for initiating BiPAP
1. Before application, gather the following baseline data:
   a. ABGs
   b. Vital capacity
   c. Maximum inspiratory pressure (MIP)
   d. Tidal volume
   e. BP
   f. Pulse
   g. Respiratory rate
   h. Auscultate chest.
   i. Inspect chest for signs of increased work of breathing, such as retractions and paradoxical chest movement, indicating diaphragmatic fatigue.
2. Select an appropriately sized nasal mask. It is very important to have a properly fitting mask. An improperly fitted mask creates excessive leaks and an inability to maintain pressure. Also, the patient should be instructed to nose-breathe as much as possible. Mouth-breathing allows the pressure to escape and reduces the pressure in the lungs.
3. Select the appropriate mode of operation. This may be based on the following patient problems:
   a. Patient's respiratory status: Can the patient move air? If not, IPAP is the important pressure for this patient. Generally, this is set higher than EPAP. IPAP, because it is similar to pressure support, provides a pressure boost during inspiration to help the inspiratory muscles overcome obstructions to create volume change. In other words, it breathes for the patient. For example, a postsurgical patient who required abdominal or thoracic surgery would benefit from IPAP. In this patient, IPAP is important to reverse the atelectasis that may have occurred during surgery.
   b. Is the patient's problem gas exchange? Is the patient hypoxemic? If so, EPAP is the important pressure to adjust because it affects the lungs in the same way as CPAP. This may be useful for a patient with asthma who is experiencing exacerbation and is not responding to oxygen therapy. In this patient the IPAP–EPAP difference would not be as large as it would be with the surgical patient.
4. Adjustment of IPAP and EPAP
   a. IPAP is started at 8 cm $H_2O$ and adjusted in increments of 2 cm $H_2O$.
   b. EPAP is started at 4 cm $H_2O$ and adjusted in increments of 2 cm $H_2O$.
5. Determining mode of operation for BiPAP
6. The following are clinical manifestations indicating the need for adjustment of IPAP:
   a. Increased work of breathing documented by retractions and paradoxical chest movement
   b. Reduced breath sounds
   c. Hypercapnia
   d. Reduced spontaneous tidal volume
   e. Reduced vital capacity
   f. Reduced mean inspiratory pressure
7. Clinical indication for the need to adjust EPAP
   a. Refractive hypoxemia as documented by an increase in $FIO_2$ with little to no change in $PaO_2$
8. Examples of settings
   a. Hypoxemic patient
      (1) Initially, set EPAP at 4 to 6 cm $H_2O$ to keep $SpO_2$ above 90%. Adjust as needed.
   b. Patient with increased work of breathing, reduced breath sounds, and hypercapnia with a stable ventilatory drive
      (1) Set in spontaneous mode
      (2) Initially, set IPAP at 8 cm $H_2O$ and EPAP at 4 cm $H_2O$ to keep $SpO_2$ above 90%. *Adjust as needed.

*In these settings, the difference is equal to 6 cm $H_2O$, which provides a pressure boost to help the spontaneous ventilation and reduce hypercapnia. If the patient still has clinical manifestations indicating no response to the settings, it may be necessary to increase IPAP to provide a greater pressure difference.

TABLE 9–7. ***Troubleshooting BiPAP Equipment Patient Complaints***

| Patient Complaint/Ventilator Problem | Solution |
|---|---|
| Patient complains of shortness of breath. | Increase IPAP.<br>Check mask for excessive leaks, appropriate fit.<br>Check to ensure patient is not breathing through the mouth. |
| Patient remains hypoxemic with increased level of $FIO_2$. | Increase EPAP.<br>Increase oxygen flowrate into the mask.<br>Check seal of mask. |
| Patient has long apneic spells. | Switch to spontaneous/time mode. |
| Breath sounds are diminished in both bases and chest radiograph shows whiting out in bases bilaterally. | Increase IPAP. |
| Patient complains of dryness in the nose or oral cavity. | Use a humidifier. |

c. Patient with increased work of breathing and reduced breath sounds with long periods of apnea
    (1) Set in spontaneous time mode. Set breaths per minute at 2 to 5 fewer than patient's spontaneous rate.
    (2) Initially, set IPAP at 8 cm $H_2O$ and EPAP at 4 cm $H_2O$ to keep $SpO_2$ above 90%. Adjust as needed.

d. Patient with increased work of breathing, reduced breath sounds, and hypercapnia with an unstable ventilatory drive and a high respiratory rate
    (1) Set in time mode. Set breaths per minute above the patient's respiratory rate.
    (2) Set percentage of inspiratory time at 33 or 50%.
    (3) Initially, set IPAP at 8 cm $H_2O$ and EPAP at 4 cm $H_2O$ to keep $SpO_2$ above 90%. Adjust as needed.

9. Once the patient is at the desired level and appropriate mode of BiPAP, obtain further data within 1 h.
    a. ABGs and $SpO_2$
    b. Capnography
    c. Reassess chest for signs of reduced work of breathing and toleration. Also check for chest discomfort, shortness of breath, headache, and eye irritation (caused by leaking around the mask).
    d. Adjust IPAP, EPAP, bpm, or percentage Itime as needed.
    e. Intolerance of the nasal mask may require switching to a full face mask. In this situation, the patient should be placed on a nothing-by-mouth (NPO) diet for at least 2 to 3 h before application.
    f. For long periods of application, humidification may be required. A heat and moisture exchanger (HME) may be added, or a humidification device may be connected to the patient's circuit (be careful not to allow occlusion of the exhalation device, which is placed proximal to the mask).
10. Other subjective findings include ear discomfort and conjunctivitis.
11. Troubleshooting equipment and patient complaints (Table 9–7)

G. Waveform for BiPAP (Fig. 9–1)
H. Disorders that benefit from BiPAP (Table 9–8)

## VI. Humidity and aerosol therapy

A. Indications for humidity and aerosol therapy
    1. Along with the administration of medical gases
    2. Along with the administration of a gas delivered to an endotracheal tube and tracheostomy tube
    3. Patients who have thick secretions
    4. With the delivery of medications to the airway
    5. When warm inspired gases are required

B. Medical gases delivered to the mouth or nose require a room temperature of 22°C and a relative humidity of 50%. When delivering a gas to the airways through an artificial airway, the gas should be heated and humidified to 32 to 35°C at 100% relative humidity.

C. Types of humidifying equipment
    1. The bubble humidifier

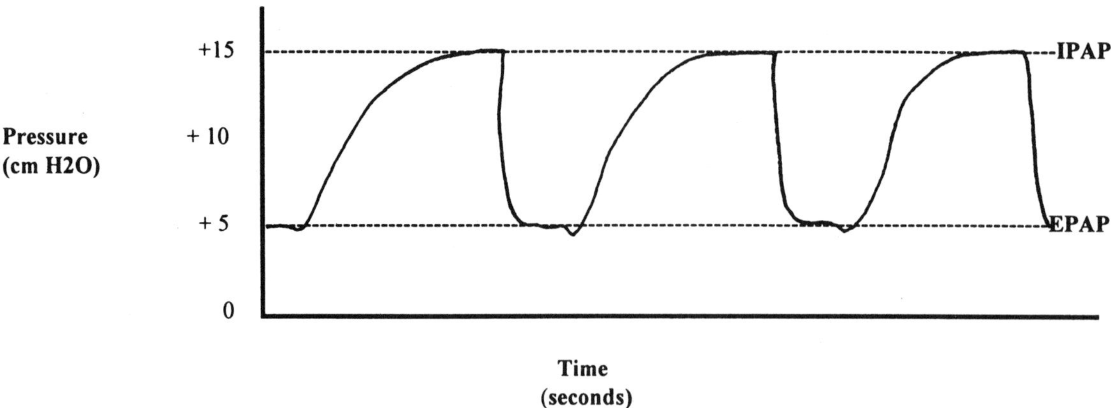


**FIGURE 9–1** EPAP pressure is 5 cm $H_2O$. With IPAP set at 15 cm $H_2O$, the pressure difference (driving pressure) is 10 cm $H_2O$.

a. Used for delivery of medical gas by way of a nasal cannula. The bubble humidifier produces a water vapor content of no more than 20 mg/L.
b. In older infants and children, a liter flow of less than 4 L/min may not require a bubble humidifier. Use a humidifier for patients complaining of dryness or irritation of the nose.

2. Pass-over humidifier
   a. This device directs gas over heated water or uses a wick-type device that draws water into a paper or cloth, which comes into contact with the stream of gas.
   c. Because it is heated, the pass-over humidifier has a water vapor output of 30 to 50 mg/L heated to at least 30°C.
   d. These devices have temperature alarms and should be set appropriately. Generally, the alarms are set to prevent overheating and underheating during operation of the heater. The heating device should initially be set up with gas flowing through the circuit. A heating device may continue heating with no gas flow and may possibly deliver extremely hot gas to the patient. A temperature monitor is placed in the inspiratory limb of the patient's circuit near the patient to provide accurate temperature monitoring. A lack of gas flow would decrease the temperature coming into contact with this probe and signal the heater to increase the temperature.
   e. Temperatures at the heating device are warmer than the temperature reaching the patient. This is caused by a cooling of the gas within the circuit by the surrounding room temperature. As much as 8°C/ft is lost. As the humidified gas cools, it forms condensation within the circuit and the gas loses its capacity to hold water (i.e., there is reduced absolute humidity).
   f. To minimize the absolute humidity loss, heating wires are placed within the circuit to decrease the difference between the humidifier and patient. Two heating elements with heating wires are used. One element monitors the temperature of the gas coming out of the humidifier, thus reducing the temperature to which the humidifier needs to be heated (32 to 36°C instead of 50°C). The other probe is in the inspiratory limb of the patient's circuit.
   g. It is important for the temperature probe closest to the patient not to be in contact with a cooling gas source (such as with in-line small-volume neb-

TABLE 9–8. ***Disorders That Benefit from BiPAP***

| Restrictive | Obstructive | Neuromuscular |
|---|---|---|
| Kyphoscoliosis | Chronic obstructive pulmonary disease | Muscular dystrophy |
| Severe obesity | Asthma | Spinal cord injury |
| | Chronic bronchitis | Quadriplegia |
| | Emphysema | Postpolio respiratory insufficiency |
| | Cystic fibrosis | |

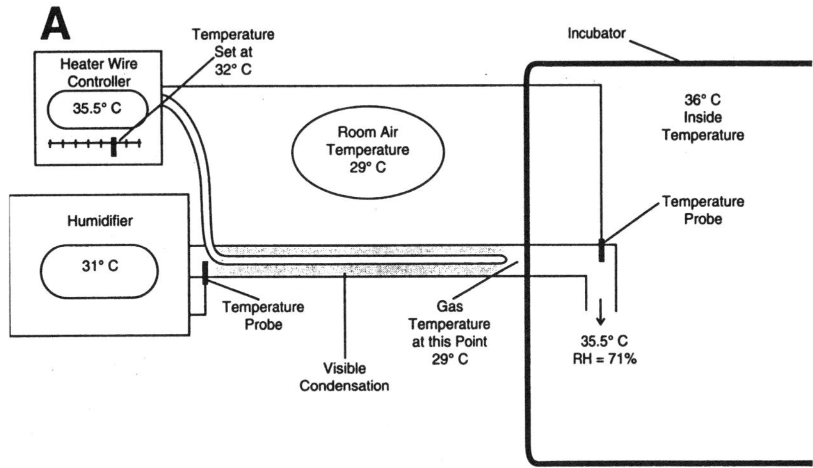


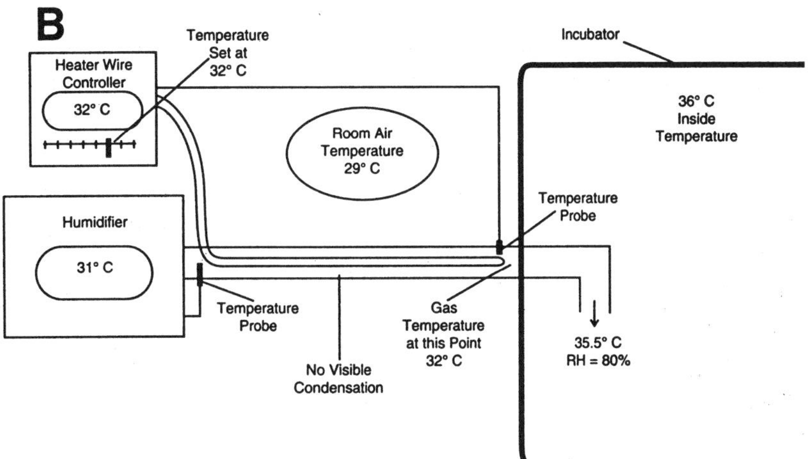


**FIGURE 9–2** Illustration of a problem encountered during the use of a patient circuit with a heated wire inside an incubator. *(A)* When the temperature probe is placed inside an incubator whose temperature is set higher than the output temperature of the humidifier, the temperature of the inspired gas increases, the temperature probe sends a signal to shut off the heating wires, condensation forms in the circuit, and the relative humidity (RH) of inspired gas drops. *(B)* When the probe is placed just outside the incubator, the heating wires function properly and the RH of the inspired gas is increased. (From Chatburn, R. [1991]. Principles and practice of neonatal and pediatric mechanical ventilation. *Respiratory Care* 36[6]:585, with permission.)

ulizers). This causes an increase in the heat provided by the unit. In this situation, place the probe proximal to the nebulizer.

h. The probe should not be enclosed in a heated environment, such as inside an incubator. If the internal temperature is higher than the set temperature on the humidifier, this will decrease the temperature output from the heating element of the humidifier. In this situation, place the probe just outside the incubator at a small distance from the patient (Fig. 9–2).
i. Set the temperature differential so that a few drops of condensate are seen in the circuit. Full saturation has now been attained.

3. Heat and moisture exchanger (HME)
   a. The heat and moisture exchanger (HME) is a device that uses the heat and moisture trapped during an exhaled breath to heat and humidify the next inspiratory breath. The device uses a hygroscopic material that traps the heat and moisture. The HME is placed between the wye adapter and endotracheal tube or tracheostomy tube. The ideal HME has little dead space, minimal compliance, and minimal weight and resistance.
   b. Contraindications include patients who are on a ventilator and who have thick, copious, or bloody secretions; patients who have either a large leak around their endotracheal tube or a bronchopleurocutaneous fistula

(below 70% of exhaled tidal volume); and patients with minute ventilation under 10 L/min and a body temperature below 32°C.

c. The HME should be removed when administering a metered-dose inhaler (MDI) or aerosol treatment unless the HME is proximal to the MDI or aerosol device.

D. Aerosol delivery devices

1. The small-volume nebulizer (SVN)

a. Indications

(1) Young patients who are unable to understand and/or are uncoordinated in the use of an MDI or dry-powder inhaler (DPI)

(2) Patients in acute distress with a reduced inspiratory flowrate

(3) Patients who are unable to perform an inspiratory hold

(4) When the respiratory pattern is unstable and/or the respiratory rate is fast

(5) When using a drug that is capable of being nebulized only in this device or that requires uncommon concentration

b. In patients over 3 years of age who are breathing spontaneously without an artificial airway and are able to cooperate, a mouthpiece and extension reservoir should be used. Face masks are used for children who are under 3 years of age or unable to negotiate a mouthpiece. An SVN can be attached to a T-piece for delivery of aerosol to patients who are breathing spontaneously; placed in line with a mechanical ventilator circuit; attached to a tracheostomy collar; or attached via a T-piece to an endotracheal tube.

c. The optimum filling volume is 3 to 4 mL run at a flowrate of 6 to 10 L/min.

d. Instruct the patient to breathe at a normal tidal volume interspersed with a slow, deep breath and an inspiratory hold.

e. Ventilators with a built-in nebulizing ability nebulize the medication during inspiration only. This lengthens the treatment. An SVN placed in line with a mechanical ventilator breathing circuit without a built-in nebulizing device requires that the SVN be powered by a blending device to achieve the same $FIO_2$ as the ventilator is providing to the patient.

f. To clean the SVN, rinse the mouthpiece and nebulizer with sterile water. Allow the device to air-dry.

g. The amount of medication that is deposited in the lungs by means of an SVN is estimated to be between 2 and 10% of the dose because of the following:

(1) Small tidal volumes (neonates), dyspneic patients

(2) Smaller-diameter airways

(3) Approximately one-half of the initial dose remaining in the reservoir

(4) Concentration of the solution increasing during nebulization and remaining in the reservoir at the end of the treatment

h. Problems associated with an SVN

(1) The continuous flow from an SVN placed in line with the patient's ventilator circuit creates a bias flow that may interfere with patient-triggered modes of ventilation.

(2) Excessive flow may be produced from the continuous flow of the in-line SVN used with a continuous-flow ventilator. This flow may create excessive PEEP, expiratory retardation, excessive airway pressure, or increased tidal volume.

(3) Inadvertent PEEP may be produced as a result of drug deposited on the exhalation valve of the ventilator.

(4) An SVN that remains in line after completion of the medication delivery can become a source of infection.

(5) Aerosol delivery with an SVN may be less effective because of the alteration in pressure, flow, and manual bagging rate.

(6) If the SVN is placed too close to the ventilated patient (6 in away from the endotracheal tube is suggested), dosage may be reduced.

2. Metered-dose inhalers (MDIs)

a. Indications

(1) Need to deliver medications in an approved MDI form

(2) Need to deliver medication only in an MDI form

(3) Need to reduce the length of time of an aerosol treatment

(4) Need for maximum portability

b. Limitations

(1) Small children under 7 years of age may have difficulty coordinating the MDI and breathing technique.

(2) Oropharyngeal impaction increases without the use of a spacer device.
(3) Inaccurate instructions may reduce the aerosol deposition (too-short period for breath holding, failure to coordinate actuation of MDI with inhalation, too-rapid inspiratory flowrate, inadequate shaking of the canister before actuation, cold Freon effect causing cessation of inspiration, exhaling during MDI actuation, turning head during actuation, or multiple firing of a single inhalation).
(4) Small dose (10 to 25%) is deposited in the lungs.

c. An MDI with a spacer device increases the dosage of drug deposited in the lungs, reduces oropharyngeal absorption, and provides coordination between firing of the canister and inhalation.
(1) Some spacer devices have a one-way valve (also called a holding chamber) in the spacer that is appropriate for infants under 3 years of age, use of corticosteroids to help reduce oropharyngeal impaction, and MDI delivery during mechanical ventilation or with a resuscitation bag.
(2) When using an MDI with a spacer device during mechanical ventilation, place the spacer in the inspiratory side of the breathing circuit connected to the wye adapter. The spacer device for neonates is placed between the endotracheal tube and the wye adapter. The MDI is actuated just before or during the flow of gas from the ventilator to the patient. An MDI actuated in line with a heated humidifier decreases the percentage of total dose to the lungs.
(3) Nonvalved spacer devices are used in older children who can coordinate inspiration and expiration and delivery of corticosteroids to reduce oropharyngeal impaction.

d. How to instruct the patient in the use of an MDI
(1) Remove the cap and insert the canister in the nozzle receptacle.
(2) Shake the canister.
(3) Exhale normally.
(4) If not using a spacer device, hold the canister 1 in from the open mouth. With a spacer device, place the mouthpiece between the lips.
(5) Actuate the canister, then breathe in slowly and completely, but not so much as to activate the flow whistle, indicating that flowrate is exceeding 30 L/min.
(6) Hold the breath for 5 to 10 s, if possible.
(7) Exhale normally and wait 30 s before taking another dose.

e. Once a day, clean the spacer device with warm water and allow the device to dry thoroughly.

3. Dry-powder inhaler (DPI)
a. Indications
(1) Need to deliver medication in DPI form
(2) Need to eliminate chlorofluorocarbon propellants

b. Limitations
(1) Children under 6 years of age may not be able to produce an adequate flow, especially during an acute exacerbation when peak flows are reduced. A flowrate of at least 60 L/min is recommended to provide deposition of the drug.
(2) Humidity may affect DPI performance.
(3) Lower airway deposition is decreased by oropharyngeal impaction (the average deposition in the lungs is 0 to 25% of the total dose average).
(4) The patient must be able to load each dose for most medications.

c. How to instruct a patient in the use of a DPI
(1) Open the device and remove used capsules of drug.
(2) Insert a new drug capsule in the holder.
(3) Close the device, which will rupture the capsule of drug.
(4) Exhale fully away from the DPI.
(5) Place the DPI in the mouth, keeping the lips firmly around the mouthpiece.
(6) Inhale as deeply and rapidly as possible.
(7) Hold the breath for a few seconds and then exhale normally.
(8) Repeat until all of the drug is evacuated from the capsule.

d. Wash the device in warm water and allow it to air-dry.

4. Large-volume nebulizers
a. Indications

(1) Delivery of continuous aerosolized medication to the lower airway of a spontaneously breathing patient without an endotracheal tube or tracheostomy tube.

b. Limitations
   (1) Children may not tolerate a cold, wet solution blowing on the face.
   (2) Lower respiratory tract deposition is decreased with nose breathing.
   (3) Used primarily in acute care; not recommended for home care.

c. Large-volume nebulizers are useful for treating severe bronchospasm when traditional dosing strategies have failed.
   (1) A common device used for continuous aerosol therapy is VORTRAN's High Output Aerosol Respiratory Therapy (HEART™) nebulizer. It has a 240-mL volume, producing a particle size between 2.2 and 3.5 μm, mean mass aerosol diameter. Over long-term nebulization, evaporation occurs and can lead to toxicity. Close monitoring with an ECG is recommended.
   (2) If the device is placed in line with the patient's breathing circuit, watch for inadvertent increases in tidal volume or airway pressures, changes in $FIO_2$, difficulty with patient-triggering and patient-ventilator synchrony, and difficulty exhaling (obstructed exhalation valve). In any of these situations, the nebulizer should be discontinued and the patient should be removed from mechanical ventilation and manually ventilated until the problem has been determined. An alteration in the aerosol delivery system may be required to avoid further complications.
   (3) A miniHEART™ nebulizer (nebulizer volume = 30 mL) can be placed in line in the patient's breathing circuit at the wye adapter (nonconstant flow ventilator) to provide continuous nebulization at a flowrate between 1 and 2.5 L/min. For a constant flow ventilator, place the nebulizer between the wye adapter and the endotracheal tube. The smaller flowrates will have less effect on delivered tidal volume as compared to the large HEART™ nebulizer.

d. Small-particle aerosol generator (SPAG) unit
   (1) This device is used to deliver ribavirin (Virazole) medication to infants with respiratory syncytial virus. The SPAG unit nebulizes the medication and then directs it into a drying chamber. The result is a drug in powder form delivered to an infant who is within a tent or head hood or on mechanical ventilation.
   (2) A scavenger system should be used with the administration of ribavirin through the SPAG system. This eliminates excessive drug within the patient environment and reduces health care personnel exposure.
   (3) It is recommended that the device not be placed in line with a mechanical ventilator because of rainout of medication into the patient's circuit and endotracheal tube, potentially causing autoPEEP or airway obstruction. However, if the drug is nebulized through the mechanical ventilator, double filters are placed on the exhalation side of the patient circuit. The filters require changing every 1 to 2 h, as does the patient's breathing circuit.
   (4) Using a SPAG unit with a volume-cycled ventilator requires alteration of mechanical tidal volume or inspiratory time or drying chamber flowrate to prevent excessive volume delivery to the patient

5. Instruction in the home use of aerosol delivery devices (also see Chapter 16)
   a. On completion of instructions on how to deliver an aerosol, assess the patient for proper technique.
   b. Family members should be taught the correct method of delivering an aerosol. Observe the family members to ensure that they can instruct the patient correctly and are able to make adjustments in technique as needed.
   c. Observe for proper preparation of medication and understanding of the medication being prepared.
   d. Observe response to medication (pulse rate, breath sounds, and peak flow) and subjective feeling of improvement. The medication dosage may require alteration if there is a poor response (peak flow) or side effects (tachycardia or bronchospasm).
   e. Ensure that the medication volume is nebulized over the desired amount of time.
   f. Record any adverse effects from the medication dose, response, and other pertinent information regarding family and patient cooperation.

D. Dosage guidelines for neonates, infants, and children (Table 9–9)
E. Drug formula for calculating drug dosages for children
   1. Young's rule (for children 2 to 12 years of age):

$$\frac{\text{Age of child} \times \text{adult dose}}{\text{Age of child} + 12}$$

   2. Clark's rule:

$$\frac{\text{Weight of child in pounds or kilograms} \times \text{adult dose}}{150 \text{ (lb) or } 70 \text{ (kg) (average adult weight)}}$$

   3. Fried's rule (for children under 2 years of age):

$$\frac{\text{Age in months} \times \text{adult dose}}{150 \text{ (lb) or } 70 \text{ (kg)}}$$

TABLE 9–9. ***Dosage Guidelines for Neonates, Infants, and Children***

| **Solutions** | **Dosage** |
|---|---|
| SYMPATHOMIMETIC BRONCHODILATORS | |
| Racemic epinephrine | Neb: 0.05 mL/kg of 2.25% solution not more frequently than q 2 h; maximum dose = 0.5 mL |
| Isoproterenol | Neb: 0.025 mL of 1:200 solution or 0.01 mL/kg; maximum dose = 0.05 mL; tid, qid |
| Metaproterenol | Neb: 0.2–3 mL of 5% solution q 4 h<br>MDI: 1–3 puffs q 3–4 h, up to 12 puffs/day |
| Albuterol | Neb: 0.05 mg/kg; minimum dose = 1.25 mg, maximum dose = 2.5 mg q 4–6 h<br>MDI: 2 puffs tid–qid and prn |
| Bitolterol | MDI: 2 puffs tid–qid and prn |
| Pirbuterol | MDI: 2 puffs tid–qid and prn |
| Salmeterol | MDI: 2 puffs q 12 h |
| ANTICHOLINERGIC BRONCHODILATORS | |
| Atropine sulfate | Neb: 0.05 mg/kg diluted in saline; maximum dose = 1 mg |
| Ipratropium | Neb: 0.25 mg q 6 h<br>MDI: 1–2 puffs q 6 h |
| MUCOLYTIC AGENT | |
| Acetylcysteine | Neb: 3–5 mL of 10 or 20% solution; tid, qid |
| rhDNase (dornase alfa) | Neb: 2.5 mg daily |
| CORTICOSTEROIDS | |
| Dexamethasone sodium phosphate | MDI: 2 puffs 3–4 times daily; maximum dose = 8 puffs |
| Becloamethasone dipropionate | MDI: Children 6–12 years: 1–2 puffs 3–4 times/day; maximum dose = 10 puffs/day |
| Flunisolide | MDI: Children 6–12 years: 2 puffs bid |
| Triamcinolone acetonide | MDI: Children 6–12 years: 1–2 puffs 3–4 times/day; maximum dose = 12 puffs/day |
| Fluticasone pripionate | MDI: Not recommended for children <12 years |
| ANTIASTHMATICS | |
| Cromolyn sodium | Neb: Children <2 years: 20 mg (1 ampule) tid–qid<br>MDI: Children ≥5 years: 2 puffs qid; <5 years: 1–2 puffs tid–qid<br>DPI: Children >5 years: 20 mg (1 capsule) qid |
| Nedocromil | MDI: 1–2 puffs bid–qid |
| ANTI-INFECTIVES | |
| Ribavirin | SPAG Neb: 6 g/300 mL (2%). 12–18 h/day |
| Pentamidine | Respirgard II Neb: ≥5 years,: 300 mg/month |

(From Rau, J.R., p. 519, with permission.)

# REVIEW QUESTIONS

1. Give two indications for oxygen therapy.

   a.

   b.

2. List two factors that contribute to retinopathy of prematurity (ROP).

   a.

   b.

3. What precautions should be taken to reduce the incidence of ROP in the newborn infant?

4. Fill in the accompanying table for oxygen delivery systems.

| System | Example | Description |
|---|---|---|
| Low-flow | | |
| Reservoir | | |
| High-flow | | |
| Enclosure | | |

5. Fill in the accompanying needs-assessment table for oxygen devices.

| Equipment | Needs Assessment |
|---|---|
| Nasal cannula | |
| Nasopharyngeal catheter | |
| Simple oxygen mask | |
| Air-entrainment nebulizers | |
| Partial rebreather | |
| Non-rebreather | |
| Air-entrainment nebulizer | |
| Hoods | |
| Tents | |
| Tracheostomy oxygen adapters | |

6. In the accompanying table, fill in the blank boxes for air-entrainment systems.

| $FIO_2$ | Flowrate of Oxygen (L/min) | Entrainment Ratio (oxygen to air) | Total Flow to Patient (L/min) |
|---|---|---|---|
| 0.24 | | 1:25 | 104 |
| 0.28 | 4 | 1:10 | |
| 0.31 | | 1:7 | 48 |
| 0.35 | 8 | | 48 |
| 0.40 | 8 | 1:3 | |
| 0.50 | 12 | | 32 |

7. Given the following two systems that combine flow, determine the $FIO_2$. (Use the tic-tac-flow method.)
   a. System A: $FIO_2$—0.60 at a flowrate of 8 L/min.
   b. System B: $FIO_2$—0.80 at a flowrate of 8 L/min.

8. Fill in the accompanying table of advantages and disadvantages for CPAP application for newborns and children.

| Device | Advantages | Disadvantages |
|---|---|---|
| Nasal prongs | | |
| Nasopharyngeal tube | | |
| Endotracheal tube | | |

9. In the accompanying table, describe how to initiate therapy with and wean patients from neonatal and pediatric CPAP.

| | Neonatal CPAP | Pediatric CPAP |
|---|---|---|
| Initiation of CPAP | | |
| Weaning from CPAP | | |

10. Describe how to determine nasal mask CPAP level for a 6-year-old child with obstructive sleep apnea.

11. What are two indications for the use of BiPAP?

    a.

    b.

12. Using a graphic illustration, identify the difference between IPAP and EPAP and label the graphs appropriately.

Pressure ($cm\ H_2O$)

+15

+10

+5

0

Time (seconds)

13. In what situation should IPAP be adjusted? In what situation should EPAP be adjusted?

14. The accompanying table lists complaints of patients while using BiPAP. List solutions to the problems given in the table.

| Patient Complaint | Solution |
|---|---|
| Patient is unable to achieve desired CPAP. | |
| Patient complains of headache and hypersomnolence. | |
| Snoring is still present. | |
| Patient complains of dryness, epistaxis of the nose. | |
| Patient complains of conjunctivitis or eye irritation. | |
| Irritation from nasal mask. | |

15. Match the following patient problems:

a. _____ Patient remains hypoxemic with increased $FIO_2$.
b. _____ Patient complains of dryness in the nose and oral airway.
c. _____ Patient complains of shortness of breath.
d. _____ Breath sounds are diminished in both bases and chest radiography shows whiting out in bases bilaterally.

1. Increase IPAP.
2. Increase EPAP.
3. Add humidity.
4. Decrease IPAP.
5. Decrease EPAP.

16. List two restrictive, two obstructive, and two neuromuscular disorders that benefit from BiPAP.

| Restrictive | Obstructive | Neuromuscular |
|---|---|---|
| a. | a. | a. |
| b. | b. | b. |

17. List two indications for humidity and aerosol therapy.

a.

b.

18. What should be the temperature range and relative humidity for medical gas being delivered to an intubated patient who is breathing spontaneously?

19. Describe the effect on delivered temperature to a newborn if the temperature probe is placed within the isolette as compared to outside the isolette.

20. List three patient conditions that would contraindicate the use of a heated moisture exchanger.

    a.

    b.

    c.

21. Give three indications in which a small-volume nebulizer may be used instead of an MDI.

    a.

    b.

    c.

22. Describe two potential problems associated with a small-volume nebulizer treatment placed in line in the patient's breathing circuit.

    a.

    b.

23. Describe how to instruct a 9-year-old child in the use of a MDI.

24. What spontaneous liter flow must be produced by a dry-powder inhaler for adequate deposition of the drug?

25. What system is used with a small-particle aerosol generator (SPAG) to reduce atmospheric contamination of ribavirin?

26. If the SPAG unit is placed in line with a volume-cycled ventilator, describe what should be done to prevent buildup of medication on the exhalation valve.

27. Using Young's rule, calculate the drug dosage of albuterol administered to a 6-year-old child with the adult dosage of 0.5 mL.

28. Using Clark's rule, calculate the drug dosage of albuterol administered to an 8-year-old child weighing 50 kg. The adult dosage of albuterol is 0.5 mL.

29. After giving a continuous aerosol of albuterol in line within the patient's breathing circuit over the last 12 h, it is noticed that the patient has difficulty exhaling and shows signs of respiratory distress. What problem could be associated with the ventilator?

30. Why should corticosteroids be used with a spacer device when administered by MDI?

## BIBLIOGRAPHY

American Association for Respiratory Care Clinical Practice Guideline. (1994). Application of continuous positive airway pressure to neonates via nasal prongs or nasopharyngeal tube. *Respiratory Care* 39(8):817.

American Association for Respiratory Care Clinical Practice Guideline. (1994). Delivery of aerosols to the upper airway. *Respiratory Care* 39(8):803.

American Association for Respiratory Care Clinical Practice Guideline. (1996). Selection of a device for delivery of aerosol to lung parenchyma. *Respiratory Care* 41(7):647.

American Association for Respiratory Care Clinical Practice Guideline. (1993). Bland aerosol administration. *Respiratory Care* 38:1196.

American Association for Respiratory Care Clinical Practice Guideline. (1991). Oxygen therapy in the acute care hospital. *Respiratory Care* 36:1410.

American Association for Respiratory Care Clinical Practice Guideline. (1996). Selection of an oxygen device for neonatal and pediatric patients. *Respiratory Care* 41(7):637.

American Association for Respiratory Care Clinical Practice Guideline. (1995). Selection of an aerosol delivery device for neonatal and pediatric patients. *Respiratory Care* 40(12):1325.

Branson, R.D., and Chatburn, R. (1993). Humidification of inspired gases during mechanical ventilation. [Editorial]. *Respiratory Care* 38:461–468.

Chatburn, R. (1991). Principles and practice of neonatal and pediatric mechanical ventilation. *Respiratory Care* 36(6):585.

Fink, J., and Jue, P. Humidity and oxygen therapy. In Barnhart, S., and Czervinske, M. (Eds.) (1995). *Perinatal and Pediatric Respiratory Care*. Philadelphia: W. B. Saunders.

Fink, J. Humidity and aerosol therapy. In Scanlon, C., et al. (Eds.) (1995). *Egan's Fundamentals of Respiratory Care*, ed 6. St. Louis: Mosby–Year Book.

Fink, J., and Cohen, N. Humidity and aerosols. In Eubanks, D., and Bone, R. (Eds.) (1994). *Principles and Applications of Cardiorespiratory Care Equipment*. St. Louis: Mosby–Year Book.

Hanhan, U., et al. (1993). Effects of in-line nebulization on preset ventilatory variables. *Respiratory Care* 38:474–478.

Harwood, R. Respiratory disorders of the pediatric patient. In Kacmarek, R., Mack, C., and Dimas, S. (Eds.) (1990). *The Essentials of Respiratory Care*, ed 3. St. Louis: Mosby–Year Book.

Kacmarek, R., Mack, C., and Dimas, S. (1990). *The Essentials of Respiratory Care*, ed 3. St. Louis: Mosby–Year Book.

Kacmarek, R., and Kratohvil, J. (1992). Evaluation of a double-enclosure double-vacuum unit scavenging system for ribavirin administration. *Respiratory Care* 37(1):37.

Rau, J. R. (1998). *Respiratory Care Pharmacology*, ed 5. St. Louis: Mosby–Year Book.

Rau, J. R. (1991). Delivery of aerosolized drugs to neonatal and pediatric patients. *Respiratory Care* 36(6): 519.

Teague, G.W. (1997). Pediatric Application of noninvasive ventilation. *Respiratory Care* 42:414–423.

Weis, C., Cox, C., and Fox, W. Oxygen therapy. In Spitzer, A. (Ed.) (1996). *Intensive Care of the Fetus and Newborn*. St. Louis: Mosby–Year Book.

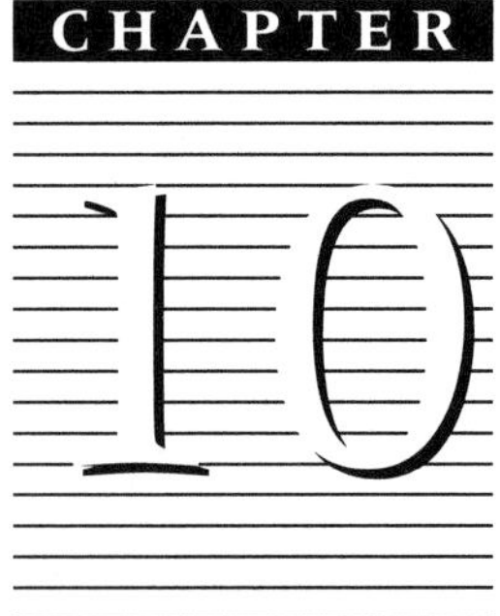

# Pediatric Diseases

## I. Overview of Upper Airway Obstructive Disorders

A. Risk of acute airway obstruction is high in childhood because of the anatomy of the pediatric airway and the activity level of the child.
   1. Infants (newborn to several months) are obligate nose breathers because of relatively large tongues and small mandibles.
   2. Absolute airway size is small, and any further reduction in airway diameter greatly increases airway resistance.
   3. The cricoid cartilage is the narrowest part of a child's upper airway until approximately 6 to 8 years of age.
   4. Abnormalities from obstruction include changes in rate and depth of respiration, inspiratory to expiratory (I/E) ratio, nasal flaring, retractions, wheezing, or stridor.
      a. Wheezing is often associated with bronchospasm but is also caused by other forms of airway obstruction.
      b. Inspiratory stridor usually indicates obstruction above the thoracic inlet.
      c. Pulmonary function testing (PFT) shows decreased flow at the highest point of the flow volume loop (peak flow) on inspiration and expiration (see Chapter 14).
      d. Expiratory or biphasic stridor usually indicates obstruction below the thoracic inlet.
      e. Thoracic breath sounds may not be audible if airflow velocity is too low to create sound.
   5. The differentiating factor for upper versus lower airway problems is stridor. Alterations in breath sounds are indicative of lower airway obstruction.

B. General etiology
   1. Acquired causes
      a. Infection is the cause of 80% of pediatric airway obstructions after the neonatal period. Common infectious problems include croup (85 to 90% of pediatric airway obstruction), epiglottitis (5 to 10% of pediatric airway obstruction), and other problems including tonsillitis and pharyngeal abscess.
   2. Neurogenic causes
      a. Altered state of consciousness
      b. Treatments include positioning patient on side or abdomen, pulling tongue forward, oropharyngeal airway, and intubation.
   3. Neoplastic causes
      a. Tumor or nodes
      b. Laryngeal papillomas
      c. Treatments include radiation, chemotherapy, surgical excision, and tracheostomy.
   4. Trauma
      a. Foreign body aspiration
         (1) Increased incidence among infants and toddlers 6 to 24 months of age
         (2) Iatrogenic causes after extubation instrumentation
      b. External trauma
      c. Burns
   5. Tracheomalacia and laryngomalacia (Table 10–1)

## II. Foreign body aspiration

A. Description
   1. Children between 8 months and 4 years of age are at the highest risk for aspiration of a foreign body.

TABLE 10–1. ***Characteristics of Tracheomalacia and Laryngomalacia***

| | Tracheomalacia | Laryngomalacia |
|---|---|---|
| Age | Birth to 3 months | Birth to several months |
| Patient presentation | Stridor, hoarseness, difficult feeding, and respiratory distress | Stridor, hoarseness, and difficult feeding |
| Physical examination | Dyspnea, respiratory distress, rhonchi, intercostal retractions, and hyperinflation | Dyspnea and respiratory distress |
| Radiologic finding | Generally need special studies | Laryngeal fullness |
| Bronchoscopy | Luminal compression | Floppy airway |
| Management | Treat underlying disease; tracheoplasty | Change feeding position, laryngoplasty, and tracheostomy |

(From Santer, D.M., p.1, with permission.)

2. Foreign body aspiration is the leading cause of death in infants less than 12 months of age.
3. Esophageal aspiration of foreign bodies is more common than tracheal or bronchial foreign body aspiration.

B. Etiology
1. Children put many objects such as toys and inappropriate food such as hard candies and uncooked food in their mouths.
2. Children may eat while walking, running, or laughing and do not concentrate on chewing or swallowing. Young children may not have coordinated swallowing or teeth to masticate the food.
3. The most frequent types of food related to asphyxia include hot dogs, nuts, grapes, and other foods that fall under the 3 S category: Small, Smooth, and Slippery.

C. Pathophysiology
1. Once the food falls past the oral cavity, it elicits a gag reflex or cough. With inspiration, the object is pulled closer to the glottic opening. If the inspiration is forceful, this may cause the food to be lodged in the glottic opening or to enter the lungs. Most foreign bodies lodge in the right main-stem bronchus. The blockage causes reduced airflow. Edema occurs (with prolonged blockage). Air trapping and emphysema can follow with incomplete obstruction.
2. Complete obstruction causes atelectasis and trapped secretions cause dilation of the bronchi and bronchioles. This leads to bronchiectasis and fibrosis. With prolonged blockage, pneumothorax, pneumopericardium, and abscess follow.

D. Clinical presentation: Signs and symptoms (Table 10–2)
1. Coughing and wheezing are the most common respiratory symptoms.
2. Also, depending on the site of enlodgement of the object, various sounds are elicited.
3. Other general respiratory signs and symptoms include reduced breath sounds, tachypnea, retractions, and cyanosis.
4. The patient may remain symptomless from hours to months following aspiration, but eventually the body begins to react to the object.
5. With the first signs and symptoms of coughing and wheezing, one needs to determine the reason.

TABLE 10–2. ***Signs and/or Symptoms of Enlodgement of a Foreign Body***

| Larynx | Trachea | Bronchus | Esophagus |
|---|---|---|---|
| Hoarseness | Cough | Cough | Refusal to eat |
| Aphonia | Hemoptysis | Hemoptysis | Vomiting |
| Drooling | Stridor | Wheeze | Drooling |
| Cough | Wheeze | Dyspnea | Pain or discomfort from swelling |
| Hemoptysis | Dyspnea | | Pain radiating to sternal or back area |
| Stridor | | | Foreign body sensation |
| Dyspnea | | | |

(Adapted from Kenna, M., and Bluestone, C., p. 27, 1988.)

6. The infant may have an acute or recurrent cough for which there is no apparent reason. Consider other pathways for coughing:
   a. Nose, sinuses (trigeminal nerve)
   b. Pharynx: Irritation causing cough through the glossopharyngeal nerve
   c. Vagus: Ear canal, tympanic membrane, larynx, trachea, bronchi, and pleura
   d. Diaphragm: Phrenic nerve

E. Diagnosis
1. History of acute distress related to aspiration or ingestion
2. Physical examination
   a. The most common symptoms at time of admission include cough, dyspnea, wheezing, tachypnea, retractions, fever, and air trapping.
   b. Listen for stridor, rales, and rhonchi in specific locations (larynx, trachea, or bronchi).
   c. Pain in oropharyngeal area may indicate sharp or pointed foreign body.
   d. Subcutaneous emphysema
3. Radiograph
   a. Perform anteroposterior and lateral radiographs

F. Treatment
1. Once the object is identified, it should be removed with rigid or flexible endoscopy. Objects lodged in the esophagus may move to the stomach and pass out of the body or may need direct removal.

## III. Viral croup

A. Etiology
1. Transmission by direct contact. Parainfluenza types 1 and 2 are the most common, but also respiratory syncytial virus (RSV) and influenza types A and B. Other forms of croup may present in the same manner as viral croup but are not as serious (Table 10–3)

B. History
1. Infants aged 3 months to 5 years often have upper respiratory tract infections (URI). Incubation period is 1 to 6 days.

C. Presentation
1. Gradual onset of symptoms from 2 to 6 days; symptoms include barking cough, hoarseness, fever, biphasic stridor, retractions, accessory muscle use, and tachypnea.

D. Laboratory
1. To rule out bacterial infection
2. If labs are done, typically the white blood cell count (WBC) is normal and blood culture shows no sepsis.

E. Diagnosis
1. Radiologic confirmation shows subglottic narrowing, thickened vocal cords, and hypopharyngeal overdistention. Frontal x-ray shows "steeple sign" or "pencil-tip" appearance.

F. Treatment
1. Humidification by mist tent. This may not help because isolation may further distress the infant. Blow-by oxygen at an $FIO_2$ of 0.30 to 0.40 with humidification while the child is being held by a parent is helpful.

TABLE 10–3. *Characteristics of Croup Syndromes*

| Characteristic | Viral Croup | Spasmodic Croup | Acute Infectious Laryngitis |
|---|---|---|---|
| Age | 3 months–5 years | 1–3 years | All ages |
| Organism | Parainfluenza type 1 and 2 | Viral-allergic | Influenza |
| Incidence | Common | Common | Common |
| Clinical presentation | Gradual onset, mild URI, barky cough, and low fever | Abrupt onset at night, no URI, no fever | Gradual onset, hoarseness, and cough |
| Physical exam | Inspiratory stridor | Inspiratory stridor | Erythematous pharynx |
| Treatment | Humidification, racemic epinephrine | Humidification | Humidification, rest voice |

(From Santer, D.M., and D'Alessandro, M.P., p. 1, with permission.)

2. Racemic epinephrine by small-volume nebulizer. Improvements from both alpha and beta effects. The dose for infants less than 6 months old is 0.25 mL in 3 mL of normal saline, and for infants greater than 6 months old it is 0.5 mL in 3 mL of normal saline of a 2.25% solution.
3. Steroids given in appropriate doses decrease inflammation, the number of racemic epinephrine treatments, and the possibility of intubation. If the infant is receiving racemic epinephrine treatments, then a trial of steroids should be started.
4. If these therapies do not control the infant and the infant deteriorates, intubation may be required. Intubation may worsen the swelling in the subglottic region because of either too large an endotracheal tube (ETT) (no leak around tube), intubation lasting longer than 5 days, or pre-existing subglottic stenosis. Intubation should be done in the operating room under controlled conditions using the nasotracheal route.
5. Extubation may be considered when:
   a. The patient is afebrile
   b. Secretions from suctioning are minimal
   c. A leak develops around the ETT when the patient is bagged with 15 to 20 cm $H_2O$ or bubbling is heard with positive-pressure ventilation. If after 5 days the infant still has not developed a leak around the ETT, a trial of extubation is done. If extubation fails, then rigid endoscopy is performed to assess the hypopharyngeal area. Once the infant is extubated, monitor for signs of distress, which include stridor, intercostal retractions, tachypnea, $SpO_2$ less than 90%, and tachycardia. For mild signs of respiratory distress, give oxygen and racemic epinephrine. Severe signs require higher $FIO_2$ and intubation.

## IV. Epiglottitis

A. Etiology
   1. Bacterial infection by *Haemophilus influenzae* type B (over 80% of children)

B. History
   1. Children 2 to 6 years of age (may be as young as 7 months)
   2. Seasonal during winter and spring
   3. Worsening symptoms after 4 to 8 h of initial symptoms

C. Presentation
   1. Quick onset of symptoms. Initial symptoms include worsening sore throat, irritability, lethargy, fever, complaint of sore throat, and dyspnea. May present as croup (Table 10–4).
   2. After initial symptoms, infant comes to ER with worsening symptoms showing:
      a. Fever greater than 100°F
      b. Marked tachypnea
      c. Child sits upright in "tripod position" with neck extended. This helps to open the supraglottic area.
      d. Severe inspiratory stridor from mucosa prolapsing into the glottis. This may lead to total obstruction.
      e. Drooling, muffled voice from partial obstruction.

TABLE 10–4. ***Comparison of Viral Croup and Epiglottitis***

| Characteristic | Viral Croup | Epiglottitis |
|---|---|---|
| Age | 3 months–5 years | 2–7 years |
| Organism | Viral | *H. influenzae* type B |
| Incidence | Common | Rare |
| Clinical presentation | Gradual onset, mild URI symptoms, barky cough, and low fever | Sudden onset, sitting forward, high fever, **D**rooling, **D**ysphagia, **D**istress, and **D**yspnea |
| Physical exam | Respiratory distress, inspiratory stridor | Toxic appearance, "Hot potato voice" |
| Radiographic appearance and projection | Steeple sign—AP view | Thumb sign—lateral view |
| Treatment | Humidification and racemic epinephrine | Take to OR and intubate under general anesthesia |

(From Santer, D.M., p. 1, with permission.)

f. The 4 D's of epiglottitis are **D**yspnea, **D**ysphagia, **D**rooling, and **D**istress.

D. Lab/Radiology
1. Lateral neck radiograph reveals enlarged epiglottis (thumb sign).
2. Increased immature WBCs. Blood culture shows *H. influenzae*.

E. Treatment
1. Once condition is diagnosed, intubate child in operating room (OR) under general anesthesia.
2. While child is in OR, endoscopy may be done to rule out other potential problems, such as foreign body aspiration of larynx or esophagus.
3. If intubation fails, attempt bag-and-mask resuscitation with 100% oxygen. Reattempt intubation. If reintubation fails, tracheotomy may be performed.
4. Twelve to 48 h of intubation are required in most cases. Sedation is required to prevent self-extubation.
5. Extubation is determined by endoscopy examination to determine whether there is reduced swelling. Extubation is also determined by listening for a leak around the ETT with 15 to 20 cm $H_2O$ applied with resuscitation bag.
6. Antibiotics are started: combination of ampicillin and chloramphenicol or third-generation cephalosporins, such as cefotaxime or ceftriaxone.
7. After extubation, provide cool aerosol, $FIO_2$ to maintain $SpO_2$ greater than 95%, and monitor infant for stridor. Treat moderate stridor with oxygen and racemic epinephrine. For severe stridor, administer oxygen and reintubate.

## V. Asthma

A. Definition
1. Regardless of its severity, asthma is a chronic inflammatory disorder of the airway.

B. Demographics
1. Asthma is the most chronic disease of childhood, affecting 4.8 million children in the United States under the age of 18. It is estimated that nearly 7% of children now have the disease.
2. Between 1982 and 1993, the prevalence of asthma in the United States increased 46% overall and 80% among those under age 18.
3. African-Americans and children are more likely to be hospitalized. African-Americans' hospitalization rate was nearly triple that of whites in 1993.
4. Death rates are the highest among African-Americans in the age group between 15 and 24 years.

C. Pathophysiology
1. Immunohistopathologic features include the following:
   a. Denudation of the epithelium of the airway. This results in the transudation of fluids, reduced clearance, and increased permeability to inhaled allergens.
   b. Edema
   c. Mast cell activation
   d. Basement membrane deposited with collagen
   e. Inflammatory cell infiltration including neutrophils, eosinophils, and lymphocytes
2. Airway inflammation contributes to the following:
   a. Airway hyperresponsiveness from the following:
      (1) Viral infections
      (2) Allergens to cat, dog dander; dust mites; cockroaches
      (3) Pollution—a growing problem
      (4) Exercise
      (5) Cold air
   b. Airflow limitation from bronchospasm, airway edema, and mucus plug formation. Bronchial smooth muscle hypertrophy causing airflow obstruction resulting in increased airway resistance. The diameter of the bronchi is influenced by edema in the wall of the bronchi, mucus production, airway smooth muscle contraction, and hypertrophy.
   c. Respiratory symptoms
   d. Disease chronicity
3. Atopy
   a. This is the genetic predisposition for the development of an IgE-mediated response to common aeroallergens. This is the strongest identifiable predisposing factor for developing asthma.

D. Childhood onset of asthma
1. Asthma frequently develops in childhood and is associated with atopy.
2. Common allergens are dust mites, animal protein (dander), and fungi.

3. A family history of allergy is strongly associated with asthma continuing through childhood.

E. Diagnosis of asthma
   1. Symptoms
      a. Symptoms of asthma include cough, wheezing, shortness of breath, chest tightness, and sputum production.
   2. Determine pattern of symptoms.
      a. Seasonal, perennial, or both
      b. Onset, duration, and frequency of symptoms
      c. Variations in sleep pattern (nocturnal or awakening in early morning)
   3. Precipitating factors
      a. Viral infection
      b. Environmental allergens
      c. Irritants (smoke, vapors)
      d. Food, food additives
      e. Weather
   4. Development of disease and treatment.
      a. Onset of disease and treatment
      b. History of medical conditions in early life
      c. Current management
      d. Drug therapy
   5. Family history
      a. History of asthma or related respiratory problems
   6. Social history (precipitate symptoms)
      a. Home environment
      b. Workplace

F. Indicators suggesting asthma
   1. Wheezing on exhalation (wheezing may be caused by other conditions)
   2. Cough, especially at night
   3. Recurrent wheezing, difficulty breathing, and chest tightness
   4. Peak expiratory flowrate (PEF) that varies 20% or more from PEF measurement in the morning (before short-acting beta-2 agonist) and in the afternoon (after taking short-acting beta-2 agonist)
   5. Worsening symptoms when associated with:
      a. Exercise
      b. Viral infection
      c. Animals with fur or feathers
      d. House dust mites (furniture, mattresses)
      e. Smoke (tobacco, wood)
      f. Pollen
      g. Strong environmental expressions (laughing or crying hard)
   6. Pulmonary function testing (spirometry)
      a. Decreased forced expiratory volume in 1 s ($FEV_1$)
      b. Decreased $FEV_1$/forced vital capacity (FVC) (less than 65%)
      c. Reversibility indicated by ≥12% and 200 mL in $FEV_1$ after inhaling a short-acting beta-1 agonist
   7. Other studies.
      a. Diffusing capacity
      b. Flow volume loops
      c. Bronchoprovocation
         (1) Methacholine challenge
         (2) Histamine challenge
         (3) Exercise challenge
      d. Chest radiograph
      e. Evaluation of sinus disease
      f. Evaluation for gastrointestinal (GE) reflux

G. Home monitoring of peak expiratory flowrate (PEF)
   1. PEF is the greatest flow velocity that can be obtained during a forced expiration (starting with fully inflated lungs).
   2. PEF meters are designed to provide ongoing monitoring, not diagnosis.
   3. Patients who benefit from PEF meters have moderate to severe persistent asthma (Table 10–5).
   4. PEF meters are used to:
      a. Determine severity and guide therapeutic decisions in the home, office, or emergency room.
      b. Detect early changes that require treatment.
      c. Evaluate responses to changes in therapy.

TABLE 10–5. *Classification of Asthma Severity (Clinical Features before Treatment*)*

| | Symptoms† | Nighttime Symptoms | Lung Function |
|---|---|---|---|
| Step 4<br>Severe persistent | Continual symptoms<br>Limited physical activity<br>Frequent exacerbations | Frequent | $FEV_1$/PEF ≤60% predicted<br>PEF variability >30% |
| Step 3<br>Moderate persistent | Daily symptoms<br>Daily use of inhaled short-acting beta-2 agonist<br>Exacerbations affect activity<br>Exacerbations ≥2 times/week; may last days | >1 time/week | $FEV_1$/PEF >60%–<80% predicted<br>PEF variability >30% |
| Step 2<br>Mild persistent | Symptoms ≥2 times/week but <1 time/day<br>Exacerbations may affect activity | >2 times/month | $FEV_1$/PEF ≥80% predicted<br>PEF variability 20–30% |
| Step 1<br>Mild intermittent | Symptoms ≤2 times/week<br>Asymptomatic and normal PEF between exacerbations<br>Exacerbations brief (from a few hours to a few days); intensity may vary | ≤2 times/month | $FEV_1$/PEF ≥80% predicted<br>PEF variability <20% |

*The presence of one of the features of severity is sufficient to place a patient in that category. An individual should be assigned to the most severe grade in which any feature occurs. The characteristics noted in this table are general and may overlap because asthma is highly variable. Furthermore, an individual's classification may change over time.

†Patients at any level of severity can have mild, moderate, or severe exacerbations. Some patients with intermittent asthma experience severe and life-threatening exacerbations separated by long periods of normal lung function and no symptoms.

d. Assess severity in patients with poor perception of airway obstruction.
e. Evaluate changes in chronic maintenance therapy.
f. Establish an individual's best PEF.

5. Establishing the individual's best PEF
   a. This requires a 2- to 3-week period, measuring PEF 2 to 4 times/day. There are normal predictive values for male and female patients (these are in the PEF package). Because predictive normal lung function varies across racial and ethnic populations, the normative standards for PEF derived from a given racial or ethnic group cannot be readily extrapolated to other groups. The most clinically useful standard for ongoing monitoring of asthma is the patient's personal best PEF value.
   b. Measure the PEF when the patient is first awakening and in the afternoon before taking a bronchodilator.
   c. Once the personal best has been established, that value is placed in the peak flow zones.
      (1) Green zone: 80% of the best PEF. Good control. Take medications as usual.
      (2) Yellow zone: 50 to 80% of the best PEF. Take short-acting beta-2 agonist right away. Consult doctor on closer day-to-day control of asthma.
      (3) Red zone: less than 50% of the best PEF. Take short-acting beta-2 agonist right away. Call doctor or Emergency Department (ED), or go to ED.
   d. The individual should use the same brand PEF meter. If another brand is used, the best PEF will need to be established again.
   e. Performing a PEF maneuver.
      (1) Move the indicator to the bottom of the numbered scale on the meter (this may be different for different PEF meters).
      (2) Stand and take a deep breath, filling the lungs completely.
      (3) Place the mouthpiece in the mouth and close the lips around it. Keep the tongue out of the mouthpiece hole.
      (4) Give one fast blast.
      (5) Write down the flowrate number from the PEF meter.
      (6) Repeat steps 1 to 5 two more times and take the best value.

f. Inaccuracies in PEF values may be caused by the following:
   (1) Breathing out through nose
   (2) Breathing out too long
   (3) Improper mouthpiece size—leaking around mouthpiece
   (4) Coughing during exhalation
   (5) Putting tongue in the mouthpiece
   (6) Spitting into PEF meter
   (7) Bending over during exhalation

g. Patients should be given an action plan based on signs and symptoms and/or PEF; this is especially important for patients with moderate-to-severe persistent asthma or a history of severe exacerbations (Table 10–6).

h. This plan should be prepared with the doctor and should include how the patient will avoid triggers, respond to early warning signs of an episode, and take medication, and the best way to reach the doctor for routine questions and urgent care.

H. Pharmacological treatment of asthma

1. Relievers

a. Beta-2 agonists are first-line-of-defense drugs. They are the drugs of choice for acute exacerbations and pretreatment of exercised-induced bronchospasm.
   (1) Albuterol (Proventil [nebulizer]), Ventolin (metered-dose inhaler [MDI]), and albuterol Rotahaler (dry-powder inhaler [DPI])
   (2) Bitolterol (Tornalate)
   (3) Pirbuterol (Maxair)
   (4) Terbutaline (Brethaire [MDI], Brethine [injection], and Bricanyl [tablets])

b. Anticholinergics
   (1) Ipratropium bromide (Atrovent) is considered the second line of defense. Atrovent enhances beta-2 agonists, blocks irritant receptors, and reduces cyclic guanosine monophosphate (cGMP). Best for large airway problems.

c. Systemic corticosteroids
   (1) Systemic corticosteroids are used for moderate to severe exacerbations and to prevent progression of exacerbation, to reverse inflammation, and to reduce rate of relapse.
   (2) Methylprednisolone
   (3) Prednisolone
   (4) Prednisone

d. Usual dosages for quick-relief medications (Table 10–7)

2. Controllers

a. Inhaled corticosteroids prevent long-term symptoms, reverse inflammation, and reduce the need for oral corticosteroids. A spacer should be used with inhaled steroids. Following the treatment, rinse the mouth to reduce the incidence of oropharyngeal candidiasis.
   (1) Beclomethasone dipropionate (Beclovent, Vanceril).
   (2) Budesonide (Rhinocort nasal inhaler).
   (3) Flunisolide (AeroBid)
   (4) Fluticasone propionate (Flovent [inhalation], Flonase [nasal spray])
   (5) Triamcinolone acetonide (Azmacort)

b. Systemic corticosteroids are given for 3 to 10 days to gain control of inadequately controlled, persistent asthma (drugs are the same as relievers).

c. Nonsteroidal anti-inflammatory agents are used to modify inflammation and are administered prior to exposure to exercise or to a known allergen.

TABLE 10–6. ***Action Plan for Patients with Moderate to Severe Persistent Asthma or a History of Severe Exacerbations***

These questions should be discussed with a doctor and answered for an asthma emergency:

- What are the signs that tell me to seek care quickly?
- What should be done if the medications I am taking do not seem to be working?
- Where should I go to get care quickly?
- Should I call the doctor first or go to the emergency department?
- What should I do if I have an asthma emergency very late at night?
- When I call, what information will my doctor want (your symptoms, what medicines you have taken, when you took them, and your peak flowrate)?

TABLE 10–7. *Usual Dosages for Quick-Relief Medications*

| Medications | Dose Form | Child Dose |
|---|---|---|
| SHORT-ACTING INHALED BETA-2 AGONISTS | MDI | |
| Albuterol | 90 µg/puff, 200 puffs | 1–2 puffs 5 min prior to exercise |
| Albuterol HFA | 90 µg/puff, 200 puffs | 2 puffs tid-qid prn |
| Bitolterol | 370 µg/puff, 300 puffs | |
| Pirbuterol | 200 µg/puff, 400 puffs | |
| Terbutaline | 200 µg/puff, 300 puffs | |
| | DPI | |
| Albuterol Rotahaler | 200 µg/capsule | 1 capsule q 4–6 h as needed and prior to exercise |
| | NEBULIZED SOLUTION | |
| Albuterol | 5 mg/mL (0.5%) | 0.05 mg/kg (min 1.25 mg, max 2.5 mg) in 2–3 mL of saline q 4–6 h |
| ANTICHOLINERGICS | MDI | 1–2 puffs q 6 h |
| Ipratropium | 18 µg/puff, 200 puffs | |
| | NEBULIZED SOLUTION | 0.25 mg q 6 h |
| | 0.25 mg/mL (0.025%) | (APPLIES TO ALL THREE SYSTEMIC CORTICOSTEROIDS) |
| SYSTEMIC CORTICOSTEROIDS | | Short-course "burst": 1–2 mg/kg/day, maximum 60 mg/day, for 3–10 days |
| Methylprednisolone | 2-,4-,8-,16-,32-mg tablets | |
| Prednisolone | 5-mg tabs, 5 mg/mL, 15 mg/mL | |
| Prednisone | 1-,2.5-,5-,10-,20-,25-mg tabs; 5-mg/mL solution | |

(1) Cromolyn sodium (Intal, Aarane)
(2) Nedocromil sodium (Tilade)

d. Long-acting beta-2 agonists are used to prevent symptoms, especially in nocturnal asthma, and are added to anti-inflammatory therapy to prevent exercise-induced bronchospasm.
   (1) Salmeterol xinafoate (Serevent)
   (2) Albuterol, sustained release
e. Methylxanthines are used to prevent symptoms and treat nocturnal symptoms.
   (1) Theophylline, sustained-release tablets and capsules

I. Stepwise approach to management of asthma in children older than 5 years of age (Table 10–8)
J. Stepwise approach to management of asthma in children younger than 5 years of age (Table 10–9)
K. Classifying severity of asthma exacerbations (Table 10–10)
L. Home treatment and management (Fig.10–1)
M. Emergency department or emergency medical care for asthma exacerbations
   1. Medications (Table 10–11)
   2. Management (Fig.10–2)
N. Criteria for admission to the hospital
   1. Distress not cleared after two to three nebulizer treatments or MDI administration.
   2. Peak expiratory flowrate (PEF) less than 50% of predicted
   3. $PaCO_2$ remains greater than 40 mm Hg.
   4. $SpO_2$ less than 90%
   5. Other repeated admissions
   6. Fever
O. Indications for continuous nebulization
   1. PEF less than 25% of predicted
   2. $PaCO_2$ greater than 40 mm Hg
   3. Poor arousal and signs of respiratory failure
P. Indications and signs for intubation and mechanical ventilation

TABLE 10–8. ***Management of Asthma in Children Older than 5 Years of Age in a Stepwise Treatment***

| Step | Quick Relief | Long-Term Control |
|---|---|---|
| Step 4: Severe persistent | Short-acting, inhaled beta-2 agonist as needed for symptoms. Long-term control may be indicated if using short-acting, inhaled beta-2 agonist on a daily basis or if the use is increasing. | Daily medications:<br>High-dose inhaled corticosteroid and long-acting beta-2 agonist and *either* sustained-release theophylline or long-acting beta-2 agonist tablets *and* corticosteroid tablets or syrup long term. |
| Step 3: Moderate persistent | Short-acting, inhaled beta-2 agonist as needed for symptoms. Long-term control may be indicated if using short-acting, inhaled beta-2 agonist on a daily basis or if the use is increasing. | Daily medications:<br>Either inhaled corticosteroid (medium dose) *or*<br>Inhaled corticosteroid (low-medium dose) with a long-acting, inhaled beta-2 agonist for nighttime symptoms.<br>Add sustained-release theophylline *or* long-acting beta-2 agonist tablets.<br>If needed, medium-high dose corticosteroid *and* long-acting, inhaled beta-2 agonist for nighttime symptoms.<br>Add sustained-release theophylline *or* long-acting beta-2 agonist tablets. |
| Step 2: Mild persistent | Short-acting, inhaled beta-2 agonist. Long-term control may be indicated if using this on a daily basis or if the use is increasing. | One daily medication:<br>Trial of cromolyn sodium or nedocromil sodium (low dose) to begin *or*<br>Inhaled corticosteroid (low dose).<br>Sustained-release theophylline is an alternative therapy (5–15 μg/mL). |
| Step 1: Mild intermittent* | Short-acting, inhaled beta-2 agonist. Long-term control may be indicated if using this more than 2 times/wk. | No daily medication required. |

*Teach basic facts about asthma. Teach inhaler-spacer-holding chamber technique. Discuss roles of medications. Develop self-management plan. Develop action plan for when and how to take rescue actions, especially for patients with a history of severe exacerbations. Discuss appropriate environmental control measures to avoid exposure to known allergens and irritants.

**Step down ↓**
Review treatment every 1–6 months. If control step is sustained for at least 3 months, a gradual stepwise reduction in treatment may be possible.

**Step up ↑**
If control is not achieved, consider step up. But first review patient medication technique, adherence, and environmental control (avoidance of allergens or other precipitant factors).

TABLE 10–9. ***Management of Asthma in Children Younger than 5 years of Age in a Stepwise Treatment Approach.***

| Step | Quick Relief | Long-Term Control |
|---|---|---|
| Step 4: Severe persistent | Bronchodilator as needed for symptoms (see Step 1) up to 3 times/day. | Daily anti-inflammatory medicine:<br>High-dose inhaled corticosteroid with spacer-holding device and face mask<br>If needed, add systemic corticosteroids 2 mg/kg/day and reduce to lowest daily or alternate-day dose that stabilizes symptoms. |
| Step 3: Moderate persistent | Bronchodilator as needed for symptoms (see Step 1) up to 3 times/day. | Daily anti-inflammatory medication. *Either*:<br>Inhaled corticosteroid (medium dose) spacer-holding chamber and face mask, *or once control is established*:<br>Inhaled corticosteroid (medium-dose) with nedocromil *or*<br>Medium-dose inhaled corticosteroid and long-acting bronchodilator (theophylline). |
| Step 2: Mild persistent | Same as for Step 1. | Daily anti-inflammatory medication. *Either*:<br>Nebulized (preferred) or MDI cromolyn sodium or MDI nedocromil sodium tid-qid. Infants and young children usually begin with a trial of cromolyn or nedocromil *or*<br>Inhaled corticosteroid (low-dose) by spacer-holding chamber and face mask. |
| Step 1: Mild intermittent | Bronchodilator as needed for symptoms < 2 times/week. Intensity of treatment depends on severity of exacerbation.<br>*Either*:<br>Short-acting, inhaled beta-2 agonist by nebulizer or face mask or spacer-holding chamber, *or*<br>Oral beta-2 agonist.<br>Infants with viral infection:<br>Bronchodilator q 4–6 h up to 24 h. Do not repeat more than once every 6 weeks. Consider systemic corticosteroids if current exacerbation is severe *or* patient has history of previous severe exacerbations. | No daily medication required. |

**Step down ↓**
Review treatment every 1–6 months. If control step is sustained for at least 3 months, a gradual stepwise reduction in treatment may be possible.

**Step up ↑**
If control is not achieved, consider step up. But first, review patient medication technique, adherence, and environmental control (avoidance of allergens or other precipitant factors).

TABLE 10–10. *Classification of Severity of Asthma Exacerbations*

| | Mild | Moderate | Severe | Respiratory Arrest Imminent |
|---|---|---|---|---|
| SYMPTOMS: | | | | |
| Breathlessness | While walking | While talking (infant—softer, shorter cry, difficulty feeding) | While at rest (infant—stops feeding) | |
| | Can lie down | Prefers sitting | Sits upright | |
| Talks in: | Sentences | Phrases | Words | |
| Altertness | May be agitated | Usually agitated | Usually agitated | Drowsy or confused |
| SIGNS: | | | | |
| Respiratory rate | Increased | Increased | Often >30/min | |
| Use of accessory muscles, suprasternal retractions | Usually not | Commonly | Usually | Paradoxical thoraco-abdominal movement |
| Wheeze | Moderate, often only end-expiratory | Loud; throughout exhalation | Usually loud; throughout inhalation and exhalation | Absent |
| Pulse/min | <100 | 100–120 | >120 | Bradycardia |
| Pulsus paradoxus | Absent <10 mm Hg | May be present 10–25 mm Hg | Often present >20–40 mm Hg | Absence suggests respiratory muscle fatigue |
| FUNCTIONAL ASSESSMENT: | | | | |
| PEF% predicted or % personal best | >80% | 50–80% | <50% predicted or personal best last <2 h | |
| $PaO_2$ (on room air) | Normal (test not usually necessary) | >60 mm Hg (test not usually necessary) | <60 mm Hg; possible cyanosis | |
| and/or $PaCO_2$ | <42 mm Hg (test not usually necessary) | <42 mm Hg (test not usually necessary) | ≥42 mm Hg; possible respiratory failure | |
| $SaO_2$ % (on room air) | >95% (test not usually necessary) | 91–95% | <91% | |

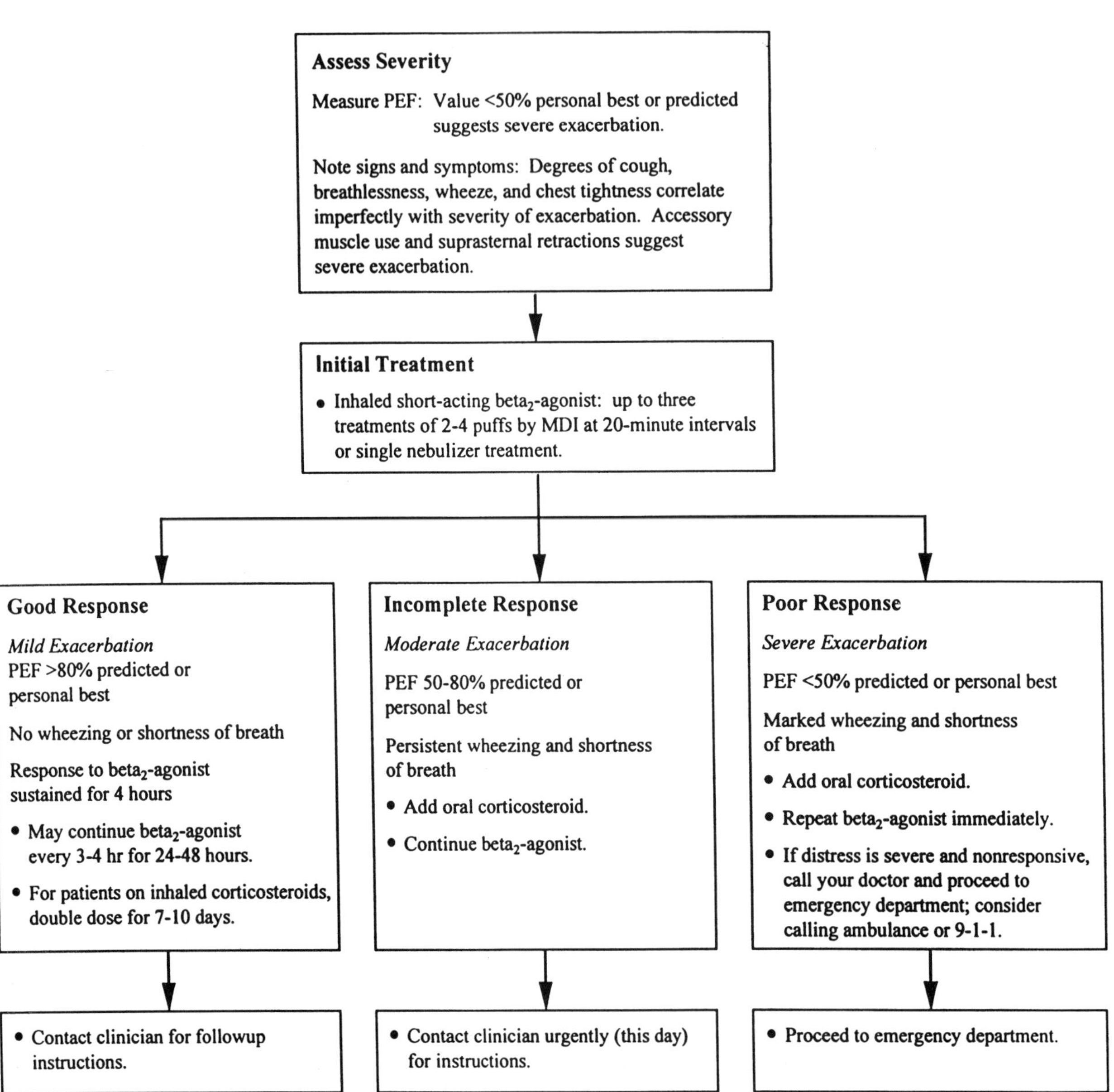


**FIGURE 10–1** Algorithm of management of asthma exacerbations through home treatment.

TABLE 10–11. ***Dosages of Drugs for Asthma Exacerbation in Emergency Medical Care or Hospital***

| Medications | Child's Dosages | Comments |
|---|---|---|
| INHALED SHORT-ACTING BETA-2 AGONISTS | | |
| Albuterol | | |
| Nebulized solution (5 mg/mL) | 0.15 mg/kg (minimum dose, 2.5 mg) every 20 min for 3 doses, then 0.15–0.3 mg/kg up to 10 mg every 1–4 h as needed, or 0.5 mg/kg/h continuous nebulization. | Only selective beta-2 agonists are recommended. For optimal delivery, dilute aerosols to minimum of 4 mL at gas flow of 6–8 L/min. |
| MDI | 4–8 puffs every 20 min for 3 doses, then every 1–4 h as needed. | As effective as nebulized therapy if patient is able to coordinate inhalation maneuver. Use spacer-holding device. |
| Bitolterol | | |
| Nebulized solution (2 mg/mL) | See albuterol dose. | Has not been studied in severe asthma exacerbations. Do not mix with other drugs. |
| MDI (370 µg/puff) | See albuterol dose. | Has not been studied in severe asthma exacerbations. |
| Pirbuterol | | |
| MDI (200 µg/puff) | See albuterol dose. | Has not been studied in severe asthma exacerbations. |
| SYSTEMIC (INJECTED) BETA-2 AGONISTS | | |
| Epinephrine 1:1000 (1 mg/mL) | 0.01 mg/kg up to 0.3–0.5 mg every 20 min for 3 doses subcutaneous. | No proven advantage of systemic therapy over aerosol. |
| Terbutaline (1 mg/mL) | 0.01 mg/kg every 20 min for 3 doses, then every 2–6 h as needed subcutaneously. | No proven advantage of systemic therapy over aerosol. |
| ANTICHOLINERGICS | | |
| Ipratropium bromide | | |
| Nebulizer solution (0.25 mg/mL) | 0.25 mg every 20 min for 3 doses, then every 2–4 h | May mix in same nebulizer with albuterol. Should not be used as first-line therapy; should be added to beta-2 agonist therapy. |
| MDI (18 µg/puff) | 4–8 puffs as needed. | Dose delivered from MDI is low and has not been studied in asthma exacerbations. |

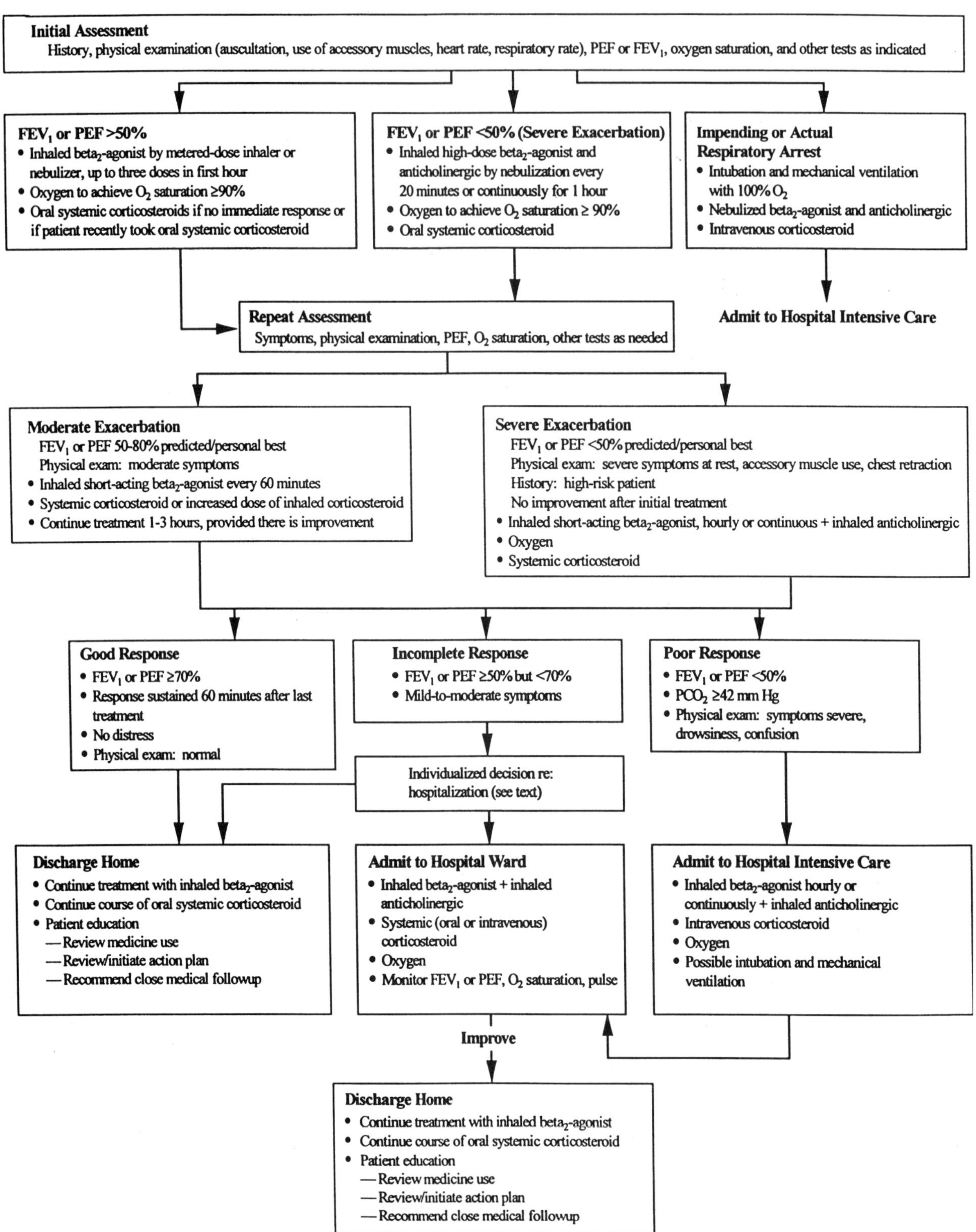


**FIGURE 10–2** Algorithm of asthma management in emergency department and hospital-based care.

1. Apnea or coma
2. $PaCO_2$: greater than 55 mm Hg
3. $PaCO_2$: increasing greater than 5 mm Hg/h
4. $PaO_2$: less than 60 mm Hg with an $FIO_2$ equal to or greater than 0.60
5. pH: less than 7.20
6. Altered sensorium
7. Apparent exhaustion
8. Markedly increased work of breathing established by the following:
   a. Retractions
   b. Nasal flaring
   c. Head bobbing
   d. Asynchronous breathing
9. Diminished or absent breath sounds
10. Fixed chest
11. Respiratory rate greater than 40 breaths per minute (bpm)

Q. Ventilator management
1. Initially permissive hypercapnia or controlled ventilation
2. Tidal volume ($V_t$) and rate appropriate to keep alveolar pressure less than 35 cm $H_2O$ (plateau pressure)
3. Accept permissive hypercapnia and acidosis. Sodium bicarbonate buffer may be necessary, but acidosis is tolerated. Permissive hypercapnia can be maintained until the alveolar pressure decreases.
4. Set I/E ratio to provide long expiratory time to help reduce hyperinflation and auto-PEEP.
5. Inspiratory flowrate should be set to provide a long exhalation time. The higher flowrates may increase PIP. PIP does not reflect hyperinflation but is a product of flowrate and increased airway resistance.
6. $FIO_2$ to achieve $SaO_2$ greater than 90%
7. Sedation and paralysis
8. Continuous aerosol in line through patient's circuit.

R. Auto-PEEP from dynamic hyperinflation
1. Hyperinflation is determined by the severity of obstruction, tidal volume, and expiratory time. Because of bronchoconstriction, auto-PEEP may occur. At this time, auto-PEEP may be helping oxygenation. Adding extrinsic PEEP ($PEEP_e$) to counterbalance the intrinsic PEEP ($PEEP_i$) may decrease venous return, decrease cardiac output, and reduce tissue oxygenation. Some use small levels of PEEP to set a new threshold when the patient assists the ventilator. But in the sedated, paralyzed patient, this is not needed. There are maneuvers to reduce auto-PEEP in the asthmatic patient on mechanical ventilation (Table 10–12).
2. As bronchospasm is relieved (reduction in PIP), auto-PEEP decreases; however, oxygenation may deteriorate, so a small level of $PEEP_e$ may help restore oxygenation.

S. Weaning
1. Indications for reversal of bronchospasm are reduced PIP (volume-cycled ventilator) and $PaCO_2$ begins to normalize.
2. Begin reversing sedation and paralyzing agent.
3. Reduce the synchronized intermittent mandatory ventilation (SIMV) rate and add pressure support ventilation (PSV) at 5 to 7 mL/kg of body weight.
4. Reduce $FIO_2$ while maintaining $SpO_2$ at greater than 90% and $PaO_2$ at 60 to 80 mm Hg. A minimum amount of PEEP may be added if $PaO_2$ begins to fall.
5. As the mechanical ventilator rate decreases, the flowrate may be decreased to provide more laminar flow and improve distribution of ventilation.
6. At a low SIMV rate, switch to CPAP and PSV to maintain a tidal volume at 5 to 7 mL/kg of body weight.

T. Home therapy
1. Before leaving the hospital, teach parents and child how to administer a proper treatment, use equipment, and develop an action plan (Table 10–13).

## VI. Bronchiolitis

A. Bronchiolitis is a diffuse inflammation of the bronchioles with airway narrowing, which is usually seen as viral bronchopneumonia in infants under the age of 1 year.

B. Epidemiology
1. Respiratory syncytial virus (RSV) is the most common causative agent in hospitalized infants under the age of 2 years. Usually seen in winter to spring.

TABLE 10–12. ***Maneuvers to Reduce Auto-PEEP***

| | |
|---|---|
| Increase Etime | Increase flowrate<br>Decrease tidal volume<br>Decrease respiratory rate |
| Bronchodilator | Continuous beta-2 agonist while on mechanical ventilation.<br>Increases chest wall compliance. |
| Sedation and paralyzation | Decrease ventilator-patient asynchrony.<br>Allow ventilation at lowest PIP. |

2. Infants at risk for severe RSV disease include the following:
   a. Infants with congenital heart disease
   b. Premature infants (less than 35 weeks' gestation)
   c. Infants with chronic lung disease (bronchopulmonary dysplasia [BPD] and cystic fibrosis [CF])
   d. Infants with immunodeficiency secondary to HIV or transplantation
   e. Otherwise healthy infants less than 2 months of age

C. Other causative agents include parainfluenza type 1, adenovirus, and *Mycoplasma* pneumonia.

D. Virus is spread by direct contact.
   1. Virus is usually caught from a brother, sister, or parent who has a cold.
   2. Handling the infant's toys can spread the disease. Babies may also be infected from contact with nasal secretions carried by hospital staff or other babies. Because viruses can remain viable for a long time on environmental surfaces, others in the room can pick it up from contact with that surface.
   3. The infection can be rubbed into the nose or eyes to cause an infection.
   4. When the adult handles the infant, the virus on the hand is spread to the infant and the infant in turn rubs the infected hand into its nose or eye. Babies shed viruses for a long time, so others who are not infected by handling the infant can become infected and pass the virus on to other infants handled by the infected staff member.
   5. Handwashing is most important for reducing the nosocomial spread of the disease, as is wearing gloves and a gown. Also, cohorting infected patients and restricting symptomatic adults and children from visitation.
   6. Course of disease (without complications) is 3 to 10 days.

E. Signs and symptoms of RSV
   1. Rhinorrhea
   2. Mild respiratory tract infection followed by 2 to 3 days of coughing and possible fever (usually less than 39.5°C)
   3. Progression of the disease results in wheezing, retractions, tachypnea, and difficulty feeding.
   4. Severe cases cause hypoxemia.

TABLE 10–13. ***Hospital Discharge Checklist for Patients with Asthma Exacerbations***

| Intervention | Dose/Timing | Education/Advice |
|---|---|---|
| Inhaled medications (MDI + spacer-holding chamber) | Select agent, dose, and frequency (e.g., albuterol). | Teach purpose.<br>Teach technique. |
| Beta-2 agonist | 2–6 puffs q 3–4 h prn. | Emphasize need for spacer-holding chamber. |
| Corticosteroids | Medium dose. | Check patient technique. |
| Oral medications | Select agent, dose, and frequency (e.g., prednisone, 20 mg bid for 3–10 days). | Teach purpose.<br>Teach side effects. |
| Peak flow meter | Measure A.M. and P.M. PEF and record best of 3 tries each time. | Teach purpose.<br>Teach technique.<br>Distribute peak flow diary. |
| Follow-up visit | Make appointment for follow-up care with primary clinician or asthma specialist. | Advise patient (or caregiver) of date, time, and location of appointment within 7 days of discharge. |
| Action plan | Before or at discharge. | Instruct patient (or caregiver) on simple plan for actions to be taken when symptoms, signs, and PEF values suggest recurrent airflow obstruction. |

F. Pathophysiology
   1. Inflammation of epithelial cells
   2. Sloughing of necrotized epithelium
   3. Plugging of bronchioles
   4. Impaired mobilization of secretions
   5. Atelectasis (secondary to poor collateral ventilation of lung units in infants)
   6. Decreased lung compliance
   7. Increased work of breathing

G. Chest radiograph
   1. Pulmonary hyperinflation
   2. Minimal infiltrates

H. Diagnosis is made by obtaining nasopharyngeal secretions by swabbing or washing the nose with saline solution. Laboratory determination is done by immunofluorescent antibody staining, which is 95% sensitive for RSV.

I. Management
   1. Isolation
   2. For mild symptoms:
      a. Humidified oxygen to keep $SpO_2$ greater than 90%
      b. Suctioning nasopharyngeal airway
      c. Using a bronchodilator
   3. For severe symptoms:
      a. Ribavirin (Virazole) aerosol to prevent intubation. This is an antiviral medication that disrupts the RNA within the virus and prevents any further transmission or shedding. It comes in a 100-mL vial, which contains 6 mg of ribavirin, and is mixed with sterile water, which will contain 20 mg/mL of ribavirin. It is administered by a small-particle aerosol generator (SPAG-2) system for 12 to 24 h, for 3 to 10 days. Generally, improvement is seen during the first day. It is recommended to use ribavirin as early as possible in patients with RSV, cyanotic heart disease, severe bronchopulmonary dysplasia, and postoperative cardiac surgery.
      b. Ribavirin may be delivered by oxygen hood, mist tent, face tent, or endotracheal tube, with or without mechanical ventilation (see Chapter 9).
      c. Ribavirin reduces antibody response by the patient and the health care personnel may be hypersensitive to the drug.
   4. Monitor $PaO_2$, $PaCO_2$, and $SpO_2$ for impending respiratory failure.
   5. Intubate and ventilate when:
      a. pH is less than 7.25
      b. $PaCO_2$ is greater than 60 mm Hg.
      c. $PaO_2$ is less than 70 mm Hg and $FIO_2$ is greater than 0.40.
      d. Breath sounds are absent.
      e. Exhaustion and lethargy are present.
   6. Monitor weight gain and hydrate adequately.
   7. A new drug, RSV-IGIV, has been approved for the prevention of serious lower respiratory tract infection caused by RSV in children less than 24 months of age with BPD or a history of premature birth (less than 35 weeks' gestation). The drug reduces the incidence and duration of RSV hospitalization and the severity of RSV illness in these high-risk infants.

## VII. Cystic fibrosis

A. Demographics
   1. Approximately 30,000 people in United States have CF; more than 12 million are symptom-free carriers of CF.
   2. One-third of the CF population is over 18 years of age. The median survival age is 29 years (male = 32 years, female = 27 years).
   3. The majority of CF patients are less than 15 years old, with more than 7% of the CF population more than 31 years old.
   4. 96% of CF patients are white, 3% are black, and 0.2% are Asian and Pacific islanders.
   5. 56% of adults with CF are men, 44% are women.
   6. Of CF adult patients, 57% are 20 to 29 years old, 23% are 30 to 39 years old.
   7. 90% of patients are diagnosed with CF by the age of 12. 4% are diagnosed first over the age of 18.
   8. The leading clinical symptom at the initial diagnosis is a persistence of acute respiratory symptoms.
   9. 60% of CF patients culture *Pseudomonas aeruginosa*. Others include *Staphylococcus aureus* and *Haemophilus influenzae*. Adults cultured *Pseudomonas* at a higher rate than other organisms.

10. The most significant complication adults experience is massive hemoptysis (greater than 240 mL blood in 24 h).
11. 82% of CF patients die of cardiopulmonary disease. 2% die of hepatic disease.
12. With continued aggressive aerosolized antibiotic therapy, chest physiotherapy, attention to nutritional status, as well as other therapies, CF patients can be expected to survive into their 40s.

B. General description
   1. CF is a mendelian recessive disorder. Inherited traits are controlled by genes, with a child inheriting two genes, one from each parent.
   2. One out of every 20 people is a CF carrier. One out of 2500 Caucasian births has CF.
   3. Both parents have to be carriers of the recessive gene.
   4. When both parents are carriers of the CF gene, each pregnancy has a:
      a. 25% chance that one child will be born with CF
      b. 25% chance that one child will not carry the gene and will not have CF
      c. 50% chance that two infants will have the gene but will not have CF
   5. In 1989 the gene that causes CF was discovered.
   6. CF screening can be done prenatally or after birth on the newborn. Population-based screening that screens extended family members of CF patients can also be performed.

C. Pathogenesis and pathology
   1. A patient with CF has a gene that disrupts a certain protein. The protein is missing one amino acid out of 1480.
   2. The protein was named cystic fibrosis transmembrane regulator (CFTR) by researchers. It is generally manufactured inside the cells lining the glands (submucosal) in the airways and the epithelia of the gut, pancreas, biliary ducts, and sperm ducts. The function of this protein is to travel to the cell's surface to control the flow of chlorine ($Cl^-$) in and out of the cell. CFTR can be thought of as a gatekeeper for salt in the cell membrane. This movement of $Cl^-$ allows the normal movement of water to maintain mucus consistency.
   3. Because the CFTR is faulty, $Cl^-$ transport does not occur. As a result, in order to maintain electroneutrality, sodium ($Na^+$) is transported into the cell along with water The accompanying water influx dehydrates the cellular surface and leads to sticky mucus, which is characteristic of the disease.
   4. Respiratory effects
      a. Because of decreased epithelial chloride permeability and thus a reduced water content, secretions thicken.
      b. These thickened secretions impair mucociliary clearance, which leads to endobronchial infection, usually caused by *Staphylococcus aureus* and *Pseudomonas aeruginosa*.
      c. Ciliary structure is normal, but function is impaired because of the thickened secretions and increased viscoelastic properties.
      d. Infections from *S. aureus* and *P. aeruginosa* become more prevalent. (Some evidence suggests that CF respiratory epithelial cells are more susceptible to *P. aeruginosa* attachment than normal cells.)
      e. Irreversible lung damage is the result of airway inflammation. Polymorphonuclear (PMN) cells enter the airway in response to bacterial infection. PMN cells release substances that cause airway damage, leading to bronchiectasis.
      f. Chronic bacterial infection persistently stimulates the immune system, releasing high levels of antibodies. These antibodies impair the phagocytosis of *Pseudomonas* by alveolar macrophages.
      g. The vicious cycle of chronic endobronchial infection, inflammation, and progressive airway obstruction eventually results in bronchiectasis and its complications: hemoptysis, pneumothorax, hypoxemia, and eventually respiratory failure.
   5. Gastrointestinal (GI) complications—Pancreas
      a. 90% of patients with CF have pancreatic involvement.
      b. As with the lungs, chloride channels are defective and the normal secretions are not made. Secretions are inspissated. Enzymes are still made within the pancreas but cannot exit; therefore, auto digestion of the pancreas occurs.
      c. Pancreatic function declines within the first year of life. Some infants develop pancreatic insufficiency (PI) within 2 years of age. As a result of PI, food, especially fats, is not broken down. Growth and development are impaired.
      d. As the CF patient gets older, the pancreas becomes fibrotic, causing greater

TABLE 10–14. ***Organ Involvement with Cystic Fibrosis***

| Organ | Manifestation |
|---|---|
| Respiratory tract | Bronchiectasis, pneumonia, sinusitis, nasal polyps |
| Pancreas | Pancreatic insufficiency |
| Liver | Biliary cirrhosis |
| Gallbladder | Cholelithiasis |
| Intestinal tract | Meconium ileus, intussusception, distal small bowel obstruction |
| Reproductive tract | Vas deferens obstruction |
| Sweat glands | Abnormal sweat electrolytes |
| Salivary glands | Abnormal salivary electrolytes |

problems with malabsorption of food. In the patient who is more than 30 years of age, pancreatitis may be seen.

6. GI complications—Liver
   a. As a result of malnutrition, liver involvement occurs.
   b. Lesions and fibrosis similar to that in the pancreas occur. Progression of liver involvement causes hepatomegaly and cirrhosis.
7. GI complications—Intestinal tract
   a. Intestinal obstruction in the newborn is called meconium ileus (MI). This is a result of inspissated meconium obstructing the distal small bowel.
   b. Approximately 16% of all newly diagnosed newborn patients with CF have MI.
8. Other problems
   a. Gastroesophageal reflux (GER)—Infants with CF who have respiratory disease tend to have GER.
   b. Distal intestinal obstruction syndrome (DIOS)—This is similar to MI, but it is usually seen in the teenager and adult CF patient. It occurs in patients with PI and may mimic symptoms similar to those of appendicitis. Diagnosis is made by abdominal x-ray.
9. Summary of organ involvement (Table 10–14)

D. Clinical manifestations
   1. Infants (newborn to 1 year)
      a. Meconium ileus—Failure to pass meconium in first 12 to 24 h of life
      b. Obstructive jaundice
      c. Failure to thrive
      d. Intussusception—Most common cause of intestinal obstruction in infants. A portion of intestine is prolapsed into the lumen of an immediately adjacent part. This may occur during the first or second year of life as a result of strong contractions. It may require surgery.
      e. Recurrent pneumonia and upper respiratory tract infections
   2. Childhood (1 to 12 years of age)
      a. *S. aureus* or *P. aeruginosa* infection
      b. Malnutrition
      c. Clubbing of the digits
      d. Esophageal varices
      e. Nasal polyps
      f. Rectal prolapse
      g. Pansinusitis
   3. Adolescence (more than 12 years of age)
      a. Recurrent pulmonary exacerbations include increased cough and sputum production, shortness of breath, decreased exercise tolerance, and weight loss.
      b. Bronchiectasis
      c. Hemoptysis
      d. Underdevelopment of growth and delayed sexual development
      e. Hypoxia and clubbing of digits
      f. Pancreatitis
      g. Chronic infection from *P. aeruginosa, Pseudomonas cepacia* (may be resistant to certain aminoglycosides)
      h. Bleb formation, pneumothorax

E. Diagnosis
   1. Clinical symptoms and family history
   2. Positive sweat chloride test

a. Test performed by collection and measurement of NaCl in sweat
b. Sweat is produced by local stimulation of sweat glands by means of pilocarpine iontophoresis or from mild electrical stimulation (2 to 3 milliamperes). Sweat is collected from the forearm, trunk, or thigh.
c. Normal NaCl in children is 45 to 60 mEq/L. More than 60 mEq/L is consistent with CF.
d. Two consecutive positive tests should be obtained.
e. Along with the sweat chloride test, protein trypsinogen is measured and found to be elevated in newborns with CF, even before symptoms appear

3. Prenatal and neonatal screening (amniocentesis, chorionic villus sampling, both with genetic analysis)

F. Laboratory findings

1. Pulmonary findings
   a. Decreased lung compliance, V/Q mismatch, and increased respiratory rate
   b. Reduced expiratory residual volume, increased residual volume
   c. Flow volume loop alteration showing reduced flowrate during exhalation
   d. Normal to decreased $PaCO_2$ in early CF; hypercapnia in older children
2. Radiologic findings
   a. Hyperinflation with flattened diaphragms and increased A-P diameter (barrel-chest appearance)
   b. Areas of atelectasis
   c. Peribronchial thickening
   d. Cystic densities

G. Treatment

1. Because there is currently no cure for CF, treatment is directed at halting or delaying the progression of symptoms.
2. Antibiotic aerosol therapy
   a. The common method of delivering medications for CF is intravenous, especially during exacerbations of pulmonary symptoms.
   b. Intravenous aminoglycosides are commonly administered for *P. aeruginosa*. Drugs such as gentamicin, tobramycin, netilmicin, and amikacin are delivered in high doses because of poor absorption by endobronchial secretions and increased clearance of antibiotics. Associated with these higher doses are concerns of nephrotoxicity and ototoxicity.
   c. Inhaled aminoglycosides are currently being used and are a way of delivering high doses of antibiotics for *P. aeruginosa* with reduced systems effects.
   d. Studies using aerosolized gentamicin, carbenicillin, and tobramycin showed:
      (1) Patients experienced subjective improvement in symptoms.
      (2) Lung function improvement measured by FVC in 1 s and PEF
      (3) Decreased frequency of hospitalizations
      (4) Improved weight gain and growth
      (5) No ototoxicity or nephrotoxicity
      (6) Reduced density of *P. aeruginosa* in sputum
      (7) Reduced pulmonary exacerbations
   e. Problems with inhaled antibiotics during these studies include the following:
      (1) *P. aeruginosa* resistant to tobramycin
      (2) Some patients showed a decline in PFTs from an initially improved level.
   f. Limitations of inhaled antibiotics include the following:
      (1) No standard aerosol delivery system for antibiotics
      (2) Chemical properties of the drug may change, which may alter the amount of active drug delivered.
      (3) Interaction between other drugs being aerosolized. For this reason, inhaled antibiotics should not be aerosolized with other drugs.
   g. Concern for family members and health care practitioners breathing exhaled aerosolized antibiotics. Drugs such as penicillin and second- and third-generation cephalosporins have a higher incidence of hypersensitivity reactions than aminoglycosides.
   h. Table 10–15 identifies aerosolized antibiotics used to treat CF.
   i. Exhaust from the nebulizer, when inhaled antibiotics are used, should be collected or vented.
3. rhDNase (Pulmozyme)
   a. Airway obstruction from purulent airway secretions is related to the viscoelastic or adhesive properties of airway mucus.

TABLE 10–15. ***Aerosolized Antibiotics Used to Treat Cystic Fibrosis***

| Name | General Information |
|---|---|
| Gentamicin | Used for *S. aureus*, resistance problem, inexpensive. |
| Tobramycin | Similar to gentamicin but better for *P. aeruginosa*, less resistance problem and less nephrotoxic. |
| Amikacin | Used when bacterial resistance is a problem with other aminoglycosides. |
| Colistin sulphomethate | Good anti-Pseudomonas, no gram + activity. |
| Ceftazidime | Good against *Pseudomonas* and *H. influenzae*, expensive |
| Amphotericin | Antifungal agent against aspergillosis. Used before and after lung transplant. |

b. The viscoelastic properties are largely due to the presence of DNA from polymorphonuclear leukocytes, which accumulate in the airway from chronic infection. This accumulation of rhDNA, along with mucus glycoproteins, increases the viscosity of mucus. Human rhDNase has been found to hydrolyze extracellular DNA in purulent secretions and reduce the viscoelastic properties in CF sputum.

c. The recommended dose is 2.5 mg once a day administered with a small-volume nebulizer.

d. Pulmozyme should coincide with the present treatment regimen.

e. Studies on aerosolized rhDNase showed:
   (1) No acute allergic or bronchospastic response
   (2) Decreased bacteria in sputum
   (3) Significant improvement in FVC and $FEV_1$
   (4) Significant decline in dyspnea
   (5) Reduction in the use of parenteral antibiotics
   (6) Improved perception of dyspnea, overall perception of well-being and CF-related symptoms
   (7) Fewer hospital days

f. Adverse effects of Pulmozyme include voice alteration from pharyngitis and laryngitis, rash, chest pain, and conjunctivitis.

g. Pulmozyme should be refrigerated and should not be exposed to room temperature for more than 24 h. The entire vial must be used once it is opened and if it has a cloudy appearance, discarded. It should not be mixed with other drugs when nebulized.

4. Positive expiratory pressure (PEP) therapy
   a. A maneuver that provides a resistance to exhalation and positive expiratory pressure to keep the airways open during exhalation, altering the I/E ratio
   b. Indications
      (1) To reduce air trapping (asthma and cystic fibrosis)
      (2) To mobilize retained secretions (cystic fibrosis and chronic bronchitis)
      (3) To prevent or reverse atelectasis
      (4) To aid in the delivery of bronchodilators
   c. Contraindications
      (1) Patients unable to tolerate increased work of breathing
      (2) Patients with intracranial pressures greater than 20 mm Hg
      (3) Trauma or surgery to the face, oral cavity, or skull
      (4) Epistaxis
      (5) Active hemoptysis
      (6) Untreated pneumothorax
   d. Hazards and complications
      (1) Hypoventilation and hypercapnia from increased work of breathing
      (2) Increased ICP
      (3) Decreased venous return, myocardial ischemia
      (4) Pulmonary barotrauma
   e. Assessment of need
      (1) Sputum retention not responsive to spontaneous or directed coughing
      (2) History of pulmonary problems treated successfully with postural drainage therapy
      (3) Secretions in airway suggested by decreased breath sounds or adventitious breath sounds
      (4) Atelectasis, mucus plugging, or infiltrates as seen on chest radiograph

f. Assessment of outcome
    (1) Change in sputum production. A patient may already be producing a large amount of sputum (more than 30 mL/day) without the use of PEP. If PEP does not increase this production, then PEP may not be indicated.
    (2) Change in breath sounds. Improved breath sounds or increased adventitious breath sounds indicate improvement if these were not present prior to the treatment.
    (3) Subjective response to therapy by patient. The patient should be questioned before, during, and after the therapy concerning any adverse reactions, including dizziness, nausea, shortness of breath, and pain. Any of these are indications to stop and re-evaluate the therapy. Changes in therapy may include a reduction in expiratory pressure, frequency of therapy, or more frequent rest periods during the procedure.
    (4) Changes in vital signs that are inappropriate for the patient. Some changes in respiratory rate and/or pulse are expected. Bradycardia, tachycardia, palpations, and significant alteration in blood pressure are indications to stop and re-evaluate therapy.
    (5) Resolution or improvement in chest radiograph
g. Equipment includes a mask or mouthpiece, T-assembly with a one-way valve, adjustable expiratory resistor, and manometer.
h. After gathering equipment, set appropriate resistance on adjustable resistor. The patient should be sitting comfortably. Apply the mask or mouthpiece to the patient. The patient, using diaphragmatic breathing, takes in a deep breath (not a total lung capacity [TLC] maneuver). Exhalation should be active but not forced, and there should be enough resistance to exhalation to produce 10 to 20 cm $H_2O$ throughout exhalation. After the patient has performed this 10 to 20 times, he or she is instructed to huff-cough to raise secretions. These steps are performed by the patient up to eight times each session.
i. Expiratory resistance should be set to achieve an expiratory pressure of 10 to 20 cm $H_2O$, and an I/E ratio of 1:3 to 1:4. An MDI or small-volume nebulizer can be attached to the PEP device to be administered along with the PEP therapy. If the patient complains about the expiratory pressure being excessive, the variable resistor can be reduced to a setting that achieves a lower expiratory pressure. Morning and evening therapy works best.
j. During periods of exacerbation, the frequency of therapy, rather than the duration, should be changed.
k. Infection control should be observed as appropriate.
    (1) Observe universal precautions as appropriate.
    (2) Disinfect any reusable equipment between patients.
    (3) Gloves, mask, and goggles may be needed to prevent transmission of tuberculosis.

5. Flutter device
    a. This device is used to loosen mucus in the airways so that it can be coughed up more easily.
    b. With the patient sitting in a comfortable position with the head slightly back, the patient is instructed to take in as large a breath as possible and to hold the breath for 2 to 3 s. With the flutter in the mouth, the patient exhales at a constant speed. The exhalation should be slow enough to get the "fluttering" sensation in the chest. Exhalation should be as complete as possible, squeezing out as much air as possible. Following this maneuver, the patient may take a deep breath and cough, or continue performing the flutter maneuver a number of times and then cough.
    c. Observe universal precautions as appropriate.
6. Bronchodilator therapy
7. Chest physiotherapy
8. Oxygen as needed during exacerbation to keep $SpO_2$ greater than 90%
9. Nutritional support
    a. Caloric increase to 150%
    b. Supplemental pancreatic enzymes to metabolize fat (streptokinase)
    c. Increase carbohydrate, protein intake.
    d. Increase water intake.
    e. May require gavage feedings via NG tube or gastrostomy tube.
    f. Vitamin supplements
10. Physical therapy

11. Supportive home care and patient-parent education
12. Lung transplantation
13. Alternate therapies and treatment
    a. Better screening
    b. Vaccine for *P. aeruginosa*
    c. Amiloride aerosolized sodium channel blocker (inhibits absorption of sodium in airway epithelium)

## VIII. Acute respiratory distress syndrome (ARDS)

A. General description
   1. Respiratory failure characterized by the following:
      a. Increased work of breathing
      b. Diffuse pulmonary infiltrates
      c. Decreased lung compliance
      d. Refractory hypoxemia
   2. Develops after an acute injury or illness
      a. Primary injury not necessarily pulmonary; could be heart (congestive heart failure [CHF]).
      b. Most common primary causes in children include the following:
         (1) Trauma
         (2) Hypovolemic or septic shock
         (3) Near-drowning
         (4) Near-strangulation
         (5) Aspiration pneumonia
         (6) Infection

B. Pathology and pathophysiology
   1. Three phases of lung changes
      a. The acute phase (within first 7 days) is associated with an influx of neutrophils, red blood cells, and fibrin in alveolar space.
      b. The subacute phase (up to 10 days) is associated with the resolution of edema and is replaced by fibrosis and increased diffusion defect.
      c. After 10 days, the disease moves into the chronic phase, in which further development of ARDS occurs with a loss of lung structure and alveolar bed and an increased pulmonary vascular resistance and pulmonary hypertension.
   2. Early phases (degree of severity variable)
      a. Microatelectasis
      b. Interstitial and alveolar edema
      c. Alveolar filling with exudate
   3. Right-to-left shunt
   4. Disease progression
      a. Atelectasis causes decreased functional residual capacity (FRC), reduced compliance, increased work of breathing, V/Q mismatch, and shunt.
      b. Hypoxic pulmonary vasoconstriction can occur and may contribute to impaired cardiac function.
   5. Recovery phase
      a. Lung fibrosis is progressive, with residual lung damage, or regressive, with return to normal lung function.

C. Elements necessary to diagnose ARDS
   1. Pulmonary or nonpulmonary event. Child does not have left heart problem or CHF and has previously healthy lungs.
   2. Respiratory distress evidenced by:
      a. Tachypnea
      b. Dyspnea
      c. Retractions
      d. Hypoxemia
      e. Reduced pulmonary compliance (less than 50 mL/cm $H_2O$)
      f. Increased shunt fraction
   3. Radiologic changes that include the following:
      a. Bilateral, diffuse pulmonary infiltrates
      b. Either interstitial or alveolar

D. Clinical features of ARDS
   1. After insult there is a latent period when the patient has little distress.
   2. Radiograph appears normal in early stages.
   3. Over the next few hours:
      a. Increased hypoxemia
      b. Cyanosis

c. Respiratory distress
d. Irritability
e. Dyspnea
4. Radiograph in later stages:
   a. Fluid in alveoli and vascular changes possibly pleural effusion
5. Hypoxemia becomes refractory to oxygen.
6. Early arterial blood gases (ABGs): hypoxemia and hypocarbia
7. Late ABGs: increased hypoxemia ($PaO_2$ less than 50 mm Hg on $FIO_2$ greater than 0.60) and hypercapnia
8. Continual reduction in compliance, often as low as 20 to 30 mL/cm $H_2O$

E. Treatment and management
   1. Treat initial injury and illness
      a. Tidal volume—7 to 10 mL/kg of body weight (high volumes may cause volutrauma). If the plateau pressure is greater than 30 to 35 cm $H_2O$, use a lower tidal volume or switch to pressure control ventilation.
      b. Use tidal volume and compliance relationship to determine the best tidal volume for the best compliance. For example:

| $V_t$ (mL/kg) | Cst (1/cm $H_2O$) |
|---|---|
| 6 | 0.030 |
| 7 | 0.048 |
| 8 | 0.041 |
| 10 | 0.036 |

      In this series, 7 mL/kg of body weight is an appropriate tidal volume to achieve the best compliance.
   2. SIMV—A higher than normal rate minimizes barotrauma. However, one needs to watch inspiratory time and expiratory time.
   3. Consider using a short inspiratory time and longer expiratory time with a high flowrate to achieve appropriate I/E ratio.
   4. Determination of optimal PEEP levels (normal blood volume is present)
      a. Increase PEEP by 3 to 5 cm $H_2O$ every 30 min
      b. Continue increasing PEEP until shunt fraction is less than 12 to 15%, oxygen consumption ($\dot{V}O_2$) is greater than 160 mL/min, and compliance increases above the previous low level. Decrease PEEP if these values show deterioration.
   5. Cardiac output
      a. Maintain pulmonary capillary wedge pressure (PCWP) at 10 to 18 mm Hg.
      b. Volume is recommended if PCWP cannot be maintained.
      c. If PCWP is still low after volume supplementation, drop PEEP level until desired PCWP is attained.
   6. Weaning
      a. Pressure support ventilation helps overcome the resistance of small endotracheal tubes and reduces muscle fatigue. Give the appropriate pressure support to maintain the appropriate tidal volume.
      b. Reduce $FIO_2$ to nontoxic levels (less than 0.50).
      c. Reduce PEEP and maintain a minimum level of 3 to 5 cm $H_2O$.
      d. Monitor ABGs, lung compliance, cardiac output, and pulmonary function parameters.

F. Other treatment recommendations
   1. Prostaglandin $E_1$ ($PGE_1$) to reduce pulmonary hypertension
   2. Pressure control or inverse I/E ratio ventilation
   3. Extracorporeal membrane oxygenation (ECMO)
   4. Surfactant administration (future research)
   5. Nitric oxide

G. Outcome
   1. 50 to 60% mortality in pediatric population

## IX. Head trauma

A. Types of head trauma
   1. Extracranial (open head injury) involving scalp lacerations and scalp hematomas
   2. Skull fracture is a linear fracture of the skull, which generally requires observation.

3. Intracranial injury (closed head injury)
   a. Mild injury—Unconsciousness for less than 5 min. Paralysis may be seen, but quickly reverses.
   b. Severe injury—Prolonged loss of consciousness for more than 5 to 10 min with the following:
      (1) Disorientation
      (2) Delirium
      (3) Seizures with vomiting and memory loss
      (4) Abnormal vital signs
      (5) Persistent headache

B. Cerebral edema, commonly seen with head trauma, is an abnormal accumulation of fluid from leaky cerebral vasculature. Increased vessel permeability causes plasma and fluid exudation to the interstitial spaces.

C. Beside trauma, poor perfusion (associated with ischemic episodes) causes cerebral edema. Generally 24 to 48 h after the insult, cerebral edema is the greatest. During this time, compression of the cerebral vessels and an increase in intracranial pressure (ICP) cause further injury.

D. Intracranial pressure
   1. ICP is the pressure exerted by the cranium on the intracranial structures.
   2. An increase in cranium volume is poorly tolerated, even by infants who have an open fontanelle or sutures not yet fused.
   3. The intracranial components are almost incompressible. If there is an increase in volume affecting an intracranial component, a reciprocal change in the volume of one of the other components is required, or intracranial pressure rises.
   4. The following are causes of increased intracranial pressure:
      a. Bleeding into the epidural, subdural, or subarachnoid spaces or into the brain; or brain edema from contusion or hematoma. Increased ICP increases the rate of reabsorption of the cerebrospinal fluid (CSF). When this fails to compensate for the raised ICP, clinical signs become evident.

E. Intracranial components
   1. CSF
   2. Brain
   3. Cerebral blood flow—Governed by CSF, pH, $PaCO_2$, $PaO_2$, BP, and neuronal activity

F. The normal ICP is <20 mm Hg. A normal ICP will provide proper perfusion, preventing brain ischemia. Normal cerebral perfusion pressure (CPP) is 50 to 60 mm Hg (CPP = mean arterial pressure [MAP] – ICP). CPP less than 50 mm Hg may result in brain ischemia. It is very important to monitor ICP and CPP to determine appropriate cerebral blood flow. Alterations in oxygen and carbon dioxide affect the cranial blood flow differently (Table 10–16).

G. Physical assessment
   1. Blood pressure, pulse, respirations
      a. Closely monitor blood pressure and pulse. A low BP and an increased pulse are more associated with shock, whereas a high BP and a decreased or increased pulse with slow or irregular respirations is associated with increased ICP.
      b. Changes in BP alter ICP (Table 10–17)
   2. Neurological exam (these signs may lag behind swelling of the brain).
      a. Assess the child's alertness, orientation, and memory.
      b. Perform an evaluation with the Glasgow Coma Scale (Table 10–18).
      c. An indication of increased ICP with the Glasgow Coma Scale is less than 5.
      d. A CT scan or MRI should be done.

TABLE 10–16. ***Effect of Oxygen and Carbon Dioxide on Cerebral Blood Flow***

| Oxygen | Carbon Dioxide |
|---|---|
| $PaO_2$ <60 mm Hg causes vasodilation, increases cerebral blood flow. Helps prevent ischemia.<br>$PaO_2$ >60 mm Hg reduces cerebral blood flow, reduces intracranial pressure. With increased ICP, keep $PaO_2$ >100 mm Hg. | $PaCO_2$ >45 mm Hg causes vasodilation. Increases in $PaCO_2$, increase cerebral blood flow.<br>$PaCO_2$ <30 mm Hg causes vasoconstriction, reducing cerebral blood flow. Optimal $PaCO_2$ to reduce ICP is 25–27 mm Hg. Greater potential of brain ischemia when $PaCO_2$ <22 mm Hg. |

TABLE 10–17. *Changes in Intracranial Pressure by Blood Pressure*

| Acutely increased blood pressure | Acutely decreased BP |
|---|---|
| ↓ | ↓ |
| Increases cerebral blood flow from increased pressure and edema. | Decreased in blow flow. |
| ↓ | ↓ |
| This increases intracranial pressure. | Decreased cerebral perfusion pressure. |
| | ↓ |
| | Increased hypoxia, hypercarbia, and acidosis. |
| | ↓ |
| | Increased intracranial pressure. |

3. Ophthalmologic assessment
   a. Size of pupils
   b. Position of pupils
   c. Doll's-head maneuver—If no neck injury is present, move the head to the left. Eyes should move to the right. If this does not occur, this may indicate brain stem dysfunction.
   d. Caloric stimulation—In a comatose patient with the head elevated 30°, the auditory channel is irrigated with 5 mL of ice water. With normal brain stem function, the eyes move toward the irrigated ear.
4. Deep pain response—No response to pain indicates lack of brain stem function.
5. Other assessments
   a. Headache
   b. Vomiting
   c. Full fontanelle, separated sutures in infants

H. Treatment
   1. If there is no neck injury, keep the head of bed elevated 30°, which will help cerebral drainage. Place the patient in a supine position if there is a neck injury or if the patient is in shock. Also, the eyes-forward head position allows jugular venous drainage. Turning the head may compress the jugular vein.
   2. No internal jugular venous catheter
   3. Hyperventilation and hyperoxygenation
      a. No PEEP during acute stages
      b. Tidal volume (7 to 10 mL/kg)
      c. Maintain a high minute ventilation (by respiratory rate) to keep $PaCO_2$ at 25 to 27 mm Hg and pH alkalotic. Maintain $PaO_2$ at greater than 100 mm Hg.
      d. An inability to reduce ICP with passive hyperventilation usually indicates a grave prognosis.
   4. Perform minimal suctioning and hyperventilate prior to suctioning. May give lidocaine down ETT to prevent coughing and Valsalva maneuver.
   5. Perform manual hyperventilation as needed when ICP is greater than 20 mm Hg.
   6. Osmotic diuretic mannitol reduces brain water by remaining in plasma and creating an osmotic gradient. It also reduces the formation of CSF. Administer when the ICP is greater than 20 mm Hg. Monitor fluid and electrolyte balance.
   7. Paralysis and sedation
   8. Reduce IV fluids to one-half to one-third maintenance.
   9. Keep BP normal, CVP low normal, and normal electrolytes.

TABLE 10–18. *Glasgow Coma Scale*

| **Best Motor Response** | **Score** | **Best Verbal Response** | **Score** | **Eye Opening** | **Score** |
|---|---|---|---|---|---|
| Obeys | 6 | Oriented | 5 | Spontaneous | 4 |
| Localizes pain | 5 | Confused conversation | 4 | To speech | 3 |
| Withdraws | 4 | Inappropriate words | 3 | To pain | 2 |
| Flexion to pain | 3 | Incomprehensible sounds | 2 | No response | 1 |
| Extension to pain | 2 | No response | 1 | | |
| No response | 1 | | | | |

10. Keep patient hypothermic (27 to 31°C).
11. The patient may benefit from barbiturate coma using phenobarbital to reduce cerebral edema and oxygen consumption.
12. Use phenytoin sodium (Dilantin) for seizures. Useful because of rapid brain entrance.
13. No percussion, vibration, and postural drainage.

**X. Neuromuscular disease and central nervous system disorders**

A. Guillain-Barré syndrome (acute infectious polyneuritis)
   1. General
      a. Inflammatory disease of the cranial nerves resulting in damage to myelin sheath
      b. Etiology unknown; likely mediated by immune system
      c. Can affect all ages
      d. Low mortality rate with early intervention
   2. Clinical manifestations
      a. Antecedent infection or vaccination seen in more than 65% is usually a viral infection (URI or GI tract).
      b. Progressive, symmetrical, ascending, with flaccid motor weakness
      c. Frequently associated with pain and paresthesia
      d. Respiratory failure occurs in 10 to 25%.
      e. Autonomic nervous system dysfunction:
         (1) Cardiac dysrhythmia
         (2) Orthostatic hypotension
         (3) Bladder dysfunction
   3. Diagnosis.
      a. CSF protein elevated
      b. Usually normal CSF pressure
      c. Must differentiate from other CNS disorders including poliomyelitis, tick paralysis, infantile botulism, and myasthenia gravis.
   4. Treatment
      a. Supportive care to prevent skin breakdown, pneumonia, urinary tract infection, and so on.
      b. Daily vital capacity (VC) measurements to determine need for mechanical support (normal VC = 40 to 65 mL/kg):
         (1) If VC = 30 to 45 mL/kg (cough reflex is decreased), treatment intervention is to cough and deep breathe.
         (2) If VC = less than 20 mL/kg, intubation should be performed.
      c. Monitor for and treat autonomic imbalance responses, especially cardiac dysrhythmia.
      d. Steroids are not indicated.
   5. Outcome
      a. Variable length of illness and outcome
      b. Recovery may take as long as 2 years.
      c. 50% have residual deficits, including weakness, sensory deficits, and absent reflexes.

B. Myasthenia gravis
   1. General
      a. Spectrum of disorders resulting from abnormal postsynaptic neuromuscular transmission.
      b. Average onset: 8 years of age
      c. Female-to-male prevalence (2:1)
   2. Clinical manifestations
      a. Descending paralysis with unequal involvement of muscle groups
      b. Slow, progressive course with relapses and remissions
      c. Early presentation: 60% ocular weakness, 40% generalized weakness
   3. Etiology
      a. May be an acquired autoimmune form or congenital.
      b. Acquired form (most common)—Results from decrease in number of acetylcholine receptors at the postsynaptic junction.
   4. Diagnosis
      a. Differentiate from numerous other neuromuscular disorders, including botulism, poisoning, sepsis, poliomyelitis, Guillain-Barré syndrome.
      b. Positive Tensilon test
         (1) Tensilon (edrophonium), an anticholinesterase, transiently improves quality at neuromuscular transmission.
         (2) Careful, objective observation required

5. Treatment
   a. Anticholinesterase therapy (neostigmine [Prostigmin] or pyridostigmine [Mestinon])
   b. Steroids
   c. Plasmapheresis
   d. Ventilatory support as necessary

## XI. Near-drowning and drowning (hypoxic encephalopathy)

A. General
   1. Second most common cause of accidental death in children (motor vehicle accident is No. 1)
   2. Common age group is 0 to 4 years of age.

B. Pathophysiology.
   1. Extremely variable outcome and pathophysiology dependent on the following:
      a. Patient condition prior to submersion
      b. Composition of water (salt, fresh, brackish)—not as important as previously thought; infection content of aspirated water is of more concern.
      c. Water temperature
   2. Pulmonary disease
      a. Large intrapulmonary shunt
      b. Change in surfactant properties (decreased compliance)
      c. Pulmonary edema
         (1) Noncardiogenic (neurogenic) pulmonary edema; caused by laryngeal spasm and increased intrathoracic pressure
         (2) Aspiration of salt water
   3. Cardiovascular changes caused by hypoxia and acid-base imbalance.
   4. CNS disease
      a. Increased ICP secondary to hypoxia (hypoxic encephalopathy)
      b. 10% of drowning victims die of acute asphyxia rather than sequelae of aspiration.
   5. Normal or near-normal serum electrolytes

C. Treatment
   1. Immediate cardiopulmonary resuscitative efforts
   2. Treat dysrhythmia
   3. Oxygen
   4. PEEP or CPAP
   5. Airway protection (risk of aspirating large quantities of water)
   6. Sodium bicarbonate ($NaHCO_3$) as needed to correct metabolic acidosis
   7. Mechanical ventilation (restore blood gas tension)
   8. If high ICP, hyperventilate ($PaCO_2$ of 25 to 27 mm Hg) to decrease ICP to less than 20 mm Hg.
   9. Bronchodilator therapy
   10. Fluid administration
   11. Monitor ABG, hematocrit (HCT), pulse (HR), respiratory rate (RR), BP, and temperature closely.
   12. Corticosteroids are of questionable benefit
   13. Antibiotics if sputum culture is positive for bacterial growth

D. Outcomes
   1. Variable outcome related to severity of hypoxic insult
   2. Mortality rates are 5 to 20%.
   3. Neurological sequelae variable
   4. Possible respiratory sequelae; airway hyperreactivity

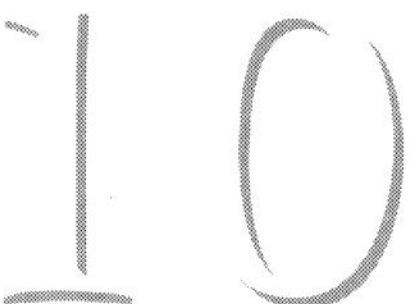

# REVIEW QUESTIONS

1. What infant age group has the highest risk for foreign body aspiration?

2. What is the difference in patient presentation between tracheomalacia and laryngomalacia?

3. In the accompanying table, fill in three signs and/or symptoms of foreign body enlodgement.

| Larynx | Trachea | Brochus | Esophagus |
|---|---|---|---|
| | | | |

4. Fill in the accompanying table comparing croup to epiglottitis.

| | Viral Croup | Epiglottitis |
|---|---|---|
| History | | |
| Organism | | |
| Presentation | | |
| Physical examination | | |
| Radiologic finding | | |
| Diagnosis | | |
| Treatment | | |

5. Place a **Y** for yes or **N** for no next to the indicator that suggests asthma in a child.

   a. _____ Cough present especially at night.

   b. _____ Peak expiratory flowrate that varies less than 20% from PEF measurement in the morning before a short-acting beta-2 agonist.

c. _____ Worsening symptoms when associated with exercise.

d. _____ Tightness in the chest and wheezing on exhalation.

6. What is the difference in PEF between step 2 Mild Persistent and step 3 Moderate Persistent?

7. Describe how you would instruct the parent of a child with asthma being discharged on determining the child's best PEF.

8. How would you instruct the same child in question 7 in performing a PEF maneuver?

9. Give four reasons why, when a child is performing a PEF maneuver, there may be inaccuracies in the value obtained.

   a.

   b.

   c.

   d.

10. Place an **R** for reliever and **C** for controller next to the medication used in the management of asthma.

    a. ______ Ipratropium bromide

    b. ______ Beclomethasone dipropionate

    c. ______ Albuterol

    d. ______ Nedocromil sodium

    e. ______ Cromolyn sodium

    f. ______ Terbutaline

    g. ______ Salmeterol xinafoate

11. What type of reliever or controller should be used for quick relief for a 7-year-old who has been classified as having moderate persistent asthma?

12. Place the correct letter next to the symptom, sign, or functional assessment to indicate if it is classified as mild, moderate, or severe exacerbation of asthma.

| | |
|---|---|
| a. Mild | _____ Patient talks in words. |
| b. Moderate | _____ Wheeze is moderate, often only end expiration. |
| c. Severe | _____ Pulsus paradoxus often present >20 to 40 mm Hg. |
| | _____ PEF% <50% |
| | _____ While walking, the child experiences breathlessness. |

13. Describe the difference between a good response and a poor response after taking three treatments of 2 to 4 puffs albuterol MDI.

| **Good Response** | **Poor Response** |
|---|---|

14. In the emergency department, what is included in the initial assessment of an asthmatic patient with exacerbation?

15. What would indicate the need to admit an asthmatic patient with exacerbation to the ICU?

16. Describe how an aerosol can be administered in line to a patient receiving volume-cycled and pressure-limited, time-cycled ventilation.

17. An asthmatic patient with exacerbation on mechanical ventilation is discovered to have auto-PEEP present. List three methods to remove auto-PEEP.

    a.

    b.

    c.

18. What are two indications that the bronchospasm is reversing in an asthmatic patient with exacerbation on mechanical ventilation?

    a

    b.

19. Fill in the accompanying table concerning bronchiolitis.

| | |
|---|---|
| Age | |
| Causative agent | |
| How is the agent spread? | |
| Signs and symptoms | |
| Chest radiograph | |
| Management | |
| Indications for ribavirin | |

20. Describe how altered cell function in cystic fibrosis causes thick secretions.

21. List the clinical presentations associated with each age group of children with cystic fibrosis.

    a. Newborn to 1 year

    b. Children (more than 1 year of age)

    c. Adolescence (more than 12 years of age)

22. What aerosolized antibiotics are used to treat cystic fibrosis?

23. What diagnostic test is used for cystic fibrosis?

24. Describe how a person should be instructed in the use of positive expiratory pressure (PEP) therapy.

25. What should be done if the patient complains of fatigue while performing PEP therapy and achieving 20 cm $H_2O$?

26. List the differences in pathological changes between acute, subacute, and chronic phases of ARDS.

    a. Acute

b. Subacute

c. Chronic

27. Fill in the ventilator settings that would be indicated for a child just intubated because of worsening symptoms of ARDS.

a. Tidal volume

b. SIMV rate

c. Inspiratory time

d. Expiratory time

e. PEEP level

f. PSV

g. $FIO_2$

28. Fill in the accompanying table concerning types of head trauma.

| | Description | Clinical Manifestations |
|---|---|---|
| Extracranial | | |
| Skull fracture | | |
| Intracranial | | |
| Mild | | |
| Severe | | |

29. What is the normal intracranial pressure (ICP)?

30. Describe the changes in ICP that occur with alterations in blood pressure?

| Increased Blood Pressure | Decreased Blood Pressure |
|---|---|
| | |

31. What three evaluations are used in the Glasgow Coma Scale?

a.

b.

c.

32. In the accompanying table, fill in the ventilator settings and ABGs that are used to reduce ICP associated with head trauma.

| | |
|---|---|
| Tidal volume (mL) | |
| Rate (bpm) | |
| PEEP (cm $H_2O$) | |
| $FIO_2$ | |
| $PaCO_2$ (mm Hg) | |
| pH | |

33. What ICP value should be the goal for a child on mechanical ventilation from head trauma?

34. Fill in the accompanying table for Guillain-Barré syndrome and myasthenia gravis.

| | **Guillain-Barré Syndrome** | **Myasthenia Gravis** |
|---|---|---|
| Description | | |
| Clinical manifestations | | |
| Diagnosis | | |
| Indication for intubation | | |
| Treatment | | |

35. Describe the pathophysiology of near-drowning.

36. What happens to ICP because of hypoxia in near-drowning victims?

## BIBLIOGRAPHY


App, E., et al. (1990). Acute and long term amiloride inhalation in cystic fibrosis lung disease. *American Review of Respiratory Diseases* 141:605.

American Association for Respiratory Care Clinical Practice Guideline. (1993): Use of positive airway pressure adjuncts to bronchial hygiene therapy. *Respiratory Care* 38:516.

Borowitz, D. (1994). Pathophysiology of gastrointestinal complications of cystic fibrosis. *Seminars in Respiratory and Critical Care Medicine* 15:391.

Burgess, W. R., and Chernick, V. (1986). *Respiratory Therapy in Newborn, Infants and Children*, ed 2. New York: Thieme-Stratton.

Burke, W., and Aitken, M. (1994). The aging cystic fibrosis patient: Presentations and problems. *Seminars in Respiratory and Critical Care Medicine* 15:383.

Busse, W. (1994). The role of respiratory infections in airway hyperresponsiveness and asthma. *American Journal of Diseases in Children* 150:577.

Coutelle, C., et al. (1993): Gene therapy for cystic fibrosis (annotations). *American Journal of Diseases in Children* 68:457.

Cunningham, J.C., and Taussig, L.M. *An Introduction to Cystic Fibrosis for Patients and Families.* Bethesda, MD: Cystic Fibrosis Foundation.

Facts and Comparisons. (1996). *Drug Newsletter* 15:17.

Fiel, S., FitzSimmons, S., and Schidlow, D. (1994). Evolving demographics cystic fibrosis. *Seminars in Respiratory and Critical Care Medicine* 15:349.

Gregory, G. A. (1981). *Respiratory Failure in the Child.* New York: Churchill Livingstone.

Goren, A., et al. (1994). Assessment of the ability of young children to use a powder inhaler device. *Pediatric Pulmonology* 18:77.

Harwood, R. (1990). Respiratory disorders of the pediatric patient. In Kacmarek, R., Mack, C., and Dimas, S. (Eds.) *The Essentials of Respiratory Care*, ed 3. St. Louis: Mosby–Year Book.

Holroyd, H. (1988): Foreign body aspiration: Potential cause of coughing and wheezing. *Pediatrics in Review* 10:59.

Hoffman, G., and Cohen, N. (1993). Positive expiratory pressure therapy. *NBRC Horizons* 19:1–3.

Kallstrom, T. J. (1997). Excerpts from *Expert Panel Report II: Guidelines for the Diagnosis and Management of Asthma. Respiratory Care* 42(5):499.

Kenna, M., and Bluestone, C. (1988). Foreign bodies in the air and food passages. *Pediatrics in Review* 10:25.

Littlewood, J. M., Smye, S. W., and Cunliffe, H. (1993). Aerosol antibiotic treatment in cystic fibrosis. *American Journal of Diseases in Children* 68:788.

Laks, Y., and Barzilay, Z. (1988): Foreign body aspiration in childhood. *Pediatric Emergency Care* 4:102.

Morray, J. R. (1987). *Pediatric Intensive Care.* Norwalk, Connecticut: Appleton & Lange.

Mahlmeister, M., et al. (1991). Positive-expiratory-pressure mask therapy: Theoretical and practical considerations and a review of the literature. *Respiratory Care* 36:1218.

MacDonnel, K. F., Fahey, P. J., and Segal, M. S. (1987). *Respiratory Intensive Care.* Boston: Little, Brown and Company.

Marshall, B. (1994): Pathophysiology of pulmonary disease in cystic fibrosis. *Seminars in Respiratory and Critical Care Medicine* 15:364.

Marshall, S., and Ramsey, B. (1994). Aerosol therapy in cystic fibrosis: rhDNase and tobramycin. *Seminars in Respiratory and Critical Care Medicine* 15:434.

McIntosh, K. (1987). Respiratory syncytial virus: Infections in infants and children: Diagnosis and treatment. *Pediatrics in Review* 9:191.

McMillan, J., et al. (1988). Prediction of the duration of hospitalization in patients with respiratory syncytial virus infection: Use of clinical parameters. *Pediatrics* 81:22.

Meissner, C. H. (1994): Prophylaxis and treatment of respiratory syncytial virus infection in high-risk infants. *Neonatal Respiratory Diseases* 4:1.

Morbidity and Mortality Weekly. (1997). Newborn screening for cystic fibrosis: A paradigm for Public Health genetics. Policy Development. Proceedings of a 1997 workshop. Atlanta: US Department of Health and Human Services, CDC.

Mylett, J., Johnson, L., and Knowles, M. (1994). Alternate therapies for cystic fibrosis. *Seminars in Respiratory and Critical Care Seminars* 15:426.

National Asthma Education & Prevention Program. Expert Panel Report. (1991). *Guidelines for the Diagnosis and Management of Asthma.* Washington, D.C.: NHLBI.

National Asthma Education & Prevention Program. Expert Panel Report II. (1997). *Guidelines for the Diagnosis and Management of Asthma.* Washington, D.C.: NHLBI.

Pollack-Latham, C. (1987). Intracranial pressure monitoring: Part I. Physiologic principles. *Critical Care Nurse* 7:40.

Rau, J. L. (1998). *Respiratory Care Pharmacology,* ed 5. St. Louis: Mosby–Year Book.

Roberts, M. (1987): *Textbook of Pediatric Intensive Car,* Vol. 1. Baltimore: Williams & Wilkins.

Rosenstein, B. (1994). Cystic fibrosis in the year 2000. *Seminars in Respiratory and Critical Care Medicine* 15:446.

Santer, D. M., and D'Alessandro, M. P. (1997, February 23). *ElectricAirway: Upper airway problems in children* [WWW document]. URL http//www.vh.org/Providers/Textbooks/ElectricAirway/Text/TracheoLaryngo.html

Santer, D. M., and D'Alessandro, M. P. (1997, February 23). *ElectricAirway: Table of characteristics of croup syndromes* [WWW document]. URL http//www.vh.org/Providers/Textbooks/ElectricAirway/TableText/TableCharCroupSynd.html

Santer D. M., and D'Alessandro, M. P. (1997, February 23). *ElectricAirway: Table of characteristics of viral croup and acute epiglottitis* [WWW document]. URL http//www.vh.org/Providers/Textbooks/ElectricAirway/TableText/TableCharCroupepi.html

Tamm, M., and Higenbottam, T. (1994). Heart-lung and lung transplantation for cystic fibrosis: World experience. *Seminars in Respiratory and Critical Care Medicine* 15:414.

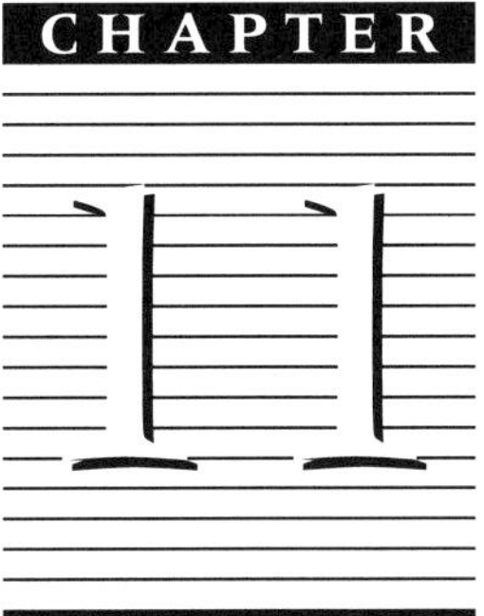


# Airway Management

**I. Causes of airway obstruction**
- A. Tongue
- B. Secretions
- C. Laryngospasm
- D. Foreign bodies

**II. Clinical indication of airway obstruction**
- A. Partial airway obstruction
  1. Stridor
  2. Poor air movement
  3. Faint or absent breath sounds
  4. Mild sternal and clavicular retractions
  5. Weak cry, ineffective cough
- B. Complete airway obstruction
  1. Marked inspiratory effort
  2. No air movement
  3. Marked sternal, intercostal, and epigastric retractions
  4. Cyanosis
  5. Unconsciousness

**III. Maneuvers to open the airway**
- A. Head tilt–chin lift maneuver
  1. Quickest method to establish a patent airway: Place one hand on the forehead and lift the chin with the other.
- B. Jaw thrust or triple airway maneuver
  1. Kneeling behind the person, place both hands on either side of the jaw and lift upward. This will pull the tongue away from the posterior pharynx. This method is also used instead of the head tilt–chin lift maneuver for infants and children with neck injuries requiring an open airway.
- C. Chin lift or mandibular displacement
  1. One hand is placed on the forehead. The other hand grabs the chin with the thumb placed behind the lower teeth and the chin is lifted upward. This is not recommended in conscious infants and children.
- D. With each maneuver, after opening the airway, the infant or child is assessed for breathing by looking, listening, and feeling for air movement.

**IV. Infant and child cardiopulmonary resuscitation**
- A. Indications
  1. Cardiac arrest, respiratory arrest, or the presence of conditions that may lead to cardiopulmonary arrest by rapid deterioration in vital signs, level of consciousness, and blood gas values
  2. Conditions
     - a. Partial or complete airway obstruction
     - b. Severe infections
     - c. Instability of the heart
     - d. Spinal cord or head injury
     - e. Drug overdose
     - f. Smoke inhalation
  3. Contraindications
     - a. The parent's desire not to have the infant or child resuscitated has been clearly expressed and documented.

b. Resuscitation has been determined to be futile because of the patient's underlying disease or condition.
4. Precautions and hazards
   a. Airway management, including failure to establish a patent airway, failure to intubate the trachea, intubation of the esophagus, aspiration, and problems with the endotracheal tube
   b. Ventilation, including inadequate delivery of oxygen, hypoventilation and/or hyperventilation, barotrauma, prolonged interruption of ventilation, and reduced venous return from high mean airway pressure
   c. Circulation, including ineffective chest compressions, fractured ribs, hypovolemia, pneumothorax, hemothorax, hypoxia, acidosis, and hypothermia
   d. Electrical therapy, including failure to defibrillate and inappropriate countershock
   e. Drug administration, including inappropriate drug or dose, allergic response to drug, or failure to deliver appropriate drug dose down the endotracheal tube (this volume should be 2 to 2.5 times the normal IV dose or intraosseous dose diluted with 10 mL of normal saline or distilled water)
5. CPR is needed when there is absence of spontaneous breathing and/or circulation due to arrest.
6. Equipment
   a. Ventilation devices, including mouth-to-mask and manual resuscitator
   b. Circulation device
   c. Airway management devices, including pharyngeal airways, endotracheal tubes, laryngoscope handle and blades, stylet, forceps, fiberoptic laryngoscope, and bronchoscope
   d. Suctioning devices
   e. Defibrillator
   f. ECG monitor
   g. $CO_2$ monitor
   h. Ventilation monitors
   i. Pulse oximeter
   j. Airway pressure monitoring
   k. Invasive cardiac monitoring devices
7. Monitoring the patient
   a. Continuous observation to assess level of consciousness, adequacy of ventilation, peripheral and apical pulse, evidence of chest and head trauma, pulmonary compliance and airway resistance, and presence of seizure activity
   b. Physiological assessment including hemodynamic data, cardiac rhythm, ventilatory rate, tidal volume and airway pressure, exhaled $CO_2$, and neurological status
8. Infant and child one-rescuer CPR (Table 11–1)

B. Infant and child foreign body airway obstruction (Table 11–2)

**V. Pharyngeal airways**

A. Oropharyngeal airway
   1. A curved airway used to insert over the tongue of an unconscious infant or child
   2. A properly placed oropharyngeal airway keeps the tongue from obstructing the posterior pharynx. It can also be used as a bite block and to facilitate oral suctioning.
   3. The proper size is determined by measuring the airway from the angle of the jaw to the lips.
   4. After inserting the airway, assess for airway patency by listening for air movement at the mouth. If no air movement is heard, remove the airway and reinsert it. A small airway will push the tongue posteriorly, causing obstruction. A large oropharyngeal airway will also obstruct the airway by obstructing the larynx.
   5. If the infant or child begins to awaken and gag, the airway should be removed.

B. Nasopharyngeal airway
   1. This is a soft, curved tube that is inserted into the nares to provide a channel of airflow between the tongue and the posterior pharynx. This device is used in conscious infants and children. The device also provides an avenue for nasotracheal suctioning.
   2. The proper length is determined by measuring from the nose to the tragus of the ear.

TABLE 11–1. *Infant and Child One-Rescuer CPR*

| Infant CPR | Child CPR |
|---|---|
| Establish unresponsiveness (activate EMS if second rescuer available). Respiratory arrest from hypoxemia more common than cardiac arrest. If the infant is lying on stomach, turn over as one unit. | Establish unresponsiveness (activate the EMS if second rescuer available). If the child is lying on stomach, turn over as one unit. |
| Open the airway with head tilt–chin lift or jaw thrust. Assess breathing by look, listen, and feel. | Open the airway with head tilt–chin lift or jaw thrust. Assess breathing by look, listen, and feel. |
| If not breathing, give *2 rescue breaths* by placing the rescuer's mouth over the infant's mouth and nose. | If not breathing, give *2 rescue breaths*, allowing for exhalation between breaths. |
| *Check brachial pulse.* If pulse is present but infant is apneic, provide breathing at a rate of 20 bpm. | *Check carotid pulse.* If pulse present but child is apneic, provide breathing at a rate of 20 bpm. |
| If no pulse, begin compressions at a rate of 100 compressions/min. One breath is interposed every 5 compressions. | If no pulse begin chest compressions at a rate of 100 compressions/minute. One breath is interposed every 5 compressions. |
| After 1 min, recheck pulse. No pulse, continue CPR. If pulse returns but patient is apneic, continue rescue breathing at a rate of 20 bpm. When breathing resumes, place infant in a recovery position. | After 1 min, recheck pulse. If no pulse, continue CPR. If pulse returns but patient remains apneic, continue rescue breathing at a rate of 20 bpm. When breathing resumes, place the child in a recovery position. |

(Adapted from American Heart Association, pp. 6–11, 1994.)

TABLE 11–2. *Infant and Child Foreign Body Airway Obstruction—Conscious and Unconscious*

| Infant Foreign Body Obstruction—Conscious | Child Foreign Body Obstruction—Conscious |
|---|---|
| 1. Assess the infant for complete airway obstruction. Look for respiratory movements without air movement, no serious cry.<br>2. Once obstruction is confirmed, give 5 back blows and then 5 chest thrusts. This is continued until the object is expelled or the infant becomes unconscious.<br>3. If the infant becomes unconscious, open the mouth with a tongue-jaw lift and look inside the infant's mouth. If the object is seen, perform a finger sweep to remove it.<br>4. Open the airway and try to ventilate. If still obstructed, reposition the infant's head and ventilate again. If still obstructed, give 5 back blows and 5 chest thrusts. Continue with this sequence (3 and 4) until the object is removed. | 1. Assess the child for obstruction. Ask "Are you choking?"<br>2. Give abdominal thrusts. Repeat abdominal thrusts until the object is expelled or the child becomes unconscious.<br>3. If the child becomes unconscious, perform a tongue-jaw lift and look into the mouth of the child. If the object is seen, perform a finger sweep to remove it.<br>4. Open the airway and try to ventilate. If the child is obstructed, reposition the head and ventilate again. If still obstructed, give 5 abdominal thrusts. Continue this sequence (3 and 4) until the object is removed. |
| **Infant Foreign Body Obstruction—Infant Found Unconscious** | **Child Foreign Body Obstruction—Child Found Unconscious** |
| 1. Establish unresponsiveness.<br>2. Open airway and try to ventilate. If still obstructed and no air enters the lungs, reposition the head and ventilate again.<br>3. If obstruction is still present, perform a tongue-jaw lift. Look into the mouth of the infant. If the object is seen, perform a finger sweep to remove it.<br>4. If the object is not seen, perform 5 back blows and 5 chest thrusts. Continue with this sequence (3 and 4) until the object is removed. | 1. Establish unresponsiveness.<br>2. Open the airway and try to ventilate. If no air enters the lungs and the child is still obstructed, reposition the head and ventilate again.<br>3. If obstruction is still present, perform a tongue-jaw lift and look into the child's mouth. If the object is seen, perform a finger sweep to remove it.<br>4. If the object is not seen, perform abdominal thrusts. Continue with this sequence (3 and 4) until the object is removed. |

(Adapted from the American Heart Association, pp. 6–11, 1994.)

3. The device should be well lubricated to ease insertion and reduce bleeding. After insertion, assess the infant for airflow by listening for air to pass through the device.
4. Assess the external nares where the device comes into contact with skin to ensure blood flow. Blanching of the skin indicates reduced blood flow. Alternating nares will help reduce this problem.

**VI. Resuscitation devices**

A. Mouth-to-mask device
   1. This device consists of a one-way valve, an oxygen nipple for supplemental oxygen, and a transparent mask with a soft transparent cuff. A filter can be placed between the one-way valve and mouthpiece.
   2. The mask is placed over the nose and mouth in a manner similar to a mask attached to a resuscitation bag. The mask is held in place by placing four fingers along the angle of the jaw and the thumbs on either side of the mask. The mandible is lifted to open the airway.
   3. As a breath is delivered through the device monitor, watch the patient's chest to ensure adequate rise. If the chest does not rise adequately, increase the breath volume delivered.
   4. Oxygen flow rate can be assessed by pulse oximetry. If oxygen is not used, the inlet should be plugged to prevent leakage of gas.

B. Bag-valve resuscitators
   1. Bag volume for children ranges from 0.2 to 0.9 L. According to the American Heart Association (AHA), a bag volume of 250 to 750 mL should be used.
   2. Infants' and children's tidal volume should be 7 to 10 mL/kg of body weight. Tidal volume delivery for child resuscitators is 70 to 300 mL and for infants is 20 to 70 mL.
   3. Bag-valve devices may be flow-inflating (see Chapter 4) and self-inflating. Generally, these devices do not use a humidifier for short-term resuscitation.
   4. The self-inflating bag without a reservoir bag can deliver from 30 to 80% oxygen at 10 L/min oxygen flow rate. With an oxygen reservoir and oxygen flow rate at 10 to 15 L/min, the oxygen delivery will be 60 to 90%. The oxygen reservoir should contain a larger volume than the resuscitation bag.
   5. Infant and child resuscitation bags may be equipped with a pressure-limited pop-off valve. This is set to release pressure at 35 to 40 cm $H_2O$. Some infants may require higher delivery pressures because of noncompliant lungs or the need for larger tidal volumes. This valve may be occluded by pressing down on the valve during inspiration. The delivery of pressure should be monitored with a pressure gauge attached to the resuscitator and observation of chest rise.
   6. To maintain positive end-expiratory pressure (PEEP), a PEEP device can be attached to the exhalation port of some resuscitators. The resuscitator with PEEP device should not be used to administer continuous positive airway pressure (CPAP) because of the increased work of breathing to open the outlet valve.
   7. Often changes in compliance of the lungs can be determined by the resistance felt by the operator during resuscitation. This may be a result of pneumothorax, right main-stem intubation, obstructed endotracheal tube, or air trapping as seen with meconium aspiration syndrome.
   8. Troubleshooting
      a. If the patient's oxygen saturation does not rise after delivering breaths with the resuscitation bag, check the oxygen connecting tube to ensure that it is connected to the bag and/or flowmeter. Also ensure that the oxygen reservoir bag is connected to the resuscitation bag and has oxygen flowing into it. The reservoir bag should be completely inflated with oxygen.
      b. If no resistance is felt while delivering a breath or no breath is delivered, check to ensure that there is a one-way valve present in the device. Placing the operator's hand over the patient outlet and squeezing the bag should prevent air from being delivered if a one-way valve is present.
      c. If there is inadequate tidal volume delivery as seen by inadequate chest rise, then increase the compression to the bag or depress the pressure-relief valve.
   9. During transport, in order to ensure adequate delivery of tidal volume, a spirometer can be attached to the bag. A pulse oximeter will provide constant monitoring of oxygen saturation during transport.

**VII. Suctioning**

A. Oral suctioning
   1. Oral suctioning in the older infant and child is accomplished by use of a tonsillar tip. This device is directly connected to a suction-regulated device. No

specific suction pressure is required. Change in the level of suction pressure is related to the thickness of secretions.
2. Oral suctioning in the newborn and small infant is performed by using a bulb syringe or small suction catheter.

B. Nasotracheal suctioning
1. Infants and children need nasotracheal suctioning when accumulated secretions, blood, vomitus, and other foreign material cannot be removed by a spontaneous cough. Nasotracheal suctioning may help avoid intubation that was solely intended for the removal of secretions.
2. Indications
   a. Inability to clear secretions
   b. Audible evidence of secretions in the large or central airways that persists in spite of the patient's best cough effort
3. Assessment of need
   a. Auscultation of chest to determine presence of secretions
   b. Assess the adequacy of the patient's cough.
4. Monitoring
   a. The patient should be monitored closely during and after the suctioning procedure. This includes breath sounds, respiratory rate and pattern, pulse rate, presence of bleeding and evidence of trauma to the nose and airway, cough, and oxygen saturation. Use ECG if the equipment is available.
   b. If, during the suctioning procedure, there is any indication of deterioration in vital signs, oxygen saturation, and hemodynamic changes, the procedure should be stopped and oxygen applied until the patient is stable.
5. Assessment of outcome
   a. Improved breath sounds
   b. Removal of secretions

C. Endotracheal suctioning of artificial airway in mechanically ventilated children
1. Indications
   a. Course breath sounds by auscultation or noisy breathing
   b. Secretions seen in the endotracheal tube
   c. Increased inspiratory pressures on a volume-controlled ventilator or decreased tidal volume on a pressure-controlled ventilator
   d. Changes in monitored flow and pressure graphics
   e. Clinically apparent increased work of breathing
   f. Deterioration of arterial blood gases
   g. Radiologic changes consistent with retention of pulmonary secretions
   h. Patient's inability to generate an effective cough
   i. Suspected aspiration of gastric or upper airway secretions
   j. The need to obtain a sputum specimen
   k. Maintain the patency and integrity of the airway
   l. Presence of atelectasis from secretion retention
2. Hazards and complications
   a. Hypoxia/hypoxemia
   b. Cardiac dysrhythmias
   c. Pulmonary hemorrhage or bleeding
   d. Tissue trauma to the tracheal and/or bronchial mucosa
   e. Bronchospasm
   f. Hypertension/hypotension
   g. Interruption of mechanical ventilation
3. Preparation of equipment
   a. Vacuum source with calibrated, adjustable regulator
   b. Collection bottle and connecting tube
   c. Sterile gloves
   d. Goggles, face shield, or other protective eye wear
   e. Appropriate size suction catheter. This is determined by the size the endotracheal tube. The catheter size should be no greater than one-half the internal diameter (ID) of the endotracheal tube (this formula may not apply to smaller endotracheal tubes, since suction catheter size is limited to 5 to 6 French).
      (1) $$\frac{\text{Internal diameter of endotracheal tube (mm)} \times 3}{2} = \text{catheter size in French}$$
      (2) A child requiring a 6-mm ID endotracheal tube will need a 9 French suction catheter.
      (3) Neonatal suction catheter selection is based on gestational age and weight (see Chapter 4).
      (4) A coudé suction catheter is used to selectively suction the left bronchus.

f. Oxygen source and resuscitation bag
g. Stethoscope
h. ECG and pulse oximeter
i. Sterile normal saline
j. Sterile water and cup

4. Suctioning the patient
   a. Patient should receive 100% oxygen for more than 30 s prior to suctioning. This can be delivered by mechanical ventilator or manual ventilation (maintain PEEP levels if PEEP is above 5 cm $H_2O$).
      (1) If a closed suction system is used, the patient can remain on the ventilator to receive oxygen. The patient should be placed on a pulse oximeter to monitor oxygen saturation levels.
      (2) Thick secretions may require instillation of normal saline before suctioning or an increase in the suction pressure (normal suction pressure is 80 to 120 mm Hg, although it should be set as low as possible to effectively remove secretions).
   b. If the suction catheter size causes deterioration in patient status because of obstruction of the endotracheal tube, use the next lower French size.
   c. The duration of the suction catheter in the endotracheal tube should be approximately 10 to 15 s. If the patient does not tolerate this time period, reduce the time. More passes may be required for adequate removal of secretions.
   d. The patient should be oxygenated for over 1 min with 100% oxygen following the suctioning pass.
   e. The duration of suction should be reduced if the patient's heart rate rises, oxygen saturation falls (because of hypoxemia), or heart rate falls (from vagal stimulation). If any of these situations arises, the suction catheter should be removed and oxygen applied to the patient until the heart rate and oxygen saturation return to the presuction level.
5. Monitoring
   a. Breath sounds
   b. Oxygen saturation
   c. Respiratory rate and pattern
   d. Pulse rate
   e. Blood pressure, ECG (if available and required)
   f. Sputum characteristics
   g. Cough effort
   h. Ventilatory parameters
6. Assessment of outcome
   a. Improved breath sounds
   b. Reduced peak inspiratory pressure on a volume-controlled ventilator with narrowing of the positive inspiratory pressure (PIP)–plateau pressure ($P_{plateau}$) or increased dynamic compliance; increased tidal volume in a pressure-limited ventilator
   c. Improvement in arterial blood gases and oxygen saturation by pulse oximeter
   d. Removal of pulmonary secretions

## VIII. Endotracheal intubation

A. Indication
   1. Ventilation
   2. Obstruction
   3. Protection
   4. Suctioning

B. Equipment required for intubation
   1. Laryngoscope handle and blades
   2. Stylet
   3. Appropriate size endotracheal tubes (extra of each size)
   4. Syringe
   5. Forceps
   6. Lubricant
   7. Extra batteries and bulb
   8. Tape or tongue blades
   9. Stethoscope
   10. $CO_2$ detection device
   11. Suction catheters
   12. Saline
   13. Alcohol wipes

C. Straight blades are preferred for infants and children since the larynx is more superior and the epiglottis is more horizontal than in adults.

D. Tube size selection is based on the child's age in years. The appropriate size can be estimated with the following formula:

1. $\dfrac{18 + \text{age (years)}}{4} = \text{ID (mm)}$
2. A 6-year-old child would require a 6.0-mm (ID) endotracheal tube. (An alternative formula substitutes 16 for 18.)
3. This formula applies to uncuffed tubes used in children from 1 year up to 8 years of age. A cuffed tube is used on children over 8 years of age. To determine the appropriate size cuffed endotracheal tube, it is suggested to follow the same formula but to use a tube one-half size smaller than calculated. Some clinicians will use the little finger as a comparison for the proper endotracheal tube size in infants under 1 year of age.
4. The appropriate size cuffless endotracheal tube is one where there is a leak at 20 cm $H_2O$.

E. Prior to intubation, the equipment should be checked to ensure proper function.

1. After attaching the blade to the laryngoscope handle, the bulb should light. If it does not, check the bulb, batteries, and blade contact with the handle. Change the bulb or batteries if needed.
2. The endotracheal tube cuff should be checked to ensure that there is no leak and the pilot balloon functions properly. With the endotracheal tube still in the sterile package, inflate the cuff and squeeze it. If the cuff deflates after squeezing, there is a leak and it should be replaced. The endotracheal tube cuff may also be placed in sterile water. After inflating the cuff, if no bubbles are seen, the cuff does not have a leak.
3. Only endotracheal tubes with high-volume, low-pressure cuffs should be used.

F. Many endotracheal tubes have an indicator line called a vocal cord guide just above the cuff. The tube should be inserted so the vocal cord guide is past the vocal cords. The distance the tube is inserted is determined by the age of the child. The following formula can be used to approximate the distance from the tip of the tube in the midtrachea to the teeth or gums for both oral and nasal endotracheal tubes:

1. Centimeter mark for an oral tube: $\dfrac{12 + \text{age}}{2}$
2. Centimeter mark for a nasal tube: $\dfrac{15 + \text{age}}{2}$
3. For example, for a 10-year-old, the centimeter mark for the oral tube would be 17, and for a nasal endotracheal tube, the centimeter mark would be 20, when positioned at the teeth or gums.

G. Before, during, and after intubation, the patient should be monitored for vital signs, oxygenation, and hemodynamic changes. A baseline for these values should be recorded prior to intubation.

H. Medications to facilitate intubation

1. Sedation and analgesia
   a. Diazepam (Valium)
   b. Midazolam (Versed)
   c. Fentanyl (Sublimaze)
   d. Morphine sulfate
2. Neuromuscular blocking agents
   a. Succinylcholine (drug of choice when rapid intubation is required)
   b. Pancuronium bromide (Pavulon)
   c. Vecuronium (Norcuron)
   d. Atracurium (Tracrium)
   e. *d*-tubocurarine (Curare)
3. Drugs to reverse the side effects of nondepolarizing neuromuscular blocking agents
   a. Neostigmine bromide (Prostigmin)
   b. Atropine sulfate
4. Topical analgesia (useful for nasal intubation)
   a. Lidocaine
5. Topical vasoconstrictor (useful for nasal intubation to reduce blood flow and thus reducing the potential for bleeding)
   a. Phenylephrine (Dristan)

b. Oxymetazoline (Afrin)
6. A sedative should be administered with a neuromuscular blocking agent.
7. Sedation is adequate when the respiratory rate decreases, the patient is resting quietly but is responsive to oral commands, blood pressure decreases, and the patient's speech is slurred. Signs of oversedation include snoring, unresponsiveness, and retractions. The oversedated patient should have the airway opened and maintained either with the head-tilt, chin-lift maneuver or immediate oral intubation.
8. If the patient shows signs of respiratory distress from airway obstruction, the patient should not be sedated, because this may increase the obstruction unless trained personnel are available and prepared to maintain a patent airway.

I. Oral intubation is the preferred route for short-term elective intubation and emergency intubation. The glottic opening is easier to view, and it is less traumatic than nasal intubation.

J. Indications for nasal intubation
1. Poor oral access because of the following:
   a. Seizures
   b. Trauma to mouth
   c. Neck fracture
   d. Prolonged intubation
   e. Surgery

K. Procedure for intubation
1. Obtain equipment.
2. Preoxygenate the patient.
3. Administer appropriate medication.
4. Place the head in the "sniffing position."
5. Insert blade (curved blade inserted into vallecula, straight blade lifts the epiglottis away from the glottis).
6. Insert the tube so the vocal cord guide passes the vocal cords.
7. Remove stylet (if used) and inflate cuff. The cuff is inflated initially until no air leak is heard with manual ventilation. Later, after the procedure is completed, cuff pressure should be measured to obtain a safe pressure.
8. Manually ventilate with oxygen and determine proper tube placement.
9. Stabilize endotracheal tube.

L. Verification of tube placement immediately following intubation
1. Lung sounds heard over trachea and lung apices
2. No breath sounds heard over epigastrium
3. Condensation on tube
4. Bilateral chest expansion
5. End-tidal $CO_2$ concentration over 4%
6. Palpation of the endotracheal tube as it passed into the trachea
7. Tube markings (centimeter marking)
8. Cuff palpation
9. Negative pressure test indicating tracheal tube placement
   a. A negative-pressure device assists in the verification of endotracheal tube placement in the trachea. The device utilizes the anatomical differences between the esophagus and trachea. If the endotracheal tube is in the esophagus, negative pressure applied to the endotracheal tube will pull in the esophageal walls, preventing air return to the device. In this case, vomit may return to the device, clinically indicating that the endotracheal tube is in the esophagus. If air does return to the device, this indicates that the endotracheal tube is in the trachea.
   b. There are two types of negative-pressure devices. One is a bulb device and the other a syringe.
   c. Lack of air return to these devices may indicate disease states that cause increased airway resistance and decreased ability to aspirate air. Also, air return may indicate that the tube is in the pharynx. If in doubt of proper placement, direct laryngoscopy should be performed.
   d. These devices are not recommended for children under 5 years of age or weighing less than 20 kg.

M. Action to take with improper endotracheal tube placement
1. Endobronchial intubation
   a. Signs of right main-stem intubation include asymmetrical chest rise, unequal breath sounds, possibly high inflation pressure with a volume-cycled ventilator, deterioration of vital signs, and desaturation.
   b. Upon these findings, the cuff (if present) is deflated and the endotracheal tube is pulled back until bilateral breath sounds are heard and symmetrical

chest expansion is seen. Improved vital signs, oxygen saturation, and inflating pressures improve if initially affected by the endobronchial intubation.

2. Esophageal intubation
   a. Signs of esophageal intubation include poor or no chest movements, failure to oxygenate with cyanosis developing within a short period after intubation, increasing abdominal distention, desaturation, and end-tidal $CO_2$ pressure near zero following ventilation.
   b. Upon these findings, deflate the cuff (if present), remove the endotracheal tube, manually ventilate and oxygenate the patient until the vital signs are stable, and reintubate with a sterile endotracheal tube.
3. After intubation, a chest radiograph is ordered to confirm proper tube placement. Proper placement of the endotracheal tube is the distance between the clavicles and 1 to 2 cm above the carina.

N. Cuff pressures
   1. Techniques to monitor and measure cuff pressure include minimal leak technique, minimal occluding volume, and direct cuff pressure measurement.
      a. Minimal leak technique requires air to be injected into the cuff until the leak stops. At peak inflation pressure, remove air until there is a small leak around the endotracheal tube. The air pushing up around the cuff will help minimize aspiration of secretions above the cuff.
      b. Minimal occluding volume requires inflation of the cuff until airflow around the cuff is no longer heard during a positive-pressure breath.
      c. Cuff pressure can be directly measured with the use of a cuff measurement device. The pilot balloon is inserted into the nipple adapter of the cuff measurement device. The manometer needle will rise to the level of the cuff pressure. If too much pressure is in the cuff, a pressure-relief device can be pressed to release the appropriate amount of pressure.
      d. An appropriate size endotracheal tube will require between 5 to 10 mL of air for the cuff to seal against the trachea. A small endotracheal tube will require a greater volume of air to seal the cuff against the trachea. Cuff pressure will be very high. In this situation, the tube should be replaced with one of appropriate size. Safe cuff pressures should be kept under 25 cm $H_2O$, or as low as possible.
      e. Document the centimeter mark at the teeth or gums in the patient's chart for future reference in case the tube changes position.

O. Following intubation, a tracheal aspirant should be obtained and the secretions tested for bacteria. Culture and sensitivity tests are performed on the sample and appropriate antibiotics are administered. Sputum is obtained in a culture trap.

P. A nasogastric orogastric tube may be inserted following intubation to remove air from manual ventilation with a mask. The appropriate length is determined by measuring the catheter from the nose to the ear and to the xiphoid process of the patient. Placement of the tip of the tube should be slightly higher than the tube that is placed for feeding. The tip of the tube should be placed just into the beginning of the stomach. If the tube is coiled in the stomach, it should be pulled back to the appropriate position. Three methods of determining proper placement are by aspirating stomach contents, by introducing a syringe to determine sounds of air in the stomach, and by using a radiograph.

Q. Proper humidification is important when bypassing the normal humidifying mechanism. In a spontaneously breathing patient, warm humidified gas between 35 and 37°C should be applied to the endotracheal tube. An appropriate fractional concentration of oxygen ($FIO_2$) should be adjusted according to blood gas values and oxygen saturation.

R. Troubleshooting endotracheal tube problems (Table 11–3)

S. Special endotracheal tubes
   1. Double-lumen endotracheal tube
      a. Several tubes are available for selective endobronchial intubation.
      b. One tube allows cannulation of the left main-stem bronchus. One lumen is labeled tracheal, and the other is labeled bronchial. Each tube has a pilot balloon attached to a cuff.
      c. After intubation, assess for proper placement. The method is similar to that for assessing proper placement of a regular endotracheal tube. If greater breath sounds are heard on the left and diminished to absent breath sounds on the right, then the tube should be assessed for proper placement. Check the centimeter mark on the tube. The tube may be down too far into the left main-stem bronchus, which requires pulling the tube back. Also, if the tube is not inserted far enough, breath sounds may still be reduced or absent on the right as compared to the left lung.

TABLE 11-3. ***Troubleshooting Endotracheal Tube Problems***

| Problem | Cause | Indication | Patient response | Treatment |
|---|---|---|---|---|
| Cuff leak. | Hole in cuff or ruptured cuff. | Spontaneously breathing patient: with manual ventilation leak heard through upper airway. Positive-pressure ventilation: Leak heard through upper airway, loss of volume or pressure with mechanical ventilation. Decreased breath sounds, reduced chest excursion. Pilot balloon will not stay inflated. | Anxiety, unstable hemodynamics, increased respiratory rate, desaturation. | Mechanical ventilation: increased tidal volume or pressure to compensate for this loss until reintubation. |
| | Insufficient air in cuff. | Same as above (except pilot balloon remains inflated). | Same as above. | Inflate cuff until leak stops. Measure cuff pressure. |
| | Leak in pilot balloon assembly. | Same as above. | Same as above. | Clamp line below leak, replace pilot balloon assembly. |
| Kinked endotracheal tube | Excessive length of endotracheal tube outside of mouth. | Spontaneously breathing patient: decreased breath sounds, reduced chest excursion, retractions. Mechanical ventilation: increased PIP, high pressure alarm, low tidal volume alarm sounds, decreased breath sounds, less chest excursion. Increased resistance to manual ventilation. | Anxiety, unstable hemodynamics, increased respiratory rate, desaturation. | After ensuring appropriate placement cut tube and leave 4–5 cm outside of mouth. |
| Obstructed endotracheal tube | Mucous plug from excessive secretions or inappropriate humidity. | Same as for kinked endotracheal tube. | Same as for kinked endotracheal tube. | Instill normal saline into endotracheal tube and suction. |
| | Lack of suctioning | Same as for kinked endotracheal tube. | Same as for kinked endotracheal tube. | Same as above. Provide more consistent suctioning. |
| | Herniated cuff over the end of the endotracheal tube from excessive volume. | Same as for kinked endotracheal tube. | Same as for kinked endotracheal tube. | Remove air from the cuff. If manual ventilator determines the obstruction is removed, inflate cuff with appropriate volume and pressure. |
| | Bevel of tube against the tracheal wall from excessive head and/or neck movement. Tube is not stabilized at the mouth or nose. | Same as for kinked endotracheal tube. | Same as for kinked endotracheal tube. | Deflate cuff and manipulate endotracheal tube. Ensure appropriate depth of insertion. Reinflate cuff and manually ventilate to ensure reduced resistance of airflow through endotracheal tube. |

2. Foam-cuffed (Kamen-Wilkinson) endotracheal tube
   a. An artificial airway that has a foam-filled cuff
   b. There is no pilot balloon because the pilot tube is left open to the atmosphere to allow the cuff to remain inflated. This cuff will expand and deflate with the change in tracheal circumference.
   c. Prior to insertion, the cuff is deflated with a syringe. After insertion, the syringe is disconnected and the cuff expands to the inner diameter of the trachea. If air is inserted, the cuff can become a high-pressure cuff. Insertion of air may be required if ventilating pressures exceed 40 cm $H_2O$. In this situation, it would be necessary to measure cuff pressures.

## IX. Extubation

A. The indication for extubation is when the indication for intubation no longer exists.

B. The procedure for extubation is the same as for oral or nasal endotracheal intubation.
   1. Prepare the equipment, which includes suctioning apparatus, humidification equipment, manual resuscitation bag and mask, small-volume nebulizer, intubation tray, and oxygen.
   2. Explain the procedure to the patient (if appropriate).
   3. Position the patient properly. Newborns and small infants may be extubated while lying supine. Older children may be placed in a semi-Fowler's position.
   4. Suction the endotracheal tube and mouth.
   5. Remove the endotracheal tube fixation device or tape.
   6. Insert a sterile suction catheter down the endotracheal tube. A meconium aspirator device can be used in place of the suction catheter. The endotracheal tube is used as a suction device as the tube is coming out of the patient.
   7. Deflate cuff (if one is present).
   8. Instruct the patient to cough (if age is appropriate), removing tube and suctioning as the tube is removed.
   9. Apply humidification and oxygen to the patient. Newborns may require an oxygen hood or tent with supplemental oxygen to keep the oxygen saturation above 90% and a heated, humidified gas source or a nasal cannula. Older children may require cool, humidified gas and appropriate $FIO_2$ to keep the oxygen saturation above 90%. The $FIO_2$ may be increased from 5 to 10% higher than the patient was receiving prior to extubation.

C. The patient is assessed for any problems following extubation.
   1. Listen to breath sounds for appropriate air movement.
   2. Listen for stridor from laryngospasm or glottic edema.
      a. One method that is used to determine whether a patient will have postextubation stridor is to perform a cuff-leak test. Prior to extubation, the cuff is deflated and the endotracheal tube is occluded in order to determine the presence or absence of a peritubular leak. A leak around the tube will indicate, but not guarantee, that postextubation stridor is unlikely.
   3. Initially, laryngospasm may last a short period of time, requiring no treatment. If it persists, racemic epinephrine treatment can be given. If symptoms become severe, reintubation may be required. A short-acting neuromuscular blocking agent may be helpful and requires controlling the airway with manual ventilation or reintubation.
   4. Children often have subglottic edema and may require reintubation.
   5. Tracheal stenosis develops as a result of the cuff, the endotracheal tube, or the bevel end of the tube rubbing against the tracheal wall. The child does well with the endotracheal tube in place. Upon extubation, the child immediately develops stridor, requiring reintubation. These patients may require a tracheostomy tube.
   6. Prior to extubation, steroids may be given to patients who have failed extubation because of inflammation in the upper airway.
   7. Tracheomalacia results from prolonged intubation related to erosion of the tracheal wall and tracheal cartilage. Diagnosis is made by bronchoscopy during spontaneous ventilation.
   8. Extubation over a bronchoscope is required when there is a possibility of vocal cord paralysis and trauma to glottic and supraglottic structures.

## X. Tracheostomy

A. Indications
   1. Long-term airway management or mechanical ventilation

2. Closing of the airway from acute laryngeal edema
3. Endotracheal tube intolerance because of severe facial or mouth trauma
4. Subglottic stenosis
5. Laryngeal fracture or destruction
6. Tracheomalacia

B. Tracheostomy is performed in an obstructed airway rather than a cricothyrotomy because of the very small cricothyroid membrane. Cutoff age for cricothyrotomy is 10 to 12 years of age.

C. Tracheostomy tubes
1. Neonatal and pediatric tracheostomy tubes do not have an inner cannula. Larger tubes used for older children and adolescent children do have an inner cannula.
2. As with endotracheal tubes, smaller-sized tracheostomy tubes do not have cuffs; therefore, an air leak will be present. It is not suggested to go to a larger tracheostomy tube to eliminate the air leak. A foam-cuffed tracheostomy tube is suggested (see Special Tracheostomy Tubes and Devices later in this chapter).
3. Tracheostomy tubes have a 15- to 22-mm adapter and an obturator to facilitate insertion through the stoma. Tracheostomy tubes with cuffs will have a pilot balloon.
4. The inner cannula can be removed when cleaning the tracheostomy tube. When replacing the inner cannula, ensure that it is locked in place. Dislocation of the inner cannula of a tracheostomy tube attached to a mechanical ventilator will cause a leak, reducing the delivered volume the patient receives.

D. After placement of a tracheostomy tube, the obturator, and extra tracheostomy tube, one of the same size currently in the patient should be placed at the bedside.

E. A newly placed tracheostomy tube should not be changed for the first 4 days to allow the tract to develop. The tracheostomy tube should be secured by ties around the neck and possibly by stay sutures.

F. Complications of tracheotomy
1. Acute
   a. Hemorrhage
   b. Pneumothorax
   c. Subcutaneous emphysema
   d. Secretion plugging
   e. Aspiration
2. Chronic
   a. Infection
   b. Tracheal stenosis
   c. Tracheoesophageal fistula
   d. Tracheomalacia
   e. Aspiration

G. Non–inner-cannula tubes may be replaced on an as-needed basis. If the tube becomes plugged because of thick secretions and the obstruction is not removed with saline instillation and suctioning, the tube should be removed and replaced immediately with a new tube.

H. A short neck or multiple skin folds can occlude the tracheostomy tube. Slight hyperextension of the neck may cause extubation that goes unnoticed until severe hypoxia develops. Carefully monitor and assess infants with short necks and skin folds.

I. The tracheostomy tube position should be assessed for patency by listening for bilateral breath sounds, by checking that air is passing through the tube, and by using a chest radiograph. Movement of the tube to one side or the other can occlude the end and cause obstruction.

J. Special tracheostomy tubes and devices
1. Fenestrated tracheostomy tube
   a. A tracheostomy tube with a hole cut in it. With the inner cannula removed, the patient can breathe through the upper airway. To assess the upper airway, remove the inner cannula, deflate the cuff, and plug the outer cannula.
   b. Care must be taken when plugging this tube to deflate the cuff; otherwise the patient will not be able to breathe through the upper airway. If the patient experiences respiratory distress, remove the plug immediately and check the cuff.
   c. It is suggested that a fenestrated tracheostomy tube not be used with mechanical ventilation.

d. Replace the inner cannula when suctioning a fenestrated tube. This will direct the catheter to the appropriate position in the trachea.
2. Tracheostomy button
    a. This is a short, straight, plastic tube inserted into the stoma that maintains the stoma. It does not occlude the trachea.
    b. Insert the hollow tube. The solid inner cannula is then inserted, causing the flange to be pushed out within the tracheal wall to secure the button.
    c. This device should not be left in place while the patient is sleeping.
3. Tracheostomy talk device
    a. This is a T-tube with a spring-loaded one-way valve that attaches to the tracheostomy tube with a suction cap. Aerosol therapy can be applied by attachment to the T-tube.
    b. During inhalation, the spring-loaded one-way valve remains open to inhalation. During exhalation the one-way valve closes, forcing air and mucus up past the vocal cords. The spring-loaded one-way valve can become clogged with secretions, making the device less sensitive to opening to inhalation. Also, infants and small children may have difficulty opening the spring-loaded one-way valve.
    c. The tracheostomy cuff is deflated when using this device.
    d. Another device, the Passy-Muir Trach Talk, which fits on the tracheostomy tube, has a membrane enclosed in a plastic case. It closes during exhalation and opens during inhalation. Oxygen or humidity devices can be attached directly to this device. Exhaled gas and secretions are directed upward through the vocal cords.
    e. The tracheostomy tube cuff should not be inflated with this device in place.
    f. This device should not be left on during sleep.

K. Troubleshooting cuffed tracheostomy tubes (Table 11–4)
L. Cleaning the tracheostomy (Table 11–5)

## XI. Postural drainage therapy

A. Postural drainage therapy consists of postural drainage, positioning, and turning and is sometimes accompanied by percussion and vibration.
B. Indications
1. Turning
    a. The inability or reluctance of the patient to change body positions because of mechanical ventilation, neuromuscular disease, or drug-induced paralysis
    b. Poor oxygenation associated with position
    c. Potential for atelectasis or patient has atelectasis
    d. Presence of an artificial airway
2. Postural drainage
    a. Presence of atelectasis as a result of mucus plugging
    b. Patients who have a large amount of mucus production and have difficulty clearing secretions
    c. Patients who have retained secretions with artificial airways
    d. Patients who have such diseases as cystic fibrosis, bronchiectasis, or cavitating lung disease
    e. Presence of foreign bodies in airway

C. Contraindications
1. Positioning
    a. Intracranial pressure over 20 mm Hg
    b. Unstable head and neck injury
    c. Active hemorrhage with hemodynamic instability
    d. Spinal injury or surgery
    e. Empyema
    f. Infants and children who are confused or anxious, or who do not tolerate position changes.
    g. The Trendelenburg position is contraindicated in patients with an uncontrolled airway who are at risk for aspiration.
    h. The reverse Trendelenburg position should be avoided in patients who are hypotensive or are receiving vasoactive medication.
2. Percussion and vibration
    a. Tender skin from grafts, surgery, infections, burns, open wounds, or chest tube insertion
    b. Lung contusion
    c. Patient intolerance to procedure
    d. Suspected pulmonary tuberculosis

TABLE 11–4. *Troubleshooting Cuffed Tracheostomy Tubes*

| Symptom | Possible cause | Action |
|---|---|---|
| Large air leak through mouth and nose. | Insufficient air in cuff. | Inflate cuff until leak stops. Measure cuff pressure. |
| | Leak in pilot balloon, pilot balloon line. | Clamp line below leak. Replace pilot balloon and one-way valve. Replace tracheostomy tube. |
| | Tube too small for trachea. | Replace tube. |
| Large air leak coming out of tracheostomy tube. | Inner cannula protruding out of trach tube. Inner cannula not locked in place. | Reinsert inner cannula and lock in place. |
| High-pressure limit alarms on the ventilator. | Mucus obstructing tube. | Instill saline and suction tube. If still obstructed, remove the inner cannula and replace with a disposable cannula. |
| | Cuff herniated over the end of the tube. | Deflate cuff, then reinflate with appropriate volume. Measure cuff pressure. |
| Unable or difficult to pass suction catheter. | Suction catheter too large for tracheostomy. | Obtain appropriate size suction catheter. |
| | Mucus blocking the inner cannula. | Suction tube. Remove inner cannula and replace with disposable cannula. |
| Difficult removal and insertion inner cannula on fenestrated tube. | Ingrowth of tissue through fenestration. | Contact physician. |
| | Kinked outer trach tube. | Change trach tube. |
| Low-pressure limit alarms on the ventilator. | Inner cannula partially out of trachea. | Reinsert inner cannula and lock in place. |
| | Leak in cuff or cuff inflation device. | Inflate cuff until leak stops. If cuff leaks again after a few breaths, change trach tube. Clamp off pilot balloon line below leak and replace pilot balloon and line. If this doesn't stop the leak, replace the tube. |

(Adapted from Mallinckrodt, p. 26, 1996.)

Table 11–5. *Tracheostomy Tube Cleaning Reference Guide*

| | Hydrogen Peroxide (half strength) | Normal Saline | Water Mild Detergent | Alcohol | Boiling | Autoclave ETO/ Gamma | Betadine |
|---|---|---|---|---|---|---|---|
| Inner Cannula | *Yes | Yes | Yes | No | No | No | No |
| Disposable Inner Cannula | No | No | No | No | No | No | No |
| Outer Cannula Cuffless | *Yes | Yes | Yes | No | No | No | No |
| Outer Cannula Cuffed | No | No | No | No | No | No | No |
| DCP | *Yes | Yes | Yes | No | No | No | No |
| DDCP | *Yes | Yes | Yes | No | No | No | No |
| Obturator | *Yes | Yes | Yes | No | No | No | No |

(From Mallinckrodt, p. 23, with permission.)
DCP—decannulation plug; DDCP—disposable decannulation plug.

Table 11–6. ***Hazards and Complications of Postural Drainage Therapy***

| Hazard and Complication | Intervention and Action |
|---|---|
| Hypoxemia | Administer 100% oxygen, stop therapy, and return patient to original resting position. Ensure effective spontaneous ventilation. Avoid hypoxemia in unilateral lung disease by placing the involved lung uppermost with the patient on his or her side. |
| Increased intracranial pressure | Stop therapy and return the patient to the original resting position. Consult physician. |
| Acute hypotension | Stop therapy and return the patient to the original resting position. Consult physician. |
| Pulmonary hemorrhage | Stop therapy and return the patient to the original resting position. Administer oxygen and maintain airway. Consult physician. |
| Vomiting and aspiration | Stop therapy, clear airway, and suction airway and mouth as needed. Administer oxygen and return patient to previous resting position. |
| Bronchospasm | Stop therapy and return patient to previous resting position. Administer oxygen and consult physician. Administer previously ordered bronchodilator. |
| Dysrhythmia | Stop therapy and return patient to previous resting position. Administer oxygen and consult physician. |

e. Recent spinal anesthesia
f. Subcutaneous emphysema
g. Untreated pneumothorax

D. Hazards and complications (Table 11–6)
E. Assessing the need for postural drainage therapy
1. Decreased breath sounds with sounds suggesting secretions in airways
2. Sputum production excessive
3. Cough effectiveness
4. Chest radiograph consistent with mucus plugging, atelectasis, or infiltrates
5. Deterioration in arterial blood gas measurements and oxygen saturation

F. Monitoring during treatment
1. Sputum production (amount, color, odor, and consistency)
2. Cough effectiveness
3. Pulse, respiratory rate, color, and oxygen saturation
4. Breathing pattern
5. Subjective response to pain, discomfort, and positioning
6. Blood pressure

G. Outcome assessment indicating successful postural drainage
1. Production of sputum is improved (if not, then the therapy is not indicated).
2. Breath sounds improved from effective coughing and decreased adventitious breath sounds
3. Chest radiograph improved from removal of secretions and improved atelectasis
4. Oxygen saturation has improved, indicating atelectasis has improved.
5. Patient's subjective response to therapy (patient complaints require adjustment of therapy).
6. Improved ventilator parameters indicating improved compliance and resistance because of removal of mucus plugging

H. Frequency
1. Turning
   a. Ventilated and critically ill patients require turning every hour. Less acutely ill patients should be turned every 2 h as tolerated.
2. Postural drainage therapy
   a. Ventilated and critically ill patients should be assessed every 4 to 6 h and reevaluated every 48 h.
   b. Spontaneously breathing patients should be assessed according to their response to therapy.
   c. Evaluate the acute care patient's orders every 72 h or with a change in status.

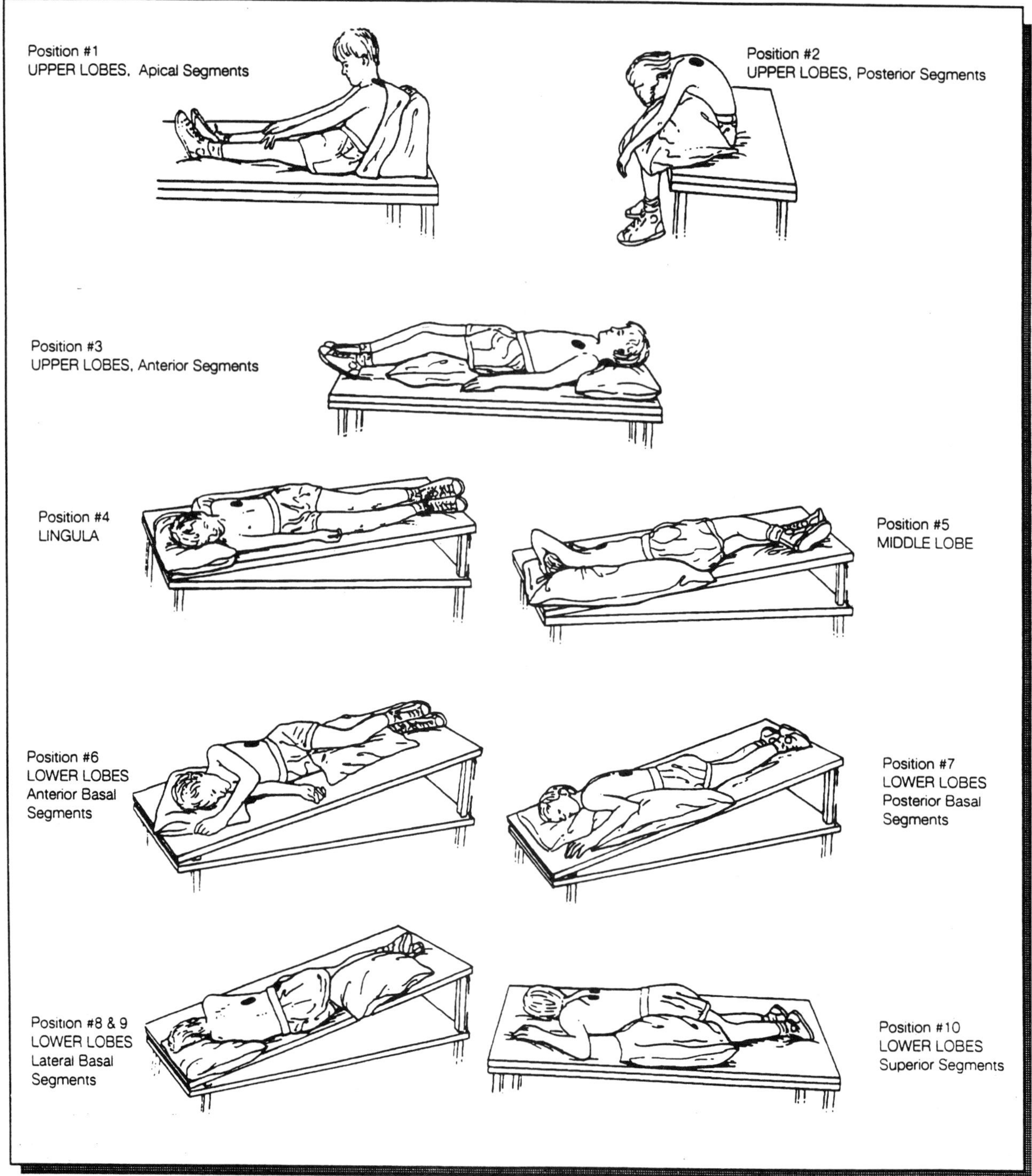


**FIGURE 11–1** Bronchial drainage positions. (From Cystic Fibrosis Foundation, Bethesda, MD, with permission.)

d. Home care patients should be reevaluated every 3 months and with a change of status.

I. Bronchial drainage positions (Fig. 11–1)

J. External percussive device
1. This device attaches to the chest by means of a vest. Small volumes of gas are alternately injected into the vest and withdrawn. This creates an oscillatory motion against the patient's thorax.
2. Optimal frequency is the one that produces the highest flows and largest volumes with each chest compression during tidal breathing. Cystic fibrosis patients seem to benefit from this device.

K. Exsufflation mechanical device
   1. This device produces extremely fast expiratory flows in patients on mechanical ventilators with neuromuscular disorders. The expiratory flows generated by this device exceed those produced by the manually assisted, directed cough.

L. Directed cough
   1. When spontaneous cough is inadequate, a forced expiratory technique or huff cough and manually assisted cough are examples of directed cough.
   2. Huff coughing consists of one or two forced expirations with the glottis open with a period of relaxed diaphragmatic breathing. This is repeated until bronchial clearance occurs.
   3. A manually assisted cough is when mechanical pressure is applied to the epigastric region with forced exhalation.
   4. Indications
      a. To aid the patient in the removal of secretions from the lower airways
      b. For patients with bronchiectasis, cystic fibrosis, neuromuscular disease, spinal cord injury, or chronic bronchitis
      c. To assist other bronchial hygiene applications such as PEP therapy or postural drainage therapy
      d. To obtain sputum sample
   5. Contraindications to huff coughing and manually assisted coughing
      a. When there is the danger of transmitting droplet nuclei pathogen.
      b. In the presence of elevated intracranial pressure
      c. When there is unstable head, neck, or spine injury
      d. When there is the possibility of regurgitation and aspiration
      e. In the presence of pregnancy or abdominal surgery
      f. When there is untreated pneumothorax
   6. Assessment of need
      a. Spontaneous cough that fails to clear secretions
      b. Ineffective spontaneous cough evidenced by atelectasis and results of pulmonary function testing
      c. Long-term-care patients who retain secretions
   7. Monitoring the patient during directed cough
      a. Observe for discomfort, dyspnea, complaint of pain, and changes in vital signs.
      b. Check breath sounds.
      c. Check consistency, color, odor, and volume of sputum produced.
      d. Assess for cardiac dysrhythmias and other hemodynamic changes.
      e. Take measures of pulmonary mechanics, such as vital capacity, peak expiratory flow, peak inspiratory pressure, and peak expiratory pressure.
   8. Outcome assessment indicating successful directed cough
      a. Presence of sputum after coughing
      b. Patient's subjective response to therapy
      c. Clinical observation of improvement
      d. Stabilization of pulmonary hygiene in patients with chronic obstructive pulmonary disease (COPD) and history of secretion retention (cystic fibrosis)
   9. Awake postoperative patients require directed cough at least every 2 to 4 h or in conjunction with other therapy
   10. Take precautions to minimize exposure to droplet nuclei during the coughing maneuver. Ask the patient to cover his or her mouth and turn his or her head away from the health practitioner. A negative-pressure room will minimize exposure to airborne pathogens.

## XII. Incentive spirometry or sustained maximal inspiration

A. Indications
   1. Presence of conditions predisposing to the development of pulmonary atelectasis, including:
      a. Upper abdominal surgery
      b. Thoracic surgery
   2. Presence of pulmonary atelectasis
   3. Restrictive lung disease associated with quadriplegia and/or dysfunctional diaphragm

B. Contraindications
   1. Patients unable to achieve a vital capacity above 10 mL/kg or inspiratory capacity below one third of predicted
   2. Patient is unable to understand instructions in the appropriate use of the device.

3. Patient has an open stoma and requires the device to be adapted to the stoma.
4. Patient does not cooperate.

C. Hazards and complications
1. Hyperventilation (allow longer rest periods and reduce the number of times a deep breath is taken)
2. Barotrauma with emphysematous lungs
3. Discomfort because of inadequate pain control
4. Hypoxia because of interruption of operation of oxygen device
5. Fatigue
6. Exacerbation of bronchospasm

D. Assessment of outcome
1. Improvement in signs of atelectasis
   a. Decreased respiratory rate
   b. Normal pulse rate
   c. Reduced fever or afebrile
   d. Improved breath sounds
   e. Improved chest radiograph
   f. Decrease in the alveolar-arterial oxygen difference (A-a$DO_2$) and increase in the $PaO_2$
   g. Increased vital capacity and peak expiratory flows
   h. Return of functional residual capacity or vital capacity to preoperative values
2. Improved inspiratory muscle performance and forced vital capacity

E. Monitoring
1. The patient should be observed to ensure mastery of technique, patient performance, and utilization. This is especially important in the young child.
2. The following should be observed and charted.
   a. Number of breaths per session (5 to 10 breaths per session every hour the patient is awake)
   b. Inspiratory volume or flow goals achieved and 3- to 5-s breath-hold maintained
   c. Effort and motivation
   d. Additional instructions if patient not compliant with technique
   e. Vital signs
   f. Increase in inspiratory volume each day

11

# REVIEW QUESTIONS

1. Give three clinical indications for partial airway obstruction and three indications for complete airway obstruction.

| **Partial Airway Obstruction** | **Complete Airway Obstruction** |
|---|---|
| a. | a. |
| b. | b. |
| c. | c. |

2. Put a T for true and F for false next to the questions concerning CPR.

   a. _______ After opening an infant's airway, you should assess breathing next.

   b. _______ The brachial pulse is checked in infant CPR.

   c. _______ The ventilation to compression ratio is 2 breaths for every 15 compressions for 2-person CPR.

   d. _______ An infant with foreign body obstruction should have five back blows and five chest thrusts performed.

   e. _______ You should perform a finger sweep even if the foreign body is not seen.

   f. _______ A child with foreign body obstruction becomes unconscious after delivering back blows and chest thrusts. You should first try to look for the foreign body.

3. Describe the way to determine the proper size for an oropharyngeal airway and nasopharyngeal airway.

4. According to the AHA, what is the resuscitation bag volume that should be used for infants and children?

5. List the assessments that would determine successful nasotracheal suctioning.

6. List two indications for endotracheal suctioning of an endotracheal tube of mechanically ventilated children.

   a.

   b.

7. What size suction catheter should be used for a 6-mm endotracheal tube?

8. What type of catheter can be used to suction the left main stem bronchus?

9. Describe what should be done in the following situations.

   a. Very thick secretions are clogging the endotracheal tube when using 80 mm Hg suction pressure.

   b. The patient's heart rate drops from 128 to 60 beats/min after passing the suction catheter down the endotracheal tube.

   c. Each time the patient is suctioned after 15 s, the patient desaturates.

10. List two assessments used to determine successful suctioning of the endotracheal tube while on mechanical ventilation.

    a.

    b.

11. List two indications for endotracheal intubation.

    a.

    b.

12. What size oral endotracheal tube is appropriate for a 6-year-old?

13. After placing the tube in question 14, at what centimeter mark should the tube be placed?

14. What signs would indicate that excessive sedation has been given prior to intubation?

15. List two signs that the endotracheal tube is in the appropriate place within the trachea.

    a.

    b.

16. List what should be done in the following situations following endotracheal tube intubation.

    a. Unequal breath sounds and asymmetrical chest rise

    b. End-tidal carbon dioxide decreases from 35 mm Hg to 0 mm Hg.

    c. Positive pressure heard over the epigastric area of the abdomen

17. What is an appropriate cuff pressure for a 6.5-mm endotracheal tube?

18. What should be done to a nasogastric tube when a chest radiograph shows it to be coiled in the stomach?

19. Describe a method to determine whether an intubated patient will have post-extubation stridor.

20. What treatment should be given for an extubated 8-year-old child who has minimal retractions, mild stridor, and no desaturation?

21. A double-lumen endotracheal tube is in place. Auscultation reveals breath sounds on the left side but not on the right. The centimeter mark is now at 15 cm from 11 cm. What should be done?

22. What are two acute complications of a tracheostomy and two chronic complications of a tracheostomy?

| **Acute** | **Chronic** |
|---|---|
| a. | a. |
| b. | b. |

23. Prior to intubating with a foam-cuffed endotracheal tube, what should be done concerning the cuff?

24. When plugging a fenestrated tracheostomy tube, describe what should be done to the cuff.

25. What is used to maintain a stomal opening?

26. List a cause of each of the following situations concerning a tracheostomy.

   a. Large air leak through the mouth and nose

   b. The high-pressure limit sounds on the ventilator.

   c. The suction catheter meets an obstruction within the tracheostomy tube.

   d. The low-pressure alarm sounds on the ventilator.

27. Give three indications and three contraindications to postural drainage.

| **Indications** | **Contraindications** |
|---|---|
| a. | a. |
| b. | b. |
| c. | c. |

28. Describe the proper drainage position for each of the following lobes or segments of the lung.

   a. Middle lobe

   b. Superior segments of the lower lobes

   c. Left lower lobe, posterior basal segment

29. List two assessments that are used to determine the successful outcome of directed cough.

   a.

   b.

30. What are two contraindications to incentive spirometry?

   a.

   b.

31. How should the patient be instructed for frequency and number of breaths per sessions concerning incentive spirometry?

## BIBLIOGRAPHY


American Association for Respiratory Care Clinical Practice Guidelines. (1995). Management of airway emergencies. *Respiratory Care* 40(7):749.

American Association for Respiratory Care Clinical Practice Guidelines. (1993). Resuscitation in acute care hospitals. *Respiratory Care* 38:1179.

American Association for Respiratory Care Clinical Practice Guidelines. (1992). Nasotracheal suctioning. *Respiratory Care* 37:898.

American Association for Respiratory Care Clinical Practice Guidelines. (1993). Endotracheal suctioning of mechanically ventilated adults and children with artificial airways. *Respiratory Care* 38:500.

American Association for Respiratory Care Clinical Practice Guidelines. (1991). Postural drainage therapy. *Respiratory Care* 36:1418.

American Association for Respiratory Care Clinical Practice Guidelines. (1993). Directed cough. *Respiratory Care* 38:495.

American Association for Respiratory Care Clinical Practice Guidelines. (1991). Incentive spirometry. *Respiratory Care* 36:1402.

American Academy of Pediatrics. (1988). *Textbook of Pediatric Advanced Life Support.* Dallas: American Heart Association.

Beattie, C. *Fiberoptic Intubation and the Difficult Airway* [WWW document]. URL http://anesthesiology.mc.vanderbilt.edu/anesth/eamg/EAMG6.htm

Benumof, J. L. (1996). *Airway Management: Principles and Practice.* St. Louis: Mosby–Year Book.

Chandra, C.N., and Hazinski, M.F. (Eds.). (1994). *Basic Life Support for Health Care Providers.* Dallas: American Heart Association.

Deshpande, J. K. *Pediatric Airway Management* [WWW document]. URL http://anesthesiology.mc.vanderbilt,edu/anesth/eamg/EAMG9.htm

Deskin, R. W. *The Management of Acute Upper Airway Obstruction* [WWW document]. URL http://www.ears.com/quinn/Airway_Obstruction.html

Feaster, W. W. (1992). Oral endotracheal intubation: Pediatric perspective. In Dailey, R. H., et al. (Eds.) *The Airway: Emergency Management.* St. Louis: Mosby–Year Book.

Finucane, B. T., and Santora, A. H. (1996). *Principles of Airway Management.* St. Louis: Mosby–Year Book.

Marik, P. E. (1996). The cuff-leak test as a predictor of postextubation stridor: A prospective study. *Respiratory Care* 41(6):509.

Mallinckrodt Medical. (1996). *A Parent's Guide to Tracheostomy Home Care for Your Child.* St. Louis: Mallinckrodt Medical, Inc.

Mallinckrodt Medical. (1996). *Tracheostomy Tube: Adult Home Care Guide.* St. Louis: Mallinckrodt Medical, Inc.

Passy-Muir, Inc. (1997). *Passy-Muir Valve Description* [WWW document]. URL http://www.acclaimedmedia.com/passy-muir/describe.html

Simmons, K: Airway care. In Scanlon, R., et al. (1995). *Egan's Fundamentals of Respiratory Care,* ed. 6. St. Louis: Mosby–Year Book.

Trauma.Org. (1997). *Trauma Anesthesia: Airway Management of the Trauma Victim* [WWW document]. URL http:www.trauma.org/anesthesia/airway.html

Walker, G. V. (1997). *The Use of Pharmacologic Agents in Airway Management* [WWW document]. URL http://anesthesiology.mc.vanderbilt.edu/anesth/eamg/EAMG7.htm

White, S. (1997). *Confirmation of Endotracheal Tube Position in Emergency Airway Management* [WWW document]. URL http://anesthesiology.mc.vanderbilt.edu/anesth/eamg/EAMG8.htm

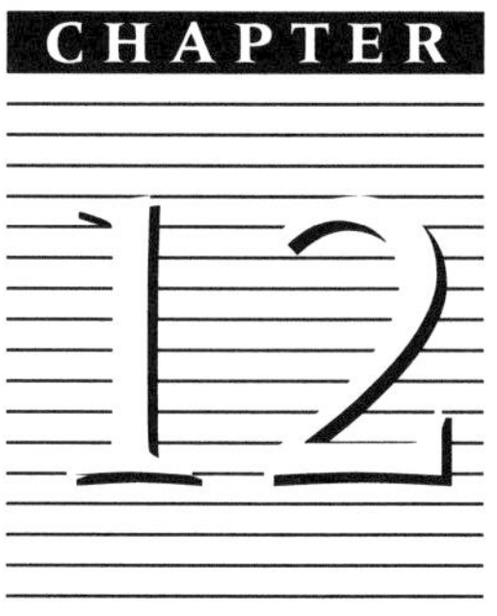

# Congenital Heart Defects

**I. General overview of heart disease**

A. If the heart fails to follow the correct sequence of development during the first trimester, abnormal or incomplete cardiac structures may result that lead to minor congenital cardiac anomalies that can be managed conservatively, or to major deformities that may require immediate medical and/or surgical intervention.

B. The majority of congenital cardiac defects (approximately 90%) are attributed to combined genetic and environmental (multifactorial) influences. Approximately 8% are attributed to genetic factors, and the remaining defects are thought to be of environmental origin.

C. Prenatal history
  1. Maternal history of heart disease and maternal illness
  2. Infection during early pregnancy with cytomegalovirus or herpesvirus
  3. Use of drugs, cigarettes, or alcohol during pregnancy

D. Birth and after birth
  1. Physical examination
    a. General behavior: irritable, flaccid, unresponsive to external stimuli, and hypotonia.
    b. The cyanotic infant may have polycythemia and hyperviscosity. Obtain hemoglobin and hematocrit (70% or greater is polycythemia).
    c. An infant with a heart defect may have longer-lasting cyanosis from crying compared to an infant with pulmonary disease.
    d. The clinical signs of a severe congenital defect do not improve with the administration of oxygen.
    e. Respirations are rapid, 40 to 50 breaths per minute (bpm). Grunting, nasal flaring, stridor, wheezing, and persistent night coughing may be signs of congestive heart failure. As a result of these problems, the infant has poor feeding habits and fails to gain weight.
    f. Venous distention may be seen in patients with right heart failure.
    g. The liver may be enlarged (hepatomegaly). The liver is a reliable indicator of cardiac function.
    h. Edema may occur as a result of heart failure (uncommon). Edema is seen in the back of hands and top of feet. (This may be normal; fat pads are found in these areas.)
    i. Murmur is often heard with heart defect. If one is heard, then it is important to obtain:
      (1) A radiograph of the chest
      (2) An ECG
      (3) The partial pressure of arterial oxygen ($PaO_2$) before discharge
    j. Anoxic spells, characterized by periods of uncontrollable crying followed by paroxysms of shortness of breath, cyanosis, and unconsciousness, are potentially fatal.
    k. Clubbing of the digits occurs from low arterial oxygen levels of long duration. Other disorders can produce clubbing of the fingers and toes.
    l. Chest deformity may suggest cardiac enlargement. A sunken chest, pectus excavatum, may interfere with cardiac performance.
    m. Palpation of pulses to determine presence of bounding pulse versus thready or absent pulse. Irregularities in the pulse while breathing, pulsus paradoxus, occur when systolic pressure decreases more than 10 mm Hg during inspiration and should be noted. The apical pulse is found in the fourth intercostal space, left of the midclavicular line, in children under 7

years of age. In children older than 7 years, it is found in the fifth intercostal space along the midclavicular line. A prolonged capillary refill time (longer than 2 s) indicates poor peripheral circulation.

n. The point of maximal impulse helps determine whether the right or left ventricle is dominant. Precordial pulse is seen or felt over the sternum and is from beating of the heart.

2. Common diagnostic tests
   a. Pulse oximetry monitors and trends oxygen saturation.
   b. Chest radiograph helps to determine pulmonary vasculature size.
   c. Two-dimensional echocardiography is the most common method for diagnosing heart defects.
   d. Doppler studies help determine pressure differences across valves.
   e. Cardiac catheterization and angiography helps assess pulmonary artery size, pulmonary artery pressure, and pulmonary vascular resistance.

E. Heart sounds
   1. The first heart sound, $S_1$, originates from the closing of the atrioventricular valves at the beginning of ventricular systole and the end of diastole. The $S_1$ sound is the result of the mitral valve and tricuspid valve closing at the beginning of systole. This is the "lubb" sound.
   2. The $S_2$ heart sound results from the closing of the aortic valve and the pulmonic valve at the end of ventricular systole and beginning of diastole. The pulmonic valve closes after the aortic valve. This is the "dup" sound.
      a. A physiological splitting of $S_2$ may occur as a result of intrapleural pressure changes during normal spontaneous inspiration. During spontaneous breathing, venous return is increased, increasing right ventricular systole and delaying the closing of the pulmonic valve.
      b. A loud pulmonic sound indicates pulmonary hypertension. A loud aortic sound indicates systemic hypertension.
   3. The $S_3$ heart sound, a normal finding in children and young adults, reflects the first phase of ventricular filling in diastole. A high-intensity $S_3$ heart sound may indicate underlying heart failure or a large left-to-right shunt.
   4. The $S_4$ heart sound, which may be generated by either the left or right atrial contraction, represents the atrial contribution of ventricular diastolic filling. It is not normal in a child. This heart sound is sometimes referred to as "atrial gallop." Characterized by high right atrial pressures, this heart sound is associated with the following disorders:
      a. Tricuspid atresia
      b. Total anomalous pulmonary venous return
      c. Pulmonic stenosis
   5. Murmur is a long heart sound generated by turbulence of blood flow. Most cardiac murmurs are caused by regurgitation or stenosis, such as in mitral valve regurgitation or as is present with patent ductus arteriosus.

F. An alteration in the fractional concentration of oxygen ($FIO_2$) and carbon dioxide is used to change vascular resistance and blood flow.
   a. An increase in $FIO_2$ or in the partial pressure of alveolar oxygen ($PAO_2$) decreases pulmonary vascular resistance (PVR) and increases pulmonary blood flow. Administration of nitric oxide, tolazoline (Priscoline hydrochloride), isoproterenol (Isuprel), and prostaglandin $E_1$ will also decrease PVR and increase pulmonary blood flow.
   b. A decrease in $FIO_2$ or $PAO_2$ increases PVR and decreases pulmonary blood flow. An increase in intrapleural pressures from positive end-expiratory pressure (PEEP), continuous positive airway pressure (CPAP), and mean airway pressure will also decrease pulmonary blood flow.
   c. Hyperventilation decreases pulmonary vascular resistance, increases pulmonary blood flow, and decreases cerebral blood flow.
   d. Hypoventilation increases pulmonary vascular resistance, decreases pulmonary blood flow, and increases cerebral blood flow.

G. Common chest radiographic appearance of heart defects
   1. A boot-shaped heart resulting from tetralogy of Fallot or truncus arteriosus
   2. An egg-shaped heart resulting from transposition of the great arteries
   3. A snowman-shaped heart resulting from total anomalous pulmonary venous return

**II. Congenital heart defects with left-to-right shunts (acyanotic and increased pulmonary blood flow)**

A. Patent ductus arteriosus (PDA)
   1. The PDA is a vascular channel that usually connects the aorta with the pulmonary arterial trunk through which pulmonary blood flow may bypass the

high-resistance, pulmonary vascular circulation and enter the descending aorta in utero (Fig. 12–1). After birth, the persistence of this vessel's patency presents varying degrees of hemodynamic demands, resulting in an instability of the cardiovascular system.

2. Signs and symptoms
   a. Murmur, which may be continuous, silent, or multiple clicks
   b. Increased pulmonary blood flow with left-to-right shunting across the PDA
   c. A fluctuating $PaO_2$ resulting from the intermittent opening and closing of the ductus
   d. Common in preterm neonates
   e. Symptoms may not show up for weeks or months; furthermore, if the ductus is small, the patient may appear well.
   f. A large PDA may produce symptoms of left ventricular failure with an $S_3$ gallop, wide pulse pressure, hyperdynamic precordium, and cardiomegaly.
   g. Right heart failure and pulmonary edema due to increased work on right heart and increased pulmonary pressure and flow
3. Diagnosis
   a. Echocardiography
   b. Use of preductal and postductal transcutaneous monitoring and/or preductal and postductal blood sample (see Chapter 5)
4. Treatment
   a. Indomethacin (Indocin), which does the following:
      (1) Promotes closure of the PDA.
      (2) Inhibits prostaglandin $E_1$ ($PGE_1$) synthesis.
   b. Action is 1 to 3 h. If, after three doses, the ductus is still patent, ligation is suggested.
   c. Increase oxygen concentration, if not at risk of RLF.

B. Atrial septal defect (ASD)
   1. ASD is a heart disease in which there is an opening in the septal wall between the right and left atrium (Fig. 12–2).
   2. Types of ASD
      a. Ostium secundum is an underdeveloped foramen ovale flap. Following birth, the flap is unable to close with pressure changes in the heart.
      b. Ostium primum is a lower interatrial septum that involves the tricuspid and mitral valves.
      c. Sinus venosus is an opening in the atrial wall found near the superior vena cava.
      d. All three types are the result of the failure of a tissue "endocardial cushion," which forms the septum, to develop.
   3. Pathophysiology
      a. Hemodynamic problems are not severe because atrial pressures are low.
      b. Left-to-right shunting occurs, causing a volume overload of the right ventricle and pulmonary circulation.
      c. The left ventricle may be smaller.
      d. Normal fetal growth
   4. Clinical presentation

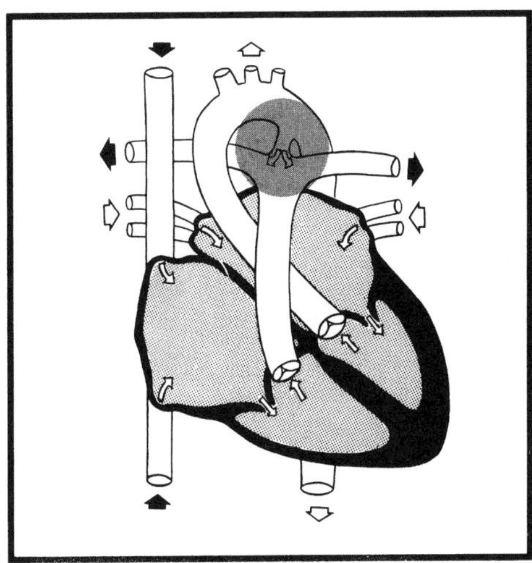

**FIGURE 12–1** Patent ductus arteriosus. (From Ross Products Division, Abbott Laboratories, Columbus, OH, with permission.)

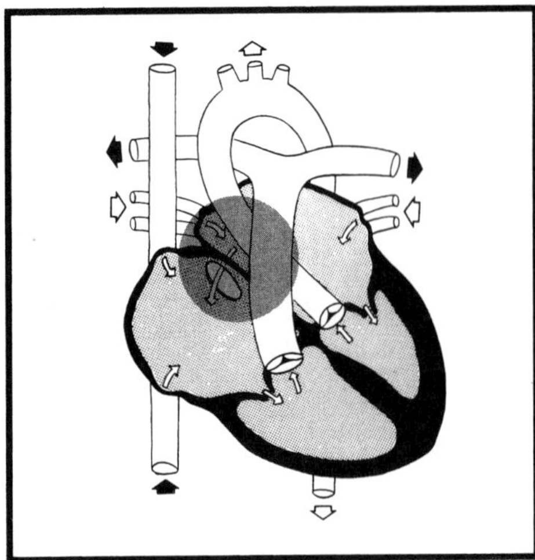

**FIGURE 12–2** Atrial septal defect. (From Ross Products Division, Abbott Laboratories, Columbus, OH, with permission.)

  a. With mild ASD, manifestations occur later in life.
  b. A large ASD will present with the following:
    (1) Cardiomegaly
    (2) Right heart failure
    (3) Enlarged pulmonary vascular markings
    (4) Dyspnea and fatigue
    (5) Failure to thrive (not gaining weight)
    (6) Murmur of pulmonary valve, which is secondary to increased pulmonary blood flow
5. Radiologic findings
  a. Depending on the size of the ASD, pulmonary vascular markings may range from normal to increased.
  b. Cardiomegaly
6. ECG
  a. Right heart enlargement
  b. Prolonged PR interval
7. Diagnosis
  a. Heart catheterization
  b. Two-dimensional echocardiography: Right atrial and ventricular enlargement can be seen, as well as the location of the ASD.
8. Treatment
  a. Supportive therapy
    (1) Digitalis
    (2) Diuretics
    (3) Oxygen
  b. Surgical treatment
    (1) Closure of the defect by open heart surgery
    (2) Usually done in childhood
    (3) Surgery will be performed earlier if the child does not respond to medical management and supportive therapy.

C. Ventricular septal defect (VSD)
1. VSD is a heart disease in which there is a septal opening of varying size and location between the right and left ventricles (Fig. 12–3). A VSD may be asymptomatic because of the small size of the opening.
2. VSD may be associated with other anomalies such as PDA and ASD.
3. An infant with a small defect will be asymptomatic, and spontaneous closure will eventually occur. Premature infants show symptoms earlier than full-term infants.
4. With a large VSD, pulmonary vascular resistance (PVR) decreases following birth. A left-to-right shunt occurs through the defect. As a result, volume and pressure overload occur in the right heart.
5. Symptoms will depend on when PVR decreases. With prematurity, PVR decreases earlier because of underdeveloped smooth muscle in the arteriolar walls of the pulmonary vasculature. There is a flood of blood into the lungs, resulting in pulmonary edema.
6. With growth of the infant, muscularization of the pulmonary vessels helps to reduce blood engorgement in the lungs.

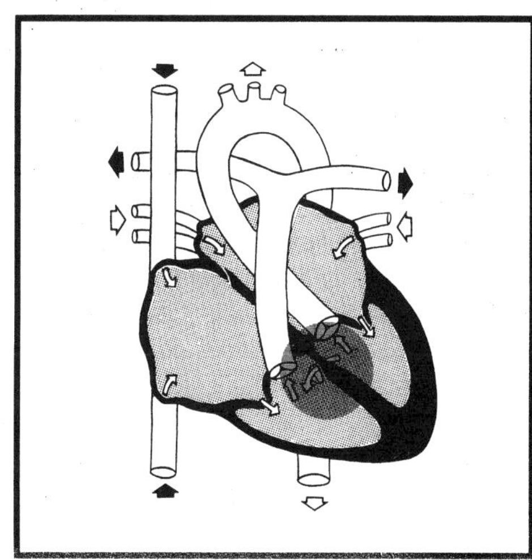

**FIGURE 12–3** Ventricular septal defect. (From Ross Products Division, Abbott Laboratories, Columbus, OH, with permission.)

7. Hemodynamic alterations include the following:
   a. Left-to-right shunt
   b. Increased pulmonary blood flow, causing congestive heart failure (CHF)
8. The amount of blood flowing through the VSD depends on the resistance of pressure between the left and right ventricles. For example:
   a. At birth, right ventricular pressures are greater than left, with minimal bidirectional blood flow.
   b. As the PVR decreases, the pulmonary venous return increases. This increases the left ventricular pressure, increasing left-to-right shunting.
   c. Pulmonary congestion occurs, causing reduced compliance, atelectasis, bronchial obstruction, and respiratory distress.
   d. Right heart failure and right heart hypertrophy result, with volume and pressure overload. Consequently, the left-to-right shunt may reverse to a right-to-left shunt.
9. Signs and symptoms (occur when PVR decreases)
   a. Small VSD
      (1) Murmur heard over lower left sternal border.
      (2) After a few months, the VSD closes.
   b. Moderate VSD
      (1) The VSD may be discovered a few weeks after leaving the hospital following birth.
      (2) Minimal tachypnea, but otherwise asymptomatic (Again, VSD will close within a few months.)
   c. Severe VSD (significant left-to-right shunting)
      (1) Loud, harsh heart sounds and murmur
      (2) Tachypnea
      (3) Tachycardia
      (4) Failure to thrive
      (5) Diaphoresis
      (6) Cyanosis: Occurs if the patient is in left heart failure or the left-to-right shunt has reversed to right-to-left shunt
      (7) Respiratory acidosis and hypoxemia resulting from pulmonary congestion
   d. Infants who go home with undetected VSD return because of the following:
      (1) Respiratory difficulties
      (2) Feeding difficulties
      (3) Failure to thrive
10. Radiologic findings
    a. Small to moderate VSD
       (1) Normal size heart and pulmonary vascular markings
    b. Large VSD
       (1) Cardiomegaly
       (2) Prominent pulmonary vasculature
11. ECG
    a. Small to moderate VSD
       (1) Normal size heart

b. Large VSD
   (1) Right ventricular enlargement
   (2) Left ventricular enlargement

12. Diagnosis
    a. Two-dimensional echocardiography allows the defect to be seen as long as blood is flowing through opening.
    b. Cardiac catheterization
13. Treatment
    a. If asymptomatic, no treatment is necessary if the infant is eating and gaining weight.
    b. Supportive therapy until surgery:
       (1) Digitalis
       (2) Diuretics
       (3) Oxygen if patient is cyanotic
       (4) Afterload reduction to reduce PVR and SVR
    c. Antibiotics for pulmonary infection.
    d. Palliative (temporary) surgery involves banding the pulmonary artery for the unstable infant. After the infant stabilizes, open heart surgery can be performed to patch the defect.

D. Endocardial cushion defect (complete or partial atrioventricular canal)
   1. The lowermost portion of the atrial septum is absent, with absence of the inlet portion of the ventricular septum. A common atrioventricular (AV) valve is present (Fig. 12–4).
   2. Signs and symptoms
      a. Failure to thrive
      b. Tachypnea
      c. Murmur
      d. CHF
      e. May have hepatomegaly
   3. Radiologic findings
      a. Cardiomegaly
      b. Increased pulmonary vascular markings
      c. Pulmonary edema
      d. Prominent main pulmonary artery
      e. Atrial enlargement
   4. ECG
      a. Left axis deviation
      b. Right ventricular hypertrophy
      c. Biatrial enlargement
      d. Prolonged PR interval
      e. Left ventricular hypertrophy
   5. Diagnosis
      a. Two-dimensional echocardiography
      b. Cardiac catheterization
   6. Treatment
      a. Medical management with digoxin and diuretics
      b. Inotropes and afterload reduction

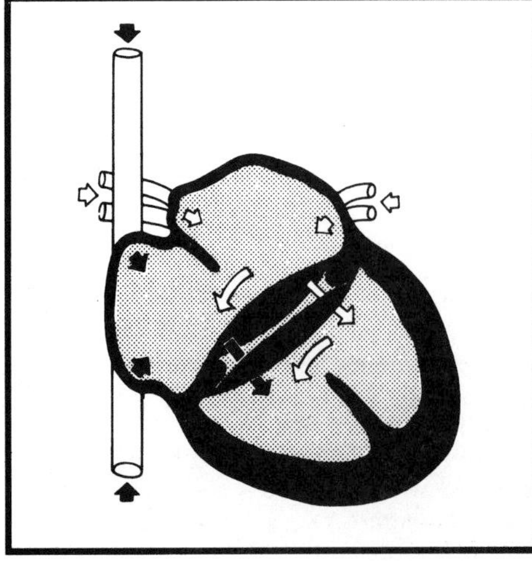

**FIGURE 12–4** Endocardial cushion defect. (From Ross Products Division, Abbott Laboratories, Columbus, OH, with permission.)

c. Surgery at approximately 6 months of age
d. Complete repair and closure of septal defects and valves if involved.
e. Pulmonary arterial banding (reduces pulmonary blood flow)

## III. Congenital heart defects with obstructive lesions (acyanotic and normal pulmonary blood flow)

A. Coarctation of the aorta

1. Coarctation of the aorta presents with a narrowed aortic lumen. It exists as a preductal obstruction in relation to the ductus arteriosus and in the area of origin of the left subclavian artery. Generally, the lesion produces an obstruction to the flow of blood through the aorta, causing an increased left ventricular pressure and workload (Fig. 12–5).
2. The narrowest portion of the aorta, it is found between the ductus arteriosus and subclavian and is a result of the fetus's normal hemodynamics.
3. It is here that the two ventricular outputs meet. A small output from the left ventricle meets the larger output from the right ventricle through the PDA.
4. The descending thoracic aorta is a continuation of the PDA and is therefore narrower than the other area of the aorta.
5. Following normal birth, the stenosis reverses as the ductus closes and more blood passes through it from the left ventricle.
6. With coarctation following birth:
   a. PVR decreases.
   b. Pulmonary congestion occurs, followed by pulmonary artery hypertension.
7. Coarctation may be complex. There may be a VSD present, which will increase the left-to-right shunt. In this case, both ventricles may fail.
8. Signs and symptoms
   a. Many infants are not diagnosed.
   b. Within days following birth, the infant presents with the following:
      (1) Tachypnea and grunting
      (2) Tachycardia
      (3) Dyspnea with feedings
      (4) Poor peripheral pulses (femoral, even brachial if severe)
      (5) Systolic pressure higher in upper extremities than in lower extremities
      (6) Reduced urine output resulting from hypoperfusion of the kidneys
      (7) Depending on the location of the defect, cyanosis may be present in the left hand and the lower body.
      (8) Shock, if ductus closes
9. Radiologic findings
   a. Cardiomegaly
   b. May see increased pulmonary blood flow
   c. Characterized by classic "E" sign as seen on a frontal view of a barium study
10. ECG
   a. Right ventricular hypertrophy
   b. In older children, left ventricular hypertrophy

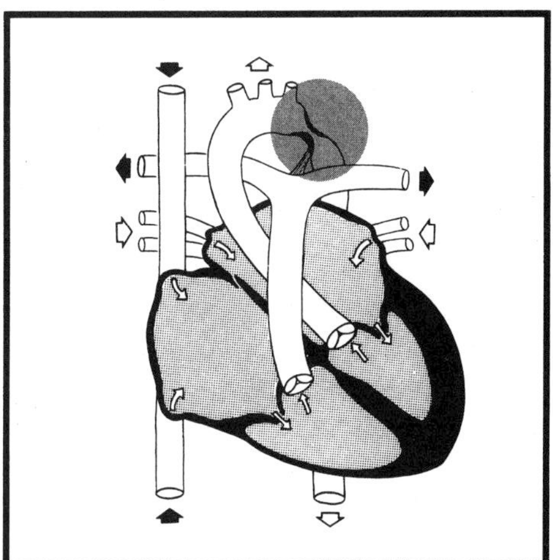

**FIGURE 12–5** Coarctation of the aorta. (From Ross Products Division, Abbott Laboratories, Columbus, OH, with permission.)

11. Diagnosis
    a. Two-dimensional echocardiography
    b. Cardiac catheterization
    c. Check blood pressure in upper and lower body in all four extremities
    d. $PaO_2$: Umbilical artery $PaO_2$ is lower than right-arm preductal $PaO_2$.
12. Treatment
    a. Restrict fluid intake
    b. Diuretics
    c. Digitalis
    d. Prostaglandin $E_1$: This will maintain the ductus opening and reduce right ventricular heart overload.
    e. Correct acidosis.
    f. Cardiac surgery

B. Aortic stenosis (AS)
1. Aortic stenosis presents as a narrowing of the aortic valve orifice. AS is usually caused by abnormal development of the aortic valve or partial fusion of the commissure, the sites of junction between adjacent cusps of the heart valves (Fig. 12–6).
2. Signs and symptoms
    a. Variable—with a mild to moderate defect, infants, older children, and adults may show no clinical signs.
    b. Severe AS shows the following:
        (1) Low cardiac output and heart failure
        (2) Respiratory distress
        (3) Tachycardia
        (4) Diminished peripheral pulses and decreased blood pressure
        (5) Poor perfusion and cool extremities
        (6) Murmur and clicks
        (7) Pale cyanosis
3. ECG
    a. Left ventricular, right ventricular, or biventricular hypertrophy
    b. Atrial enlargement is possible.
    c. ST-segment and T-wave changes
4. Radiologic findings (depending on the degree of obstruction)
    a. Normal or cardiomegaly
    b. Pulmonary vascular markings may be normal or increased.
5. Diagnosis
    a. Two-dimensional echocardiography
    b. Cardiac catheterization
    c. Clinical examination
6. Treatment
    a. In critical or severe AS, $PGE_1$ is used to keep the ductus arteriosus patent, allowing an increased blood flow to the body.
    b. Until surgery can be performed, the treatment of symptoms includes the following:
        (1) Digitalis

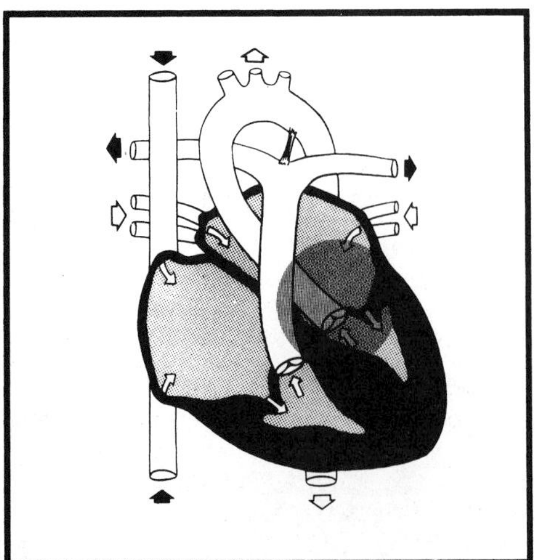

**FIGURE 12–6** Aortic stenosis. (From Ross Products Division, Abbott Laboratories, Columbus, OH, with permission.)

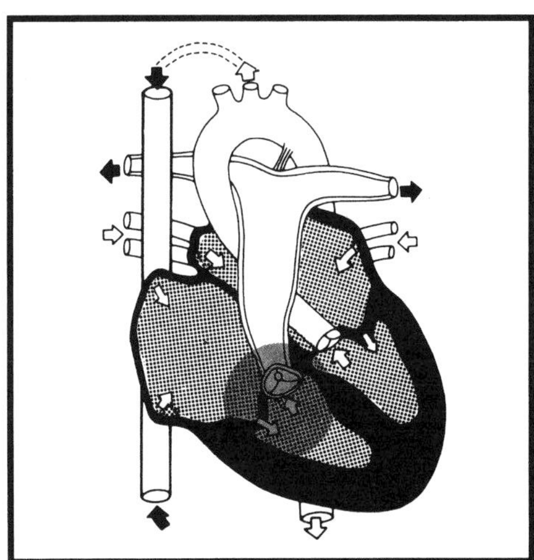

**FIGURE 12–7** Pulmonary stenosis. (From Ross Products Division, Abbott Laboratories, Columbus, OH, with permission.)

(2) Inotropic support
(3) Treatment of acidosis
(4) Electrolyte balance
c. Surgical valvotomy
d. Aortic balloon valvuloplasty
e. Valve replacement
f. Surgical resection of subaortic obstruction or patching a supravalvular obstruction

C. Pulmonary stenosis (PS)
1. PS presents with obstruction of the pulmonary arterial tree, which may involve the right ventricular outflow tract, the pulmonary valve, and the pulmonary arterial branches. A hypoplastic right ventricle may also be present (Fig. 12–7).
2. Signs and symptoms
a. The majority of patients are asymptomatic.
b. Upper left sternal border murmur
c. Cyanosis may be present; the severity depends on the obstruction.
d. Tachypnea
e. Right ventricular pressure is elevated, and pulmonary artery pressure is reduced (from reduced blood flow entering the pulmonary vasculature).
f. Mild exertional dyspnea
g. CHF
3. ECG (depending on the amount of obstruction)
a. Normal to right ventricular hypertrophy
b. Right heart enlargement, enlarged P wave
4. Radiologic findings (depending on the amount of obstruction)
a. Normal or slightly enlarged heart
b. Normal or decreased vascular marking
c. A prominent main pulmonary artery or a right atrial segment may be present.
5. Diagnosis
a. Two-dimensional echocardiography
b. Cardiac catheterization
6. Treatment
a. $PGE_1$
b. Pulmonary valvotomy
c. Shunting procedure to increase pulmonary blood flow
d. Reconstruction of right ventricular outflow tract

## IV. Congenital heart defects with admixture lesions (cyanosis and increased pulmonary blood flow)

A. Complete transposition of the great arteries (TGA)
1. With this anomaly, there is an abnormal anatomic relationship among the great arteries. The aorta originates from the right ventricle, and the pulmonary artery originates from the left ventricle (Fig. 12–8).
2. Pathophysiology

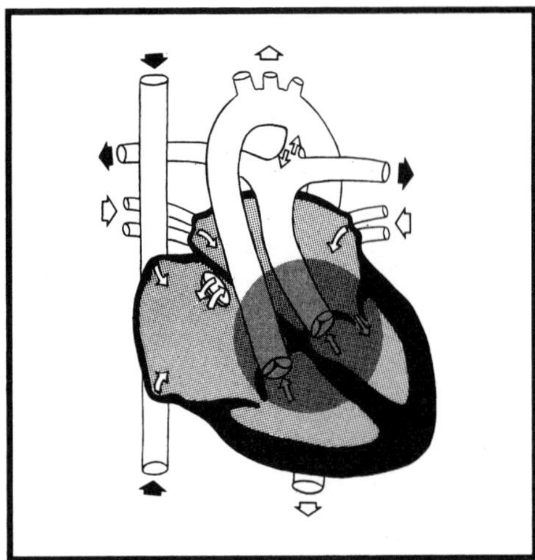

**FIGURE 12–8** Transposition of the great vessels. (From Ross Products Division, Abbott Laboratories, Columbus, OH, with permission.)

a. Oxygenated blood from the pulmonary veins enters the left atrium and left ventricle and is brought back into the lungs by the misplaced pulmonary artery.
b. At the same time, systemic venous return enters the right atrium from the SVC and IVC, enters the right ventricle, and is brought back to systemic circulation by the misplaced aorta.
c. Consequently, oxygenated blood returns to the lungs, and unoxygenated blood returns to systemic circulation.
d. In order for these two blood supplies to mix, a shunt must be present, such as a PDA, VSD, or ASD.

3. Signs and symptoms
   a. The infant is normal at birth because fetal circulation may still be present.
   b. However, as fetal circulation changes to newborn circulation, and in the absence of other defects, the infant suddenly deteriorates, becoming severely cyanotic and hypoxemic.
   c. Severity of cyanosis:
      (1) Mild to moderate with VSD
      (2) Moderate with ASD and PDA
      (3) Severe with intact septum
   d. Poor response to oxygen therapy:
      (1) $PaO_2$ hovers around 25 to 35 mm Hg on room air, with minimal changes on 100% oxygen.
   e. Tachypnea
   f. Murmur depends on presence of ASD or VSD. May have soft ductal murmur.
   g. Tachycardia
4. Radiologic findings
   a. Narrow mediastinum
   b. Normal pulmonary vascular markings
   c. Increased pulmonary vascular markings with VSD
   d. Egg-shaped cardiac silhouette
5. ECG
   a. TGA with intact septum from a normal or right ventricular hypertrophy
   b. TGA with VSD from biventricular and biatrial enlargement
6. Diagnosis
   a. TGA should be suspected when an infant presents with:
      (1) Severe cyanosis
      (2) No obvious pulmonary disease
      (3) No murmur
   b. No change in $PaO_2$ given 100% oxygen. For example:
      (1) No significant difference between preductal and postductal blood gases. (With PDA, with normal placement of the aorta and pulmonary artery, the preductal is higher than the postductal value.)
   c. Two-dimensional echocardiography
   d. Cardiac catheterization
   e. Clinical findings
7. Treatment

a. $PGE_1$ for an infant with a $PaO_2$ less than 20 mm Hg. This will relax the ductus arteriosus and improve pulmonary blood flow.
b. Atrial balloon septostomy (Rashkind procedure)
   (1) A balloon-tipped catheter opens the foramen ovale, allowing a mixture of blood (right-to-left shunt). With this opening, the $PaO_2$ will increase to approximately 35 to 50 mm Hg and $SaO_2$ will increase to 50 to 80%.
c. Correct the pH and provide oxygen.
d. Further surgery

B. Total anomalous pulmonary venous return (TAPVR)
1. TAPVR presents with pulmonary venous blood, which normally enters the left atrium, returning to the right heart by means of anomalous venous connections emptying indirectly or directly into the right atrium, vena cava, or coronary sinus connections (Fig. 12–9).
2. Anomalous pulmonary venous drainage will follow one or more of these aberrant routes.
   a. Nonobstructive types
      (1) All four pulmonary veins may drain by means of a common vessel entering into the superior vena cava.
      (2) Pulmonary veins may return to an enlarged coronary sinus.
      (3) Pulmonary veins may empty into the left innominate vein.
   b. Obstructive type
      (1) There may be a portal system below the diaphragm that will return pulmonary blood flow to the right atrium via the inferior vena cava.
3. Signs and symptoms
   a. The infant may be asymptomatic at birth except for cyanosis.
   b. Tachypnea
   c. Fatigue and dyspnea
   d. Tachycardia
   e. Right heart failure
   f. Hepatomegaly
   g. Protrusion of left side of the chest
   h. Feeding difficulty
   i. Prominent $S_1$, systolic click, and widely split $S_2$ heart sounds
4. Radiologic findings
   a. "Snowman" appearance of heart from contour-shaped enlarged ventricle, and superior vena cava from increased pulmonary blood flow
   b. Heart size may be normal at birth, but weeks later, shows "snowman" appearance.
   c. Pulmonary edema with obstructive type
5. ECG
   a. Right ventricular hypertrophy
   b. Right atrial hypertrophy
   c. Incomplete right bundle branch block
6. Diagnosis
   a. Two-dimensional echocardiography
   b. Cardiac catheterization

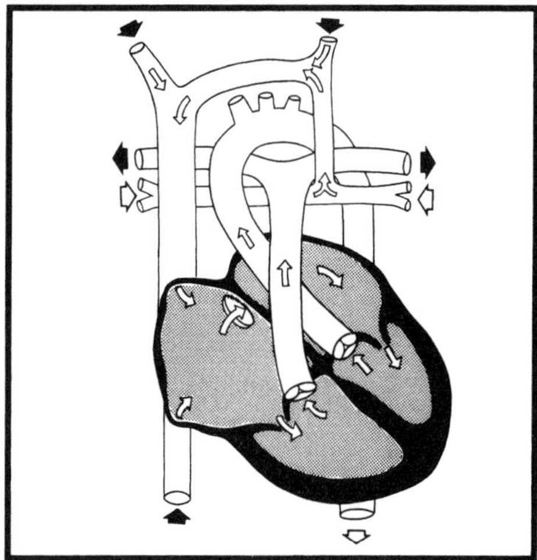

**FIGURE 12–9** Total anomalous pulmonary venous return. (From Ross Products Division, Abbott Laboratories, Columbus, OH, with permission.)

7. Treatment
   a. $PGE_1$
   b. Until surgery is performed, supportive therapy that includes digoxin and diuretic
   c. Surgical repair to redirect pulmonary venous drainage into the left atrium
   d. Balloon atrial septostomy at catheterization

C. Truncus arteriosus (TA)
1. TA presents as a single arterial trunk resulting from failure of the aorta and the pulmonary artery to separate during embryo myologic development. The truncal root overrides the ventricular septal defect (Fig. 12–10).
2. The coronary arteries arise normally from the truncus.
3. To be compatible with life, a VSD must be present. The entire pulmonary and systemic circulation leaves the heart through the VSD by way of a single trunk.
4. The valve is a single semilunar valve with two to six cusps.
5. The pulmonary arterial connections to the truncal vessel are variable.
6. Signs and symptoms
   a. Acyanotic if pulmonary arteries arise from the truncus
   b. Increased pulse pressure with bounding pulses
   c. Hyperactive precordium
   d. Dyspnea
   e. Increased PVR
   f. CHF if pulmonary blood flow is unobstructed
   g. Murmur, ejection click, and thrill along left sternal border may be present.
   h. Mild desaturation that is not usually responsive to oxygen
   i. Failure to thrive
7. ECG
   a. Biventricular hypertrophy or left ventricular hypertrophy
   b. Biatrial enlargement of left atrial enlargement
   c. Depressed ST segment
   d. Inverted T waves
8. Radiologic findings
   a. Narrow mediastinum with cardiomegaly
   b. May have variable pulmonary blood flow indicated by pulmonary vascular markings
   c. A right aortic arch may be present.
   d. Pulmonary artery shadow may be absent.
9. Diagnosis
   a. Two-dimensional echocardiography
   b. Cardiac catheterization
10. Treatment
   a. Medical management for CHF with cardiac glycosides and diuretics
   b. Surgical correction with possible valve replacement

## V. Congenital heart defects with intracardiac defect and obstruction to pulmonary blood flow (cyanosis and decreased pulmonary blood flow)

A. Tetralogy of Fallot (TOF)

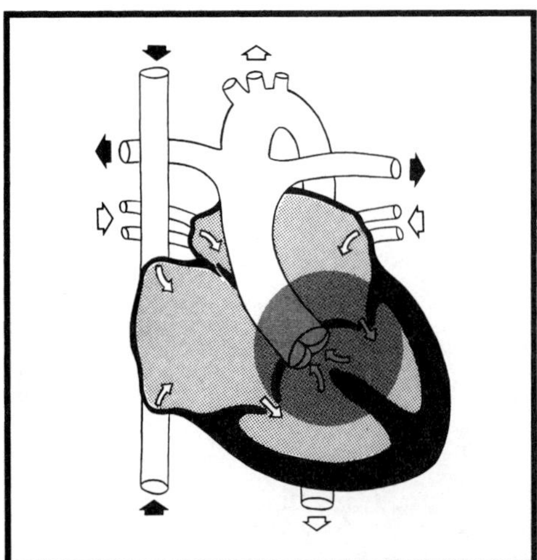

**FIGURE 12–10** Truncus arteriosus. (From Ross Products Division, Abbott Laboratories, Columbus, OH, with permission.)

1. TOF is characterized by four abnormalities (Fig. 12–11).
   a. Pulmonary stenosis or obstruction of the outflow tract of the right ventricle
      (1) The pulmonic valve may be bicuspid or constricted in or just below the location of the pulmonic valve.
      (2) The pulmonary annulus (a small ring or encircling structure) is hypoplastic (incomplete development of this tissue).
      (3) The infundibulum (a funnel-shaped passageway), the subvalvular portion of the right ventricle, may be hypoplastic or severely hypertrophic.
   b. Ventricular septal defect
   c. Overriding aorta
   d. Right ventricular hypertrophy
2. Pathophysiology
   a. Severe cyanosis and hypoxemia because of right-to-left shunt
   b. The right-to-left shunt is caused by reduced left heart pressures from a decreased pulmonary venous return.
   c. This shunt will increase as the following happen:
      (1) Pulmonary artery pressure increases.
      (2) Pulmonary venous return decreases.
      (3) Systemic blood pressure decreases because of reduced cardiac output.
   d. If the ductus arteriosus closes, further hypoxemia and reduced systemic circulation will occur.
3. Signs and symptoms
   a. Variable cyanosis: The incidence of cyanosis is greater in the following instances:
      (1) With a greater degree of pulmonary valve stenosis
      (2) With right-to-left shunting
      (3) When the infant is crying and feeding
      (4) With spasming of the infundibulum intermittent, severe cyanosis and hypoxemia result; this is referred to as a "TET" spell (see Treatment later in this section).
   b. Mild tachypnea
   c. Arterial blood gases show metabolic acidosis with severe hypoxemia.
   d. Practitioner should become suspicious when the infant receives oxygen and the $PaO_2$ stays at 30 to 40 mm Hg.
   e. Polycythemia
   f. Systolic ejection murmur
4. Radiologic findings
   a. Mild TOF
      (1) Normal heart size
      (2) Reduced pulmonary vasculature
   b. Severe TOF
      (1) Boot-shaped heart caused by the enlarged right heart pushing up the smaller left ventricle
5. ECG
   a. Increased right heart that persists with age
   b. Right atrial enlargement may also be present.

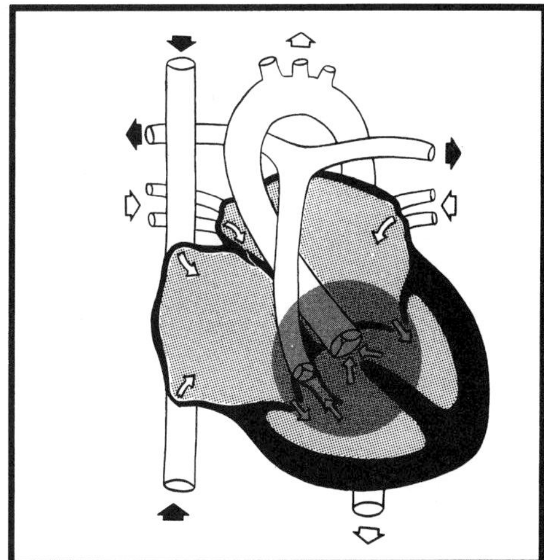

**FIGURE 12–11** Tetralogy of Fallot. (From Ross Products Division, Abbott Laboratories, Columbus, OH, with permission.)

6. Diagnosis
   a. Two-dimensional echocardiography
   b. Cardiac catheterization
   c. Clinical history and physical
7. Management
   a. Two objectives for management:
      (1) To increase pulmonary blood flow
      (2) To maintain ductal blood flow
8. Treatment
   a. $PGE_1$ in patients with cyanosis who are ductal-dependent
   b. Oxygen
   c. Sodium bicarbonate to correct metabolic acidosis if it is persistent
   d. Initially, surgery is performed to increase pulmonary blood flow. Later, between the age of 12 to 18 months, complete repair is done.
   e. Treatment of "TET" spell:
      (1) The patient's knees are pulled to the chest in order to increase venous return.
      (2) 100% oxygen is administered.
      (3) Morphine sulfate is administered.
      (4) Methoxamine or phenylephrine (alpha-adrenergic agent) is administered.
      (5) Beta-blocker (propranolol)
      (6) Emergency surgical intervention if severe

B. Tricuspid atresia
1. Tricuspid atresia is a defect with an absence, or agenesis, of the tricuspid valve (Fig. 12–12).
2. Blood from the right atrium cannot directly enter the right ventricle. If no ASD or patent foramen ovale is present, the patient does not survive. The atrial communication allows blood to enter the left atrium, the left ventricle, and, subsequently, the systemic circulation. Blood flows to the lungs through a PDA or, if a VSD is present, through the right ventricle (RV) cavity and then through the RV outflow tract. The RV may be hypoplastic or may appear normal in size.
3. Signs and symptoms
   a. Cyanosis is usually severe (present in 50% of patients at 1 day of life).
   b. Hypoxemia
   c. Acidosis
   d. Tachypnea
   e. Normal pulse
   f. Quiet precordium
   g. Systolic murmur with VSD
   h. No diastolic murmur
   i. A prominent $S_4$ gallop may be present if a restrictive atrial opening is present.
4. Radiologic findings
   a. Normal or slightly enlarged heart

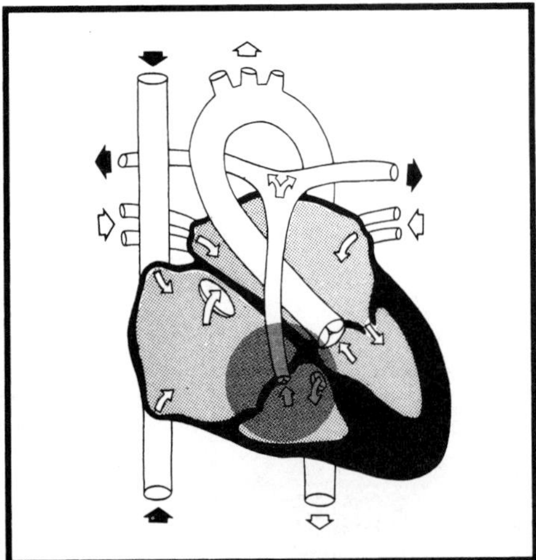

**FIGURE 12–12** Tricuspid atresia. (From Ross Products Division, Abbott Laboratories, Columbus, OH, with permission.)

b. Decreased pulmonary vascular markings
c. Concave pulmonary artery segment may be present.
5. ECG
a. Right atrial hypertrophy (peaked P wave)
b. Left ventricular hypertrophy
c. Diminished right ventricle force
6. Diagnosis
a. Two-dimensional echocardiography
b. Cardiac catheterization
c. Little change in $PaO_2$ with oxygen administration
7. Treatment
a. $PGE_1$
b. Shunt procedure to increase pulmonary blood flow
c. At 2 to 5 years of age, surgery is performed to anastomose the pulmonary artery to the right atrium to direct right atrial blood flow to the pulmonary circulation. The VSD and ASD are patched.
8. Ventilator consideration
a. Preoperative
(1) Low positive inspiratory pressure (PIP)
(2) Low PEEP
(3) Low mean arterial pressure (MAP)
(4) Higher mechanical rate
b. Following the shunt procedure, extubate the patient as soon as possible because positive pressure may not be tolerated. Until extubation is accomplished, the ventilator settings should be managed so as to use little or no PEEP and to keep MAP as low as possible.

## VI. Hypoplastic left ventricle (increased pulmonary venous markings)

A. Hypoplastic left ventricle
1. Hypoplastic left ventricle presents with an underdevelopment (hypoplasia) of the left ventricle, left heart valves, and the aortic arch. Complete atresia or severe stenosis of the mitral and aortic valve may occur. No survival if, after closing the PDA, there is no atrial septal opening (Fig. 12–13).
2. Signs and symptoms
a. The infant may be asymptomatic at birth until the ductus begins to close. Then the infant deteriorates quite suddenly and presents with shocklike symptoms such as:
(1) Respiratory distress
(2) Tachycardia
(3) Decreased blood pressure and cardiac output
(4) Weak or absent pulses in all extremities
(5) Slow perfusion and cold extremities
b. Murmur
c. Cardiomegaly
d. Cyanosis with a low $PaO_2$ and $SaO_2$
e. CHF
3. ECG

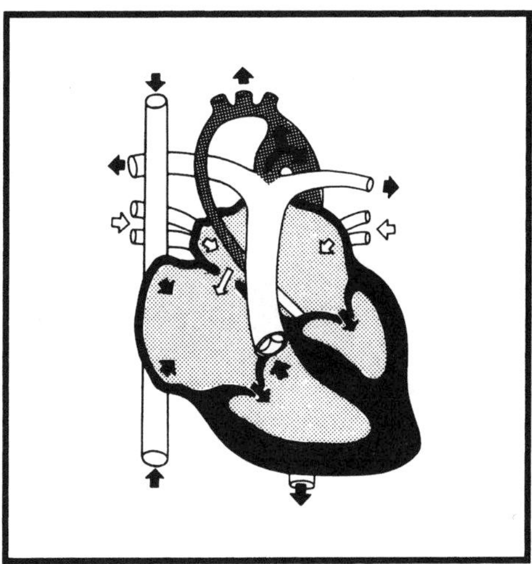

**FIGURE 12–13** Hypoplastic left heart. (From Ross Products Division, Abbott Laboratories, Columbus, OH, with permission.)

   a. Sinus tachycardia
   b. Right ventricular hypertrophy with ST-segment and T-wave changes
   c. Atrial enlargement
4. Radiologic findings
   a. Cardiomegaly
   b. Increased pulmonary markings
   c. Right atrial enlargement
5. Severe pulmonary edema if restrictive atrial opening is present with mitral stenosis
6. Diagnosis
   a. Two-dimensional echocardiography
   b. Cardiac catheterization
7. Treatment
   a. $PGE_1$ and supportive therapy until either a heart transplant or a procedure to route blood flow to systemic circulation can be arranged
   b. $CO_2$ or nitric oxide therapy
   c. Inotropic agents for shock

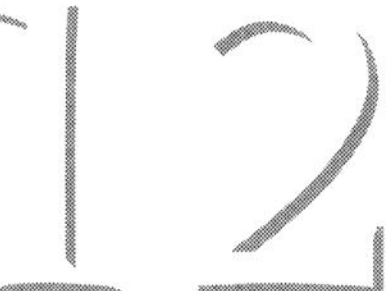

# REVIEW QUESTIONS

1. In the accompanying table, fill in the identifying congenital heart defects, the appearance of the heart on chest radiograph, and treatments.

| Congenital Heart Defect | Description of Defect(s) and Chest Radiographic Appearance (if present) | Treatment |
|---|---|---|
| Patent ductus arteriosus | | |
| Atrial septal defect | | |
| Ventricular septal defect | | |
| Endocardial cushion defect | | |
| Coarctation of the aorta | | |
| Aortic stenosis | | |
| Pulmonary valvar stenosis | | |
| Complete transposition of the great vessels | | |
| Total anomalous pulmonary venous return | | |
| Truncus arteriosus | | |
| Tetralogy of Fallot | | |
| Tricuspid atresia | | |
| Hypoplastic left ventricle | | |

2. Describe the following heart sounds.
   a. $S_1$
   b. $S_2$
   c. $S_3$
   d. $S_4$
   e. Murmur

3. What is pulsus paradoxus?

4. Where is the apical pulse found in a newborn?

5. What common tests are performed to determine cardiac defects?

6. What is a precordial pulse and where is it found?

7. List five findings on physical examination of a newborn that would indicate congenital heart defect.
   a.
   b.
   c.
   d.
   e.

## BIBLIOGRAPHY

Adams, H. F., Emmanouilides, G. C., and Riemenschneider, T.A. (1980). *Heart Disease in Infants, Children and Adolescents,* ed. 4. Baltimore: Williams & Wilkins.

Edwards, J. E., et al. (1990). The pathology, abnormal physiology, clinical recognition, and medical and surgical treatment of congenital heart disease. In Hurst, J. W., et al. (Eds.) *The Heart,* ed. 7. New York: McGraw-Hill.

Elliot, L. P., and Schiebler, G. L. (1979). *The X-ray Diagnosis of Congenital Heart Disease in Infants, Children, and Adults.* Springfield, IL: Charles C Thomas.

Emmanouilides, J. H., and Neal, W. A. (1988). *Neonatal Cardiopulmonary Distress.* Chicago: Year Book Medical.

Gates, P. C. (1983). *Clinical Cardiology: A Bedside Approach.* Chicago: Year Book Medical.

Gussenhoven, E. J., and Becker, A. E. (1983). *Congenital Heart Disease: Morphologic Echocardiographic Correlation.* Edinburgh: Churchill Livingstone.

Lehrer, S. (1992). *Understanding Pediatric Heart Sounds.* Philadelphia: W. B. Saunders.

Long, W. A. (1990). *Fetal and Neonatal Cardiology.* Philadelphia: W. B. Saunders.

Moller, J. H., and Neal, W. A. (1990). *Fetal, Neonatal, and Infant Cardiac Disease.* Norwalk, Connecticut: Appleton & Lange.

Park, M. K. (1988). *Pediatric Cardiology for Practitioners,* ed. 2. Chicago: Year Book Medical.

Pawlak, R. P., and Herfect, L. T. (1988). *Drug Administration in the NICU: A Handbook for Nurses.* Petaluma, CA: Neonatal Network.

Rowe, R. D., Freedom, R. M., and Mehrizi, A. (1981). *The Neonate with Congenital Heart Disease,* ed 2. Philadelphia: W. B. Saunders.

Ross Laboratories and Clinical Education Aid. (1992). *Congenital Heart Abnormalities.* Columbus, OH: Abbott Laboratories.

Silber, E. N. (1987). *Heart Disease,* ed. 2. New York: Macmillan.

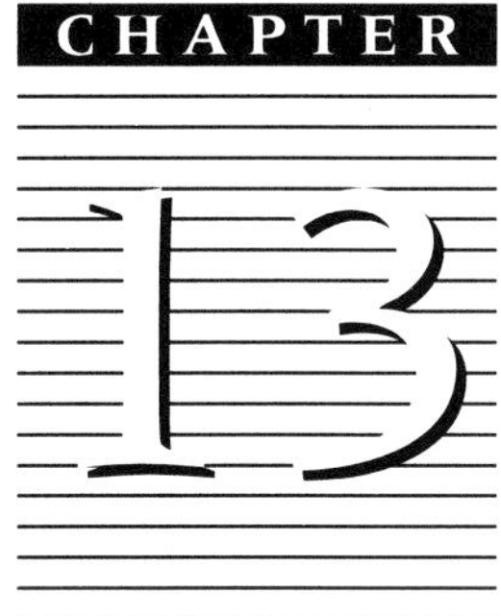

# Mechanical Ventilation

## I. Classification

A. Triggering mechanisms (begin inspiration)

1. Time-triggered ventilation, also called controlled ventilation, refers to ventilation provided in a time-controlled manner. The patient receives the set number of breaths regardless of the inspiratory effort.
2. Pressure-triggered, or assisted, ventilation occurs when changes in pressure in the upper airway are sensed by the ventilator as the patient inspires. An assisted breath is delivered when the machine detects this pressure change.
3. Flow-triggered ventilation, also called flow-by ventilation, occurs when the ventilator senses a change in inspiratory flow effort and delivers a flow to the patient. Ventilators may deliver a flow to augment the breath or actually deliver a pressure-limited or volume-limited breath.
4. With patient-triggered ventilation, the ventilator delivers a positive-pressure breath when a sensing device detects a patient effort. The sensing device detects the patient's effort and synchronizes the breath in the assist-control and/or synchronized intermittent mandatory ventilation (SIMV) mode. Sensing devices include the following: the Graseby capsule, which senses abdominal movements; the hot wire anemometer, which senses flow; the variable-orifice pneumotachometer flow sensor; and the chest lead impedance. The response time of the system has to be less than 100 ms in order to avoid stimulating active expiration. Flow sensors placed between the endotracheal tube and the patient circuit require low dead space to prevent $CO_2$ retention in small infants.

B. Cycling mechanisms (end inspiration)

1. Pressure-cycled ventilation terminates inspiration when a preset pressure is reached.
   a. The volume delivered will depend on the flow pattern, the length of inspiration, and the lung characteristics.
   b. Estimating tidal volume using flowrate and inspiratory time:

$$\begin{aligned}
\text{Tidal flow} &= \text{flowrate (mL/s)} \times \text{inspiratory time (s)} \\
&= 8 \text{ L/min} \times 0.6 \text{ s} \\
&= 8000 \text{ mL/min} \times 0.6 \text{ s (convert 8000 mL/min to mL/s by dividing by 60)} \\
&= \frac{8000 \text{ L/min}}{60} = 133 \text{ mL/s} \\
&= 133 \text{ mL/s} \times 0.6 \text{ s} = 80 \text{ mL}
\end{aligned}$$

   c. Pressure-cycled ventilators are specifically designed to have multipurpose and multimodal capabilities. They are constant-flow, time-cycled, pressure-limited devices. The continuous flow supplies a fresh gas source to the spontaneously breathing infant. Pressure-limited ventilation meets pressure early in inspiration but another parameter, such as time, determines expiration. Common neonatal ventilation is pressure-limited, time-cycled ventilation.
   d. An advantage to a pressure-cycled ventilator is that it limits pressure that may be damaging to the lungs. Pressure remains constant in spite of changing compliance and airway resistance. Constant flow allows the patient to take spontaneous breaths easily.
   e. A disadvantage to pressure-limited ventilation is that as compliance decreases and airway resistance increases, the delivered tidal volume decreases. If compliance improves, from surfactant administration, the ventilator does not detect the increase in tidal volume.

2. Volume-cycled ventilation terminates the inspiratory phase after the set volume has been delivered.
   a. Volume delivered to the patient must be measured at the exhalation side of the patient circuit since some of the delivered volume remains in the patient circuit due to expansion of the circuit, compression of the gas, or leakage around the endotracheal tube.
   b. Correcting for tubing compliance (this is for older children with tidal volumes greater than 200 mL)
      (1) If tubing compliance is unknown (commonly 3 mL/cm $H_2O$), then set the ventilator at a low volume such as 200 mL. Occlude the patient outlet on the ventilator circuit. Record the peak inspiratory pressure (the pressure limit alarm will need to be set at maximum). Divide tidal volume of 200 mL by the peak inspiratory pressure.
      (2) Tubing compliance = $\dfrac{200 \text{ mL}}{67 \text{ cm } H_2O}$ = 2.9 mL/cm $H_2O$ or 3.0 mL/cm $H_2O$
   c. Determine volume lost to gas compression (patient connected to ventilator).
      (1) Peak inspiratory pressure × tubing compliance
      20 cm $H_2O$ × 3 mL/cm $H_2O$ = 60 mL
   d. Determine actual delivered volume if the set volume is 300 mL.
      (1) Set volume – lost volume = actual delivered volume
      300 mL – 60 mL = 240 mL
   e. An advantage of volume-cycled ventilation is that with cuffed endotracheal tubes, tidal volume remains constant with changing lung compliance and resistance.
   f. A disadvantage of volume control ventilation is that tidal volume is maintained at the expense of peak airway pressure. As compliance decreases and airway resistance increases, peak airway pressure increases, possibly causing barotrauma. Leaks around the endotracheal tube can result in a loss of volume, causing hypoventilation. When ventilating a neonate with volume-cycled ventilation, maintain a tidal volume in the range of 5 to 8 mL/kg.
3. Time-cycled ventilation terminates inspiration after a predetermined time has been met. Inspiratory time is determined by a time mechanism in the ventilator and is not determined by lung characteristics.
4. Flow-cycled ventilation terminates inspiration after a predetermined flow has been achieved.
   a. Pressure support ventilation flow-cycles out of inspiration. Termination of flow varies between ventilators, but it may be as a result of reaching a percentage of peak flow (25% of peak inspiratory flow), a specific flowrate value (5 L/min), or a pressure above the set pressure support (3 cm $H_2O$ above the set pressure support). Volume and flowrate are determined by patient demand and lung characteristics.

## II. Modes of ventilation

A. Continuous positive-pressure ventilation (see Chapter 8)
B. Intermittent mandatory ventilation (IMV)
   1. This mode provides either a demand flow or a continuous gas flow for infants to breathe at their own rate and tidal volume. Mandatory breaths are delivered at a set rate. This may be a pressure-cycled or volume-cycled breath.
   2. Because the mandatory breaths are time-triggered, asynchronous breathing is a problem with small neonates. Often the infant's spontaneous exhalation is interfered with by a positive-pressure breath called "phase locking," which prolongs exhalation and reduces effective ventilation. Increased tidal volume occurs when a positive-pressure breath is delivered on top of a spontaneous breath. Problems such as pneumothorax, hyperventilation, or cerebral blood flow alteration can occur. Synchronizing the patient with the ventilator may require respiratory rates of greater than 60 breaths per minute (bpm) and adjusting the inspiratory time close to 0.3 s. To synchronize breathing, sedation and paralysis may also be required.
   3. There is greater variation in tidal volume using IMV versus SIMV.
C. SIMV or patient-triggered ventilation
   1. Mandatory positive-pressure breaths are synchronized with spontaneous breaths. Because the breaths are synchronous, there are fewer cardiovascular side effects, pulmonary complications, and cerebral blood flow problems.
   2. SIMV systems provide breath synchronization by means of pressure, flow, and motion sensors (see patient triggering).
   3. Pressure support ventilation can be used for spontaneous breaths to augment ventilation.

D. Pressure support ventilation (PSV)
1. PSV is a form of pressure-triggered or flow-triggered, pressure-limited ventilation where the ventilator provides a specific pressure once the patient has made an inspiratory effort.
2. The pressure reached during inspiration is set by the operator. The volume the patient receives is determined by the preset pressure, the lung characteristics, and the patient's inspiratory effort.
3. Cycling occurs when a predetermined decelerating flow (such as 5 L/min) has been reached or a percentage of peak inspiratory flow (such as 25% of peak flow) has been reached.
4. PSV may be added to IMV, SIMV, and CPAP. It also may be used as a standalone mode.
5. PSV is used to help overcome the endotracheal tube's resistance, to improve patient comfort, and to reduce the patient's work of breathing.
6. Different methods have been used to determine the amount of PSV to use (Table 13–1).
7. Adding PEEP or CPAP to pressure support will adjust the peak airway pressure to reflect both PEEP or CPAP and PSV level. If pressure support is initially 10 cm $H_2O$, adding (+) 5 cm $H_2O$ PEEP or CPAP will result in a peak inspiratory pressure of 15 cm $H_2O$.

E. Pressure control ventilation (PCV)
1. PCV provides the patient with constant air pressure during inspiration.
2. The pressure, rate, and inspiratory time are set by the operator. The inspiratory time may be provided by setting a specific time in seconds or by setting a constant I:E ratio.
3. This mode may be used with control, assist-control, SIMV, and PSV.

TABLE 13–1. ***Methods to Determine Pressure Support Levels to Overcome Endotracheal Tube Resistance***

**Method 1**

Determine the level of PSV by the amount of airway resistance ($R_{aw}$) created by the endotracheal tube.

$$R_{aw} = \frac{\text{PIP} - \text{plateau pressure}}{\text{flow}}$$

$$= \frac{30 - 20 \text{ cm } H_2O}{40 \text{ L/min}}$$

$$= \frac{10 \text{ cm } H_2O}{0.66 \text{ L/s}}$$

$$= 15 \text{ cm } H_2O\text{/L/s}$$

PSV is initially set at 15 cm $H_2O$. Changes in this level will depend on patient tolerance.

**Method 2**

Determine the patient's spontaneous tidal volume before adding PSV.

Increase PSV by increments of 1 to 2 cm $H_2O$ until the PSV volume is the same as the spontaneous volume before adding PSV.

Spontaneous volume before PSV was 150 mL.

PSV of 10 cm $H_2O$ achieved a pressure-supported volume of 250 mL.

**Method 3**

Determine the patient's spontaneous tidal volume using 5–7 mL/kg of body weight. Increase PSV until the tidal volume is equal to this volume.

Patient weighs 110 lb.

Patient's weight in kg:

$$= \frac{110 \text{ lb}}{2.2 \text{ kg/lb}} = 50 \text{ kg}$$

$$= 50 \times 5 - 7 \text{ mL} = 250 - 350 \text{ mL}$$

PSV is added to achieve 250 to 350 mL of tidal volume.

**Method 4**

Using the following formula to estimate PSV:

$$P_{psv} = \frac{\text{peak pressure} - \text{plateau pressure}}{\text{flowrate}} \times \text{insp. flow}$$

$$= \frac{40 \text{ cm } H_2O - 30 \text{ cm } H_2O}{60 \text{ L/min or } 1 \text{ L/s}} \times 30 \text{ L/min or } 0.5 \text{ L/s}$$

$$= \frac{10 \text{ cm } H_2O}{1 \text{ L/s}} \times 0.5 \text{ L/s}$$

$$= 5 \text{ cm } H_2O$$

4. Expiration is time-cycled.
5. Flow is adjusted by the ventilator to meet the patient's inspiratory flow demand.
6. Adding PEEP to PCV does not change the preset pressure. If the initial pressure is set at 30 cm $H_2O$ and (+) 10 cm $H_2O$ PEEP is added, the pressure limit is still 30 cm $H_2O$. However, the driving pressure difference is now 20 cm $H_2O$ instead of 30 cm $H_2O$. This may cause reduced tidal volume delivery and hypoventilation.
7. The preset pressure should be set to deliver a volume that is appropriate for the ideal body weight (IBW) of the patient. Exhale volumes should be monitored to determine changes in the pressure.

## III. Indications for mechanical ventilation

A. Apnea
B. Respiratory or ventilatory failure, despite the use of CPAP and an $FIO_2$ greater than or equal to 0.60
   1. Respiratory acidosis with a pH less than 7.20 to 7.25
   2. $PaO_2$ less than 50 mm Hg
   3. A physical examination that shows increased inspiratory effort, including nasal flaring, grunting, and sternal and intercostal retractions
   4. Agitation, pale color, or cyanosis
C. Alterations in neurological status, such as congenital neuromuscular disorders and intracranial hemorrhage, that compromise the central drive to breathe
D. Impaired pulmonary function caused by decreased compliance and increased airway resistance, causing a decrease in functional residual capacity due to the following:
   1. RDS
   2. Meconium aspiration syndrome
   3. Pneumonia
   4. BPD
   5. Sepsis
   6. Bronchiolitis
   7. Congenital diaphragmatic hernia
E. Impaired cardiovascular function resulting from the following:
   1. Persistent pulmonary hypertension
   2. Shock
   3. Congenital heart defects
   4. Conditions following resuscitation
F. Impaired pulmonary function leading to respiratory failure. Physiological measurements needed to determine respiratory failure and the need for mechanical ventilation are given in Table 13–2. Some of these measurements may only be obtained in older children.

## IV. Hazards and complications of mechanical ventilation

A. Barotrauma and/or volutrauma causing air leak syndromes, including the following:
   1. Pneumothorax
   2. Pneumomediastinum
   3. Pneumopericardium
   4. Pneumoperitoneum
   5. Pulmonary interstitial emphysema
B. Bronchopulmonary dysplasia from chronic prolonged mechanical ventilation and oxygen administration
C. Endotracheal intubation causing airway problems, including the following:
   1. Laryngotracheobronchomalacia
   2. Damage to upper airway structures from malpositioned endotracheal tube (ETT) and intubation equipment
   3. Mucus plugging the ETT
   4. Kinking of the ETT
   5. Self-extubation
   6. Air leakage around ETT
   7. Subglottic stenosis
   8. Main-stem intubation
   9. Small ETT causing increased work of breathing as a result of the small diameter increasing airway resistance
D. Pneumonia
E. Application of positive pressure to the thorax
   1. Decreased cardiac output

TABLE 13–2. ***Physiologic Measurements to Determine the Need for Mechanical Ventilation from Respiratory Failure***

| Physiologic Measurement | Normal Value | Abnormal Value |
|---|---|---|
| Maximum inspiratory pressure (MIP) | > (–) 20 cm $H_2O$ | < (–) 20 cm $H_2O$ |
| Vital capacity | 65–75 mL/kg of body weight | < 15 mL/kg of IBW |
| Tidal volume | 5–7 mL/kg of body weight | < 5 mL/kg of IBW |
| Forced expiratory volume in 1 s | 50–60 mL/kg of body weight | < 10 mL/kg of IBW |
| Respiratory rate | Newborn: 40–60/min<br>Infant (up to 1 year): 20–25/min<br>Child (1–12 yr): < 20/min<br>> 12 yr: 12–18/min | Newborn: > 60/min<br>Infant (up to 1 year): > 25/min<br>Child (1–12 years): > 20/min<br>> 12 years: > 20/min |
| $P(A\text{-}a)O_2$ difference:<br>$PAO_2 = Pb - PH_2O(47\text{ mm Hg}) \times FIO_2 - \frac{PaCO_2}{0.8}$<br>$PaO_2$ = arterial blood gas value | Newborns: 40–50 mm Hg for several days following birth.<br>Infants and children: < 25 mm Hg. | Newborn: > 300 mm Hg on oxygen.<br>Infants and children: > 450 mm Hg on oxygen. |
| Arterial/alveolar $PO_2$<br>$PaO_2 \div PAO_2$<br>100 mm Hg ÷ 125 mm Hg = 0.80 | > 0.75 | < 0.15 |
| Oxygenation index:<br>Mean airway pressure × $FIO_2 \div PaO_2$ | < 25: Used for postsurfactant response and to evaluate infants before ECMO therapy. | 25–40: 50% mortality<br>> 40: 80% mortality |
| Pulmonary shunt:<br>$Q_s/Q_T = \frac{(PAO_2 - PaO_2)\ (0.003)}{(PAO_2 - PaO_2)\ (0.003) + a\text{-}vDO_2}$<br>$CaO_2 = Hb \times SaO_2 \times 1.34 + PaO_2 \times 0.003$<br>$CvO_2 = Hb \times SvO_2 \times 1.34 + PvO_2 \times 0.002$ | Infants and children: 2–5% (no cardiac anomalies).<br>Newborn's shunt will normalize after a few days following birth. | Infants and children: > 15% (no cardiac anomalies).<br>Newborn shunt may increase because of PDA reopening or cardiac anomalies present. |

2. Decreased venous return
3. Increased intracranial pressure
4. Decreased blood flow to kidney, reducing urine output

F. Retinopathy of prematurity from increased $FIO_2$

G. Inappropriate ventilator settings causing the following:
1. Auto-PEEP
2. Reduced alveolar ventilation
3. Hyperventilation
4. Increased work of breathing
5. Patient-ventilator asynchrony

H. Ventilator dysfunction
1. Ventilator alarm failure
2. Loss of gas supply
3. Excess condensation in ventilator circuit
4. Humidifier failure

## V. Neonatal ventilator management (pressure-targeted ventilation using pressure-limited, time-cycled ventilation)

A. Oxygen
1. The goal in selecting a specific $FIO_2$ is to achieve a clinically acceptable $PaO_2$ value of between 50 and 70 mm Hg in the newborn.
2. If the $FIO_2$ is achieving the clinically acceptable value before putting the patient on the ventilator, then use the same $FIO_2$ setting when initiating mechanical ventilation.
3. Oxygen should be adjusted according to the pulse oximeter to maintain a saturation greater than 90%. The high saturation alarm is set at 95 to 97% on an $FIO_2$ greater than 0.21; when on an $FIO_2$ of 0.21, the alarm is set at 100%.
4. Blending devices should be used to deliver manual ventilation during suctioning to prevent the abrupt changes in $PaO_2$. These devices provide specific

$FIO_2$ by precisely mixing oxygen and air. A high-pitched alarm will sound if oxygen and/or air pressure decreases below a set level. A flowmeter attached to the blender provides flow with a specific $FIO_2$. Generally, the same $FIO_2$ as the ventilator $FIO_2$ is used when manually ventilating a newborn, unless the clinical status requires a higher $FIO_2$ (desaturation during suctioning).

5. Improvement in oxygenation has been found to occur when patients are placed in the prone position. This may have to do with this position generating a transpulmonary pressure sufficient to exceed airway opening pressure in dorsal lung regions, such as in regions where atelectasis, shunt, and ventilation-perfusion mismatch are most severe.

B. Peak inspiratory pressure (PIP) and tidal volume
   1. With pressure-limited, time-cycled ventilators, the primary determinant of tidal volume is PIP. Changes in PIP will alter the tidal volume delivery. As compliance and resistance in the lungs change, this will change tidal volume. This is difficult to monitor without a device to measure exhaled tidal volume.
   2. Because pressure is limited, adding PEEP will change the driving pressure and alter the tidal volume. For example, in a patient receiving 25 cm $H_2O$ without PEEP, the driving pressure is 25 cm $H_2O$. If (+) 5 cm $H_2O$ PEEP is added, the difference is 20 cm $H_2O$ (25 minus 5), thus reducing the driving pressure. When adding PEEP, it is important to observe expired tidal volume to ensure an appropriate tidal volume range. Hypercarbia may develop because of the drop in driving pressure. A reduction in PEEP, an increase in PIP, or an increase in mechanical respiratory rate may reverse the hypercarbic state.
   3. With pressure-limited, time-cycled ventilation, changes in lung compliance are often unnoticed if a bedside graphics monitor with pressure volume loops is not available. This is especially important after surfactant delivery, when an acute increase in lung compliance occurs. As compliance increases, delivered tidal volume increases, potentially leading to pneumothorax. Exhaled tidal volume should be monitored closely when delivering surfactant, and changes in PIP should be made as compliance changes. Also observe for the rise and fall of the chest to help determine excessive volume delivery.
   4. Various levels of PIP are used depending on the patient's compliance, gestational age, weight, airway resistance, airway graphic analysis, and time constant of the lungs.
      a. A time constant is the product of airway resistance and lung compliance. It is the time necessary for pressure within the alveolus to reach the total airway pressure change during positive-pressure ventilation. In other words, the amount of time needed for proximal airway pressure to equilibrate with alveolar pressure is a time constant.
         (1) One time constant allows 63% of pressure change in the lung.
         (2) Two time constants allow 86% of pressure change in the lung.
         (3) Three time constants allow 95% of pressure change in the lung.
         (4) Four time constants allow 98% of pressure change in the lung.
         (5) Five time constants allow 99% of pressure change in the lung.
      b. A time constant is the product of compliance times resistance. For example, if an infant's compliance is .004 L/cm $H_2O$ and airway resistance is 30 cm $H_2O$/L/s, then the time to deliver 63% of the PIP is 0.12 s. The recommendation is to have 3 to 5 time constants. Five time constants would be 0.6 s (0.12 × 5 time constants).
      c. Patients with reduced compliance and increased airway resistance have decreased time constants, and the movement of gas in and out of their lungs occurs more quickly. If the compliance of an RDS lung is 0.001 L/cm $H_2O$ and airway resistance is 60 cm $H_2O$/L/s, then 1 time constant is 0.06 s. Five time constants is 0.30 s. Changes in ventilator settings should be made to reflect this shorter amount of available time to move air into and out of the lungs. Allowing less than 3 time constants may not provide an appropriate change of pressure in the lungs.
   3. Setting PIP (Table 13–3)

C. Respiratory rate, minute ventilation, and I:E ratio
   1. Rate times tidal volume determines minute ventilation.
   2. Rate is made up of inspiratory time ($T_I$) and expiratory time ($T_E$). The length of $T_I$ and $T_E$ determines the I:E ratio.
   3. The interrelationship of $T_I$, $T_E$, TCT, respiratory frequency, and tidal volume (this tidal volume is what enters the patient's lungs, not the expired tidal volume)
      a. TCT = 60 s ÷ rate, or $TCT = T_I + T_E$

TABLE 13–3. ***Comparison of Peak Inspiratory Pressure***

| Level of PIP | Rationale for Use | Problems Associated with This Level of PIP |
|---|---|---|
| ≤ 25 cm $H_2O$ | Fewer problems associated with BPD and pulmonary air leak syndromes (PALS). | May not be enough pressure to maintain appropriate ventilation ($PaCO_2$). Atelectasis may develop if PIP too low. Difficult to maintain appropriate $PaO_2$ with low PIP level. |
| ≥ 25 cm $H_2O$ | Open areas of atelectasis. Reduce $PaCO_2$ and increase $PaO_2$ (increase mean airway pressure). Improve compliance. | Greater incidence of BPD and air leak syndromes. Alteration in cerebral blood flow. Reduced venous return and cardiac output. |

b. $T_I = TCT - T_E$
c. $T_E = TCT - T_I$
d. Determining $T_I$ and $T_E$ given I:E ratio and rate:
   (1) Rate = 10/min = 6 s TCT
   (2) I:E ratio is 1:2 = 3 total parts
   (3) 6 s ÷ 3 parts = 2 s $T_I$
   (4) 6 s – 2 s = 4 s $T_E$
e. Determining tidal volume from inspiratory time and flowrate: $V_T = T_I \times$ flowrate.
   (1) $T_I$ = 0.5 s and flowrate = 8 L/min
   (2) 0.5 s × 8000 mL/min (convert this to mL/s: 8000 mL /60 s = 133 mL/s)
   (3) 0.5 s × 133 mL/s = 67 mL
f. Determining $T_I$ from tidal volume and flowrate: $T_i$ = tidal volume ÷ flowrate
   (1) Tidal volume = 67 mL and flowrate = 8 L/min or 133 mL/s
   (2) 67 mL ÷ 133 mL/s = 0.5 s
g. Determining flowrate from $T_I$ and tidal volume: Flowrate (L/min) = $V_T \div T_I$
   (1) Tidal volume = 67 mL and $T_I$ = 0.5 s
   (2) 67 mL ÷ 0.5 s = 133 mL/s
   (3) 133 mL/sec × 60 s = 8000 mL/min or 8 L/min
h. With pressure-limited ventilation, tidal volume is not set, but is a function of PIP, compliance of the lungs, resistance of the lungs, and PEEP. Monitoring volume on pressure-limited ventilation is important because as compliance decreases and airway resistance increases, tidal volume will decrease. Changes in ventilator settings will be required if these lung conditions change. PIP, PEEP, and inspiratory time help to increase tidal volume.

4. Rate setting (Table 13–4)

D. Flowrate

TABLE 13–4. ***Ranges of Ventilator Rate Setting***

| Rate Setting | Rationale | Problems Associated with This Level of Rate |
|---|---|---|
| ≥ 40/min | Increase minute ventilation (may allow reduction in PIP and mean airway pressure). Decrease in $PaCO_2$. Improves acidosis. Higher rates > 60/min may cause auto-PEEP and increase mean airway pressure. Used for persistent pulmonary hypertension. To synchronize patient with time-controlled ventilation. | May cause auto-PEEP, increase mean airway pressure, and cause problems, such as decreased venous return, reduced cardiac output, increased pulmonary vascular resistance, and reduced cerebral blood flow. Increased $V_D/V_T$ ratio, reduced effective alveolar ventilation, and decreased compliance. |
| ≤ 40/min | Used for weaning. Less pressure in lung in a given amount of time, reducing positive-pressure effects on the heart, cerebral blood flow, and pulmonary vasculature. | May require higher PIP and PEEP. Asynchronous ventilation with time-controlled ventilation requiring sedation and paralysis. |

1. The typical flowrate during mechanical ventilation is 4 to 10 L/min.
2. Set the flowrate to achieve a least 2 times the minute ventilation and to maintain a pressure plateau. Low flowrates cause inspiratory pressure to be reached late in inspiration. Also, a low flowrate may not meet the patient's inspiratory demand and may cause the infant's inspiratory work of breathing to increase. Because of the increased resistance, excessive flowrate may also increase the infant's work of exhaling.

E. Mean airway pressure
   1. Pressure- and volume-limited ventilators do not have a mean airway pressure control so that a specific mean airway pressure cannot be chosen.
   2. Increasing mean airway pressure will help improve oxygenation because of the factors that make up mean airway pressure. Mean airway pressure times $FIO_2$ is proportional to oxygenation.
   3. Factors that make up mean airway pressure include PIP, PEEP, inspiratory and expiratory time, flowrate, and the flow waveform. To determine mean airway pressure, use the following formula:
      a. $$\frac{(T_I \times PIP) + (PEEP \times T_E)}{T_E + T_I}$$
   4. The area under the pressure curve is the mean airway pressure.
   5. Increasing the mean airway pressure may be accomplished by the following methods:
      a. Increase tidal volume by increasing tidal pressure.
      b. Increase respiratory frequency by reducing $T_E$, producing auto-PEEP.
      c. A decrease in the inspiratory flowrate increases $T_I$, leading to dynamic hyperinflation (not done with a pressure-limited, time-cycled ventilator).
      d. Adding an end-inspiratory pause (inspiratory hold or inspiratory plateau) creates similar conditions as decreasing inspiratory flowrate.
      e. Adding PEEP increases airway pressure during exhalation.
      f. Using a decelerating flow ramp causes a greater proportion of average flow earlier in inspiration.

F. PEEP
   1. PEEP helps improve alveolar stability, preventing collapse during exhalation and improving the inflation of the alveoli. Keeping the alveoli open improves lung compliance, reduces shunt, and increases $PaO_2$.
   2. PEEP is indicated with a $PaO_2$ less than 50 mm Hg on an $FIO_2$ greater than 0.60. PEEP is instituted at 3 to 5 cm $H_2O$ and titrated upward to achieve a 50- to 70-mm Hg $PaO_2$.
   3. Excessive PEEP, upwards of 10 cm $H_2O$, can cause overdistention of the lungs and reduced compliance. Patients may develop hypercarbia because the chest is in a "fixed position." The chest radiograph will show the diaphragm to be below rib 9 and the diaphragm flattened. PEEP should be reduced in this condition.
   4. With pressure-targeted ventilation, the driving pressure will be decreased as PEEP is increased and PIP will remain constant.
   5. The hazards of PEEP include reduced venous return, decreased cardiac output, increased pulmonary vascular resistance, alteration of cerebral blood flow, and barotrauma.
   6. Optimal PEEP is the least amount of PEEP needed to produce the largest increase in $PaO_2$. As levels of PEEP are increased, the $PaO_2$, compliance, cardiac output, and $SpO_2$ are monitored. Excessive PEEP has occurred when the $PaO_2$, compliance, cardiac output, and $SpO_2$ fall. PEEP is adjusted back to the previous setting.

G. Interrelationship of factors affecting pressure-targeted ventilation (Fig. 13–1)

## VI. Pediatric mechanical ventilation

A. Volume-targeted ventilation is indicated when consistent minute ventilation is required because of changes in compliance and resistance.

B. Tidal volumes are set to deliver approximately 7 to 10 mL/kg of IBW, the respiratory rate needed to deliver an appropriate minute ventilation.

C. Minute ventilation can be determined by using the following formula, which uses body surface area (BSA). After finding the BSA, multiply this value by the minute ventilation required for this patient.
   1. For infants weighing 2.5 kg to 20 kg
      $$BSA = \frac{(3.6)\ (\text{weight}) + 9}{100}$$
   2. For children weighing more than 20 kg to 40 kg

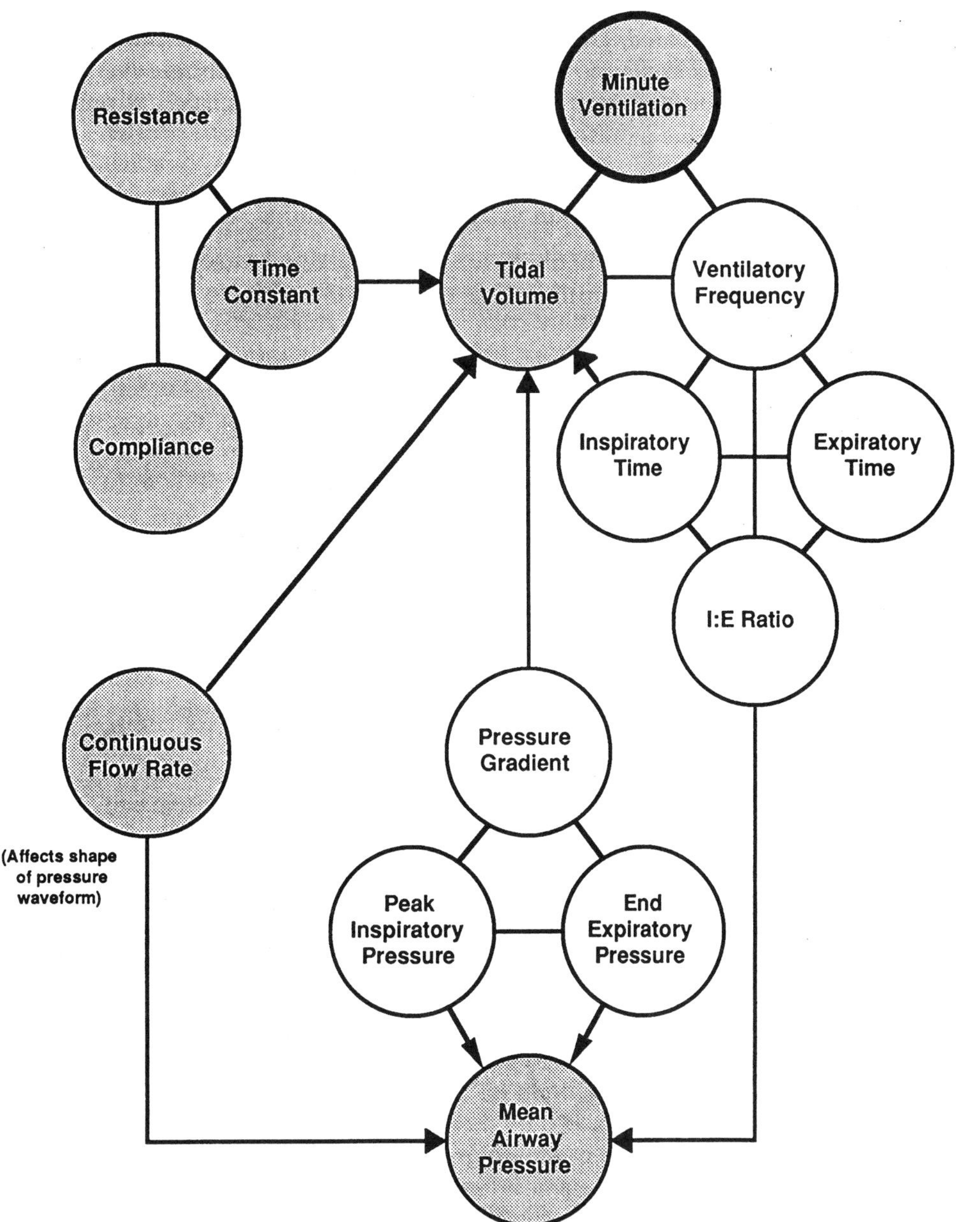


**FIGURE 13–1** Diagram illustrating the interrelationship of factors that affect pressure-targeted ventilation. (Pilbeam, S. [1992]. *Mechanical Ventilation*. St. Louis: Mosby–Year Book, p. 555, with permission.)

$$\text{BSA} = \frac{(2.5)\ (\text{weight}) + 9}{100}$$

3. For patients weighing more than 40 kg, determine the minute ventilation as follows:
   a. Male minute ventilation = BSA × 4.
   b. Female minute ventilation = BSA × 3.5.

D. Setting tidal volumes can be determined by using the following formula, which is based on the patient's $PaCO_2$ (this may be useful for patients with tidal volumes that are within adult tidal-volume limits):
   1. $$\text{Desired } V_T = \frac{\text{known } PaCO_2 \times V_T}{\text{desired } PaCO_2}$$
   2. A patient is being mechanically ventilated with a tidal volume of 300 mL. ABGs show that the pH is 7.27, $PaCO_2$ is 60 mm Hg, and $PaO_2$ is 50 mm Hg. The goal is to get the $PaCO_2$ to 40 mm Hg. At what should the tidal volume be set?

$$\text{Desired } V_T = \frac{60 \times 300}{40} = 450 \text{ mL}$$

E. Setting the appropriate respiratory rate with a patient in the control male or assist-control mode (not assisting) can be determined by the following formula:
   1. $$\text{Desired rate} = \frac{\text{known rate} \times \text{known } PaCO_2}{\text{desired } PaCO_2}$$
   2. A patient being mechanically ventilated in the assist-control mode has a machine rate of 12 breaths per minute (bpm) with no assisted breaths. Blood gas analysis shows that pH is 7.50, $PaCO_2$ is 30 mm Hg, and $PaO_2$ is 77 mm Hg. The goal is to correct the $PaCO_2$ to 40. What is the desired rate to achieve this goal?
   $$\text{Desired rate} = \frac{12 \times 30}{40} = 9 \text{ bpm}$$
F. SIMV may be beneficial to these infants to allow them to set their own $PaCO_2$ level with the assistance of pressure support ventilation (PSV). Because of the high resistance from the artificial airway, PSV levels may be instituted at 8 to 10 cm $H_2O$ and increased from there, depending on the airway resistance and returned tidal volume. Airway resistance is determined by the following formula:
   1. $$\frac{\text{PIP} - \text{plateau pressure}}{\text{flowrate (constant flow setting)}}$$
   2. A 12-year-old asthmatic is on mechanical ventilation. The PIP is 35 cm $H_2O$ and the plateau pressure is 25 cm $H_2O$. The flowrate is set on 60 L/min. At what should the pressure support be set?
      a. $$\text{Airway resistance } (R_{aw}) = \frac{35 - 25 \text{ cm } H_2O}{60 \text{ L/min or } 1 \text{ L/s}} = 10 \text{ cm } H_2O/L/s$$
      b. Set the PS at 10 cm $H_2O$ and monitor the exhaled tidal volume.
      c. Widening of PIP and plateau pressure (remains constant) indicates increased airway resistance.
G. Static lung compliance can be determined with volume-targeted ventilation.
   1. $$C_{ST} = \frac{\text{change in volume (tidal volume)}}{\text{plateau pressure} - \text{extrinsic PEEP} - \text{auto-PEEP}}$$
   2. A 10-year-old is receiving 400 mL tidal volume. PIP is 30 cm $H_2O$, plateau pressure is 25 cm $H_2O$, PEEP is 5 cm $H_2O$, and auto-PEEP is 0. What is the static compliance?
      a. $$C_{ST} = \frac{400 \text{ mL}}{25 - 5 \text{ cm } H_2O} = 20 \text{ mL/cm } H_2O \text{ or } 0.02 \text{ L/cm } H_2O$$
      b. A decrease in static lung compliance would indicate the need for an increase in PEEP. Optimal PEEP is determined by serial measurements of static lung compliance. A decrease in static lung compliance as PEEP is increased would indicate that optimal PEEP has been exceeded and the PEEP level returned to the previous setting.
      c. With PIP remaining constant, a narrowing between PIP and plateau pressure indicates a decrease in lung compliance.
   3. Because PIP will vary as the lung's compliance and resistance change, other modes of ventilation may be helpful in controlling the rise in pressure.
   4. Switching to pressure-controlled ventilation is recommended when alveolar pressure is greater than 30 cm $H_2O$. This pressure can be determined by obtaining a plateau pressure. Initially, pressure is set at one-half the alveolar pressure; then the pressure is adjusted to deliver a tidal volume of 7 to 10 mL/kg of IBW. PEEP is adjusted to deliver the appropriate $PaO_2$ with the lowest possible $FIO_2$.
H. The following equation can be used to determine desired $FIO_2$.
   1. If a patient's $PaO_2$ is 40 mm Hg on an $FIO_2$ of 0.40, what $FIO_2$ would be required to achieve a $PaO_2$ of 80 mm Hg?
      a. $$\text{Desired } FIO_2 = \frac{\text{desired } PaO_2 \times \text{known } FIO_2}{\text{known } PaO_2} = \frac{80 \text{ mm Hg} \times 0.40}{40 \text{ mm Hg}} = \frac{32}{40} = 0.80$$
I. Volume-targeted ventilation factors (Fig. 13–2)

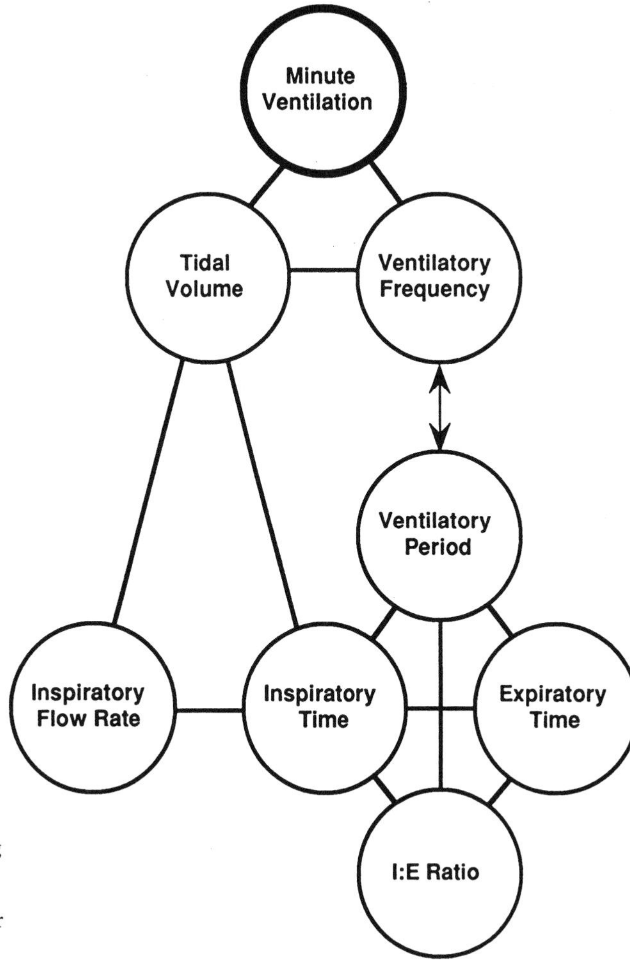


**FIGURE 13–2** Factors affecting volume-targeted ventilation. (Pilbeam, S. [1992]. *Mechanical Ventilation*. St. Louis: Mosby–Year Book, p. 556, with permission.)

J. Alarms (Table 13–5)

**VII. Instituting mechanical ventilation**

A. Recommended equipment
 1. Commercially available ventilator equipped with the appropriate modes, alarms, and limits
 2. Servo-regulated humidifier with low compressible volume chamber and a continuous water source
 3. Low-compliance ventilator circuit with heated inspiratory and expiratory wires with a servo-regulated humidification system with drainage capability
 4. Suction source, suction catheters, and normal saline
 5. Resuscitation device with manometer, mask, and oxygen connected to blender
 6. ETT with equipment to intubate and secure ETT
 7. Continuous noninvasive monitoring of oxygenation by either transcutaneous monitor or pulse oximetry with high- and low-alarm capabilities
 8. Continuous noninvasive monitoring of carbon dioxide by either transcutaneous monitor or end-tidal $CO_2$ with high- and low-alarm capabilities
 9. Continuous ECG and respiratory rate device with high- and low-alarm capabilities
 10. Graphic display of airway pressure, flow, and tidal volume, if available

B. Initial settings for pressure-targeted ventilation (Table 13–6)

C. Initial settings for volume-targeted ventilation (Table 13–7)

D. After placing the infant on the ventilator, obtain a blood gas and adjust ventilator settings to maintain pH greater than 7.25, $PaO_2$ greater than 50 mm Hg, and $PaCO_2$ at 40 to 50 mm Hg.

E. The patient-ventilator system should be checked at regular intervals (every 2 h) as well as following any change in ventilator settings, prior to obtaining blood gas samples, prior to obtaining hemodynamic or pulmonary function data, and

TABLE 13–5. *Common Ventilator Alarms, Settings, and Reasons for Activation*

| Alarm | Setting and Reason for Activation |
|---|---|
| Low tidal volume | Set below exhaled tidal volume (ventilator delivered or spontaneous). Activation of alarm indicates exhaled volume is less than set tidal volume on machine. This alarm may be the result of patient disconnection from the ventilator or because there is a leak in the patient circuit or around the endotracheal tube. |
| Low minute volume alarm | No set value but should be set appropriately so that if minute ventilation drops because of disconnection or apnea, the alarm will activate. |
| High pressure alarm | Set 10–15 cm $H_2O$ above PIP on volume-cycled venilators. Activation of alarm indicates the PIP has exceeded the set alarm value, and this ends inspiration. Activation of this alarm may be the result of patient coughing, buildup of pressure in the lungs from excessive secretions or pneumothorax, reduction in compliance, or increase in airway resistance. With pressure-controlled ventilation, the PIP level is the high pressure limit. Also on pressure-cycled ventilators, a pop-off pressure is set to prevent high pressure delivery to the infant in case of the circuit becoming occluded or dysfunctional exhalation valve. When the PIP has been set, the pop-off can be set by occluding the patient circuit at the wye adaptor and adjusting the pressure pop-off to 5 cm $H_2O$ above the PIP. This will require adjustment if the PIP is changed. |
| Low pressure alarm | Set at a level where, with each positive pressure breath, the manometer passes this level. For example, if the PIP is 20 cm $H_2O$, the low pressure alarm may be set at 5–10 cm $H_2O$. Activation of this alarm would be the same as for low tidal volume. |
| Low PEEP/CPAP | Set 5 cm $H_2O$ below the PEEP level. If PEEP $< 5$ cm $H_2O$, set 2–3 below PEEP level. Activation of this alarm indicates PEEP/CPAP has dropped below the set value, possibly due to a leak. |
| Apnea | Alarm activation indicates apnea and is set so the patient will not miss breaths, such as when the patient is receiving a low SIMV rate or is in the CPAP mode. Settings may include apnea time (depending on the respiratory rate), tidal volume, rate, $FIO_2$. On some ventilators, if apnea vetilation is activated, after sensing a number of spontaneous breaths by the patient, the ventilator switches back to the previous mode before apnea occurred. |
| High respiratory rate | No specific value, but alarm should be set to detect a rise in respiratory rate out of the normal range for the age of the patient. Activation of this alarm generally indicates the need for assessment of the patient to determine the reason for the rise in respiratory rate. |

as soon as possible following an acute deterioration of the patient's condition, particularly when this occurs after violation of a ventilator alarm threshold. Documentation of the patient's response to mechanical ventilation is performed:

1. To verify that the ventilator is functioning properly and is correctly connected to the patient
2. To verify that the inspired gas is correctly heated and humidified
3. To verify that the alarms are activated
4. To verify and document that the inspired oxygen concentration is measured with every change in $FIO_2$ or at least every 24 h
5. To verify and document that the ventilator settings comply with the physician's orders

F. All patient-ventilator system checks are to be recorded on official hospital forms and placed in the patient's medical record. At the time of the check, the following information should be documented as having been observed on the ventilator:

1. Name, hospital number, and diagnosis of patient
2. ETT or tracheostomy size and position
3. Date and time of last patient-ventilator system check
4. Current ventilator settings
   a. Set oxygen concentration and humidifier temperature setting.
   b. Mode of ventilation
   c. Set ventilator frequency.
   d. Peak, mean, baseline pressures, and presence of auto-PEEP
   e. Set PIP and pressure support level.
   f. Set tidal volume and delivered tidal volume.
   g. Set minute ventilation.
   h. Set inspiratory flowrate.
   i. Set continuous flowrate.
   j. Set I:E ratio, percentage inspiratory and expiratory time.
   k. Set sensitivity level (flow or pressure triggering).

TABLE 13–6. ***Pressure-Targeted Ventilation Settings for Infants***

| Ventilator Setting | Value for Noncompliant Lung | Value for Compliant Lung | Rationale |
|---|---|---|---|
| PIP (cm $H_2O$) | 20–25 | <20 | Larger pressure needed to overcome airway resistance and reduced compliance in the noncompliant lung such as an RDS infant. Increased pressure may improve oxygenation by increasing mean airway pressure. Monitor the postsurfactant patient and adjust pressure to prevent overdistention. |
| Respiratory rate (bpm) | 40–60 | <40 | To keep PIP low, the rate is increased to provide appropriate minute ventilation and $PaO_2$. Monitor exhaled tidal volume to maintain 5–7 mL/kg of body weight. |
| PEEP (cm $H_2O$) | 5–10 | ≤5 | PEEP improves lung stability. Increased PEEP improves mean airway pressure, improves compliance. Watch the level of $PaCO_2$ with increased levels of PEEP. Driving pressure is reduced as PEEP is increased, possibly reducing alveolar ventilation (PIP – PEEP = driving pressure). |
| Inspiratory time (s) | 0.3–0.5 | 0.4–0.6 | Time constant requires low inspiratory time based on the compliance and resistance of RDS lungs. As compliance improves, time constant changes, allowing inspiratory time to be adjusted. |
| $FIO_2$ | Adjust $FIO_2$ to maintain $PaO_2 \geq 50–70$ mm Hg. | Adjust $FIO_2$ to maintain $PaO_2 \geq 50–70$ mm Hg. | Improve $PaO_2$, reduce $A\text{-}aDO_2$, increase $PaO_2/PAO_2$ ratio, reduce pulmonary shunt. |
| Flow rate (L/min) | 4–10 | 4–10 | Provide constant flow through circuit to achieve pressure plateau before ventilator cycles. |
| I:E ratio | 1:2, 1:1 | 1:3, 1:4 | Increased I:E ratio (1:1, 1:2) shortens expiratory time, increases inspiratory time, allowing time for pressure to plateau in lung, and increased mean airway pressure. More potential problems with cardiovascular, renal, and cerebral systems. Less pressure time during inspiration with I:E ratio of 1:3, 1:4. |

5. Current alarm and alarm settings
6. Description of any problems with the proper functioning of the equipment
7. Signature of person performing patient-ventilator check with initials and credentials

G. On the patient record, the physician orders should state the ventilator variables to initiate in order to achieve the desired blood gas range. This includes mode, rate, pressure, tidal volume, pressure support, and delivered oxygen concentration.

H. Observations and evaluation of the patient should be documented and recorded. These include the following:
1. Breath sounds
2. Color
3. Chest movement
4. Level of consciousness
5. ETT cuff pressure and stability of the tube (if present)
6. Presence of resuscitation bag and mask at the bedside
7. Vital signs
8. ABG; glucose; $SpO_2$; transcutaneous, end-tidal $CO_2$ measurements

I. Tubing should be changed according to hospital policy or if there are conditions that obviously warrant the change. Condensation in the ventilator tubing is considered infectious waste and should be disposed of appropriately.

**VIII. Pharmacological agents used during mechanical ventilation (Table 13–8)**

**IX. Adjusting ventilator setting based on arterial blood gas analysis**

A. $PaO_2$ (Table 13–9)

B. $PaCO_2$ (Table 13–10)

TABLE 13–7. *Volume-Targeted Ventilation Settings for Infants and Children*

| Ventilator Setting | Value | Rationale for Setting |
|---|---|---|
| Tidal volume (mL/kg) | 7–10<br>Tidal volume is compensated for tubing volume loss. | Low volumes to reduce incidence of volutrauma/barotrauma but enough volume to maintain minute ventilation. If tidal volume causes high PIP, may reduce tidal volume and provide minute ventilation with rate. |
| Respiratory rate (bpm) | Infants: 20–40<br>Children: <20 | Maintain appropriate minute ventilation based on BSA. Minute ventilation may be achieved with rate to maintain low PIP. Excessive rate may create dynamic hyperinflation leading to auto-PEEP. |
| PEEP (cm $H_2O$) | 5–10 | Establish baseline to provide lung stability and increased compliance and increased mean airway pressure. Possibly, PIP may increase when increasing PEEP. |
| $FIO_2$ | Adjust to maintain $PaO_2$ for infants 60–80 mm Hg, children 80–100 mm Hg. | Improves $PaO_2$, reduces A-$aDO_2$, increases $PAO_2/PaO_2$ ratio. |
| Pressure support ventilation | Adjust to maintain a spontaneous tidal volume of 5–7 mL/kg. | Overcomes resistance created by small endotracheal tube, and supports spontaneous breath to help reduce the work to breath. Patient may tolerate stand-alone PSV if asynchronous with the ventilator. |
| I:E ratio | 1:2, 1:3, 1:4 | Longer expiratory time helps venous return, reduces incidence of auto-PEEP. Increased inspiratory time will increase mean airway pressure to improve oxygenation. |

C. Assessment of the patient after making ventilator adjustments. Improvement is noted by the following:
   1. Patient's work of breathing is reduced. This is assessed by observing a reduction in the respiratory rate, a reduction in the severity of retractions, and improved lung volume.
   2. Radiographic evidence of improved lung volume
   3. Increased chest excursion and aeration of the lungs assessed by chest auscultation
   4. Improved gas exchange as evidenced by an increased $PaO_2$ of greater than or equal to 50 mm Hg; an increased pH of greater than 7.25; and a decrease in grunting, nasal flaring, sternal and intercostal retractions, and respiratory rate

D. Monitoring the patient-ventilator system should be done every 2 to 4 h and should include the following:
   1. ABG or venous or analysis
   2. Continuous monitoring of ECG and respiratory rate
   3. Blood pressure by indwelling catheter or cuff measurements
   4. Mean airway pressure, PIP, and PEEP
   5. Inspiratory time, expiratory time, I:E ratio
   6. Inspiratory flowrate and the demand flowrate
   7. Alarms
   8. Periodic assessment of chest excursion and breath sound
   9. Periodic evaluation of chest radiographs to compare disease progression and ETT placement

## X. Weaning (see Managing $PaO_2$ and $PaCO_2$ by Ventilator Setting)

A. Pressure-targeted ventilation
   1. Decreased $FIO_2$
   2. Decreased PIP
   3. Decreased rate
   4. Decreased PEEP
   5. These settings are decreased until minimal settings are achieved. Switch to CPAP when the following settings have been achieved:
      a. $FIO_2$: less than 0.30
      b. PIP: less than 20 cm $H_2O$
      c. Rate: less than 15 bpm
      d. PEEP: less than or equal to 5 cm $H_2O$
   6. Monitor the patient for fatigue and increased work of breathing, which would require switching the infant back to mechanical ventilation.

TABLE 13–8. *Medications Used in ICU for Patients on Mechanical Ventilation*

| Medications | Comments |
|---|---|
| SEDATIVES | Induce amnesia and patients remain responsive and cooperative. |
| Benzodiazepines: | |
| Diazepam (Valium) | Used for status epilepticus. Metabolites prolong sedation. |
| Lorazepam (Ativan) | Drug of choice for status epilepticus; no active metabolites that prolong sedation. |
| Midazolam (Versed) | Ideal for short-term sedation during procedures; active metabolite prolongs sedation |
| Barbituates: | Negative effects on cardiovascular and respiratory effects. |
| Thiopental | Anesthesia for intubation. |
| Mexohexital | Anesthesia for intubation. |
| Phenobarbital | Used for status epilepticus and intracranial hypertension. |
| OTHER AGENTS | |
| Propofol (Diprivan) | Respiratory and cardiovascular depressant. Intravenous sedative-hypnotic allows patients to awaken quickly even after long use (although it is not approved for long-term use in PICU). Used during painful procedures, for children not tolerating mechanical ventilation. |
| Ketamine | Causes high level of sedation and analgesia. Rapid onset and short duration. It has bronchodilatory effects with no respiratory depressant effects. Has direct negative inotropic effects. |
| Chloral hydrate (Noctec, Somnos) | No analgesic effect and produces a metabolite that prolongs its effect. Sedation for agitation that interferes with ventilation. |
| ANALGESICS | Medications that relieve pain. Often administered to patients on mechanical ventilation, during procedures to relieve pain. |
| Morphine sulfate | Slow onset, delayed drug elimination and formation of metabolite that prolongs drug effect. Used with infants receiving higher rates and pressures. |
| Meperidine (Demerol) | Similar to morphine but not as potent. |
| Fentanyl (Sublimaze) | Short onset and short duration. Causes respiratory depression with minimal cardiovascular side effects. Rapid drug tolerance in newborns because of drug accumulation in fatty tissue. |
| NEUROMUSCULAR BLOCKING AGENTS | Short-term use during surgery and long-term use for mechanical ventilation to synchronize assisted ventilation breaths, especially in the newborn population. Monitor the effects by a peripheral nerve stimulator. |
| D-Tubocurarine (Curare) | Bolus administration causes histamine release and hypotension, which can lead to either tachycardia or bradycardia. These side effects are minimized with constant infusion. |
| Pancuronium (Pavulon) | Most common drug used with children on mechanical ventilation. More potent than D-tubocurarine. Side effects include tachycardia, increased blood pressure and cardiac output, and norepinephrine release (these side effects may help patients who are hypotensive and bradycardic because of analgesics and sedatives). Reversed by neostigmine and atropine. |
| Doxacurium (Nuromax) | Most potent neuromuscular blocking agents. Slower onset, lower dosage, and longer duration. No histamine release; minimal cardiovascular side effects. |
| Atracurium (Tracium) | May cause hypotension, increased bronchial secretions, and wheezing, if rapidly injected. Released from the body regardless of organ function. |
| Vecuronium (Norcuron) | Lack of cardiovascular effects. Longer duration of effect in infants <12 months old. Reversed by neostigmine and atropine. |
| Rocuronium (Zemuron) | Cardiovascular stability and no histamine release. Younger patients take longer to clear the drug. |

a. Increased periods of apnea and bradycardia
b. Increased heart rate
c. Intercostal and substernal retractions
d. Desaturation
e. Increased respiratory rate
f. Pallid color
g. Increased $PaCO_2$, decreased $PaO_2$, and acidosis

B. Volume-targeted ventilation
1. Decreased $FIO_2$
2. Decreased rate. Switch to SIMV/IMV and add PSV.
3. Decrease in PEEP down to less than or equal to 5 cm $H_2O$
4. Switch to CPAP/PSV when minimal settings have been achieved.

TABLE 13–9. *Managing $PaO_2$ by Ventilator Settings*

| $PaO_2$ (mm Hg) | Ventilator Changes during Pressure-Targeted Ventilation | Ventilator Changes during Volume-Targeted Ventilation |
|---|---|---|
| <50 | Increase $FIO_2$ in increments of 5–10%.<br>Increase PEEP/CPAP to 5 cm $H_2O$, if not already at this level. Check for changes in $PaCO_2$. If $PaCO_2$ is increased, PIP may need to be increased to provide appropriate driving pressure.<br>Monitor with ABGs every 20 min until appropriate $PaO_2$ is achieved.<br>Continuous monitoring with pulse oximeter to keep $SpO_2 > 90\%$. | Increase $FIO_2$, PEEP, and rate the same as for pressure ventilation.<br>(With volume ventilation, PIP will adjust to the compliance and resistance of the lung.) |
| 50–70 | Maintain settings. If stable after a period of time, consider decreasing $FIO_2$. | Same as for pressure ventilation. |
| >70 | Decrease $FIO_2$ in increments of 1-2% until it is <0.40.<br>Decrease PEEP in increments of 1 cm $H_2O$. | Same as for pressure ventilation. |

a. $FIO_2$: less than 0.30
b. Rate: no specific value but spontaneous rate should be within appropriate range for patient in SIMV/ IMV
c. PSV: no specific value but should be at a range where the patient is getting appropriate spontaneous tidal volume with normal work of breathing (5 to 7 mL/kg IBW)
d. PEEP: less than or equal to 5 cm $H_2O$
e. Switch to CPAP/PSV. Both pressures remain the same as the patient was receiving on volume ventilation.

**XI. Difficulty ventilating an intubated, mechanically ventilated patient (Fig. 13–3)**

TABLE 13–10. *Managing $PaCO_2$ by Ventilator Settings*

| $PaCO_2$ (mm Hg) | Ventilator Changes during Pressure-Targeted Ventilation | Ventilator Changes during Volume-Targeted Ventilation |
|---|---|---|
| >50 | Increase IMV or SIMV rate in increments of 5/min.<br>Increase PIP in increments of 1–2 cm $H_2O$.<br>Obtain blood gases every 20 min until appropriate $PaCO_2$ is achieved. | In assist-control mode (patient is not assisting), increase rate by using the formula:<br>$\text{Desired rate} = \frac{\text{known rate} \times \text{known } PaCO_2}{\text{desired } PaCO_2}$<br>If the patient in assist-control is breathing at a higher rate than the set rate on the ventilator, adjusting the set rate will not change the $PaCO_2$.<br>In SIMV/IMV, increase the rate. Add PSV to assist spontaneous breaths.<br>Adjust tidal volume, maintaining a 7–10 mL/kg IBW range.<br>Obtain blood gases every 20 min until appropriate $PaCO_2$ is achieved. |
| 40–50 | Maintain settings. Repeat blood gases in 2 h. | Maintain settings. Repeat blood gases in 2 h. |
| <50 | Decrease PIP in increments of 1–2 cm $H_2O$.<br>Decrease rate in increments of 5 bpm.<br>Obtain blood gases every 20 min until appropriate $PaCO_2$ value is achieved. | In assist-control mode (patient is not assisting), decrease rate by using the rate formula above.<br>If the patient in assist-control is breathing at a higher rate than the set rate on the ventilator, switch to SIMV.<br>In SIMV/IMV, decrease the rate. Add PSV to assist spontaneous breaths.<br>Decrease tidal volume, maintaining a 7–10 mL/kg IBW range.<br>Obtain blood gases every 20 min until appropriate $PaCO_2$ is achieved. |

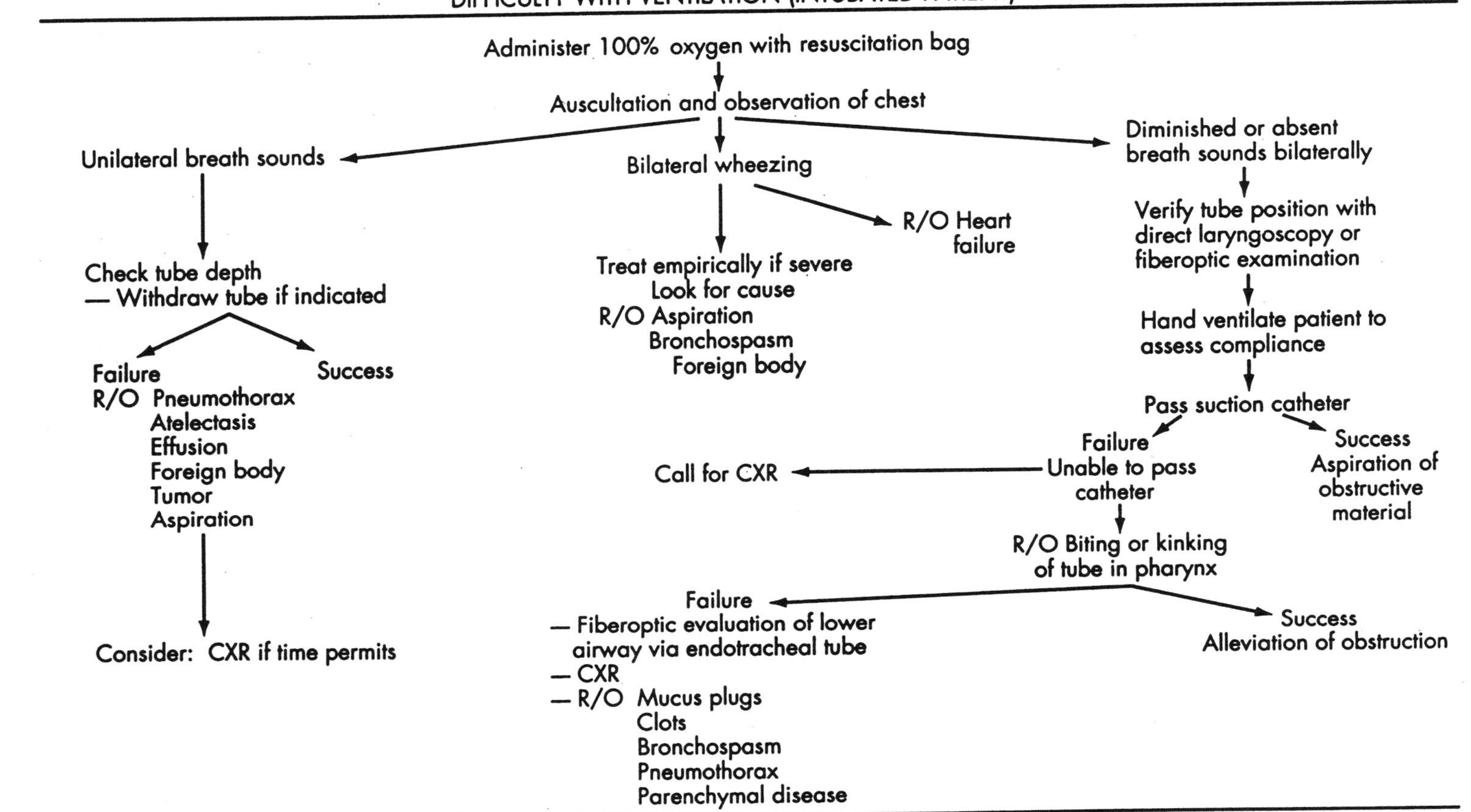


**FIGURE 13–3** A difficulty-with-ventilation algorithm for the intubated patient. (Finucane, B.T., and Santora, A.H. [1996]. *Principles of Airway Management,* ed. 2. St. Louis: Mosby–Year Book, p. 331, with permission.)

## XII. High-frequency ventilation (HFV)

A. High respiratory rate, low tidal volume (may be close to, or less than, dead space), and low peak inspiratory pressures are used.
B. Frequency is measured in hertz. One hertz (Hz) is equal to 60 bpm.
C. The magnitude of the chest rise is amplitude.
D. Indications for HFV
   1. Diffuse alveolar disease: respiratory distress syndrome
   2. Pulmonary air leak syndrome: pulmonary interstitial emphysema, bronchopleural fistula
   3. Nonhomogenous lung disease: meconium aspiration syndrome
   4. Pulmonary hypoplasia: diaphragmatic hernia, Potter's syndrome (undersized lung)
   5. During and after cardiac surgery
E. Types of high-frequency ventilation
   1. High-frequency positive-pressure ventilation (HFPPV)
      a. Utilizes a respiratory frequency of 60 to 150 bpm
      b. Tidal volume is less than 5 mL/kg.
      c. A conventional ventilator applies HFPPV or pneumatic valve systems with bulk gas flow.
      d. Exhalation is passive and no additional gas is entrained.
      e. Gas trapping may occur because of the relatively large tidal volume and short exhalation time.
   2. High-frequency flow interruption (HFFI)
      a. High-frequency flow interrupters deliver high-pressure, small tidal volume breaths in conjunction with mechanical ventilation. The pressure changes are monitored proximal to the ETT.
      b. Respiratory rates range from 120 to 1680 bpm (2 to 28 Hz).
      c. Frequency is adjusted by controlling the time the high-frequency breath is off. This in combination with a fixed breath determines the I:E ratio.
      d. Pressure amplitude is the result of end-expiratory pressure and mean airway pressure delivered by the mechanical ventilator settings.
   3. High-frequency jet ventilation (HFJV)
      a. HFJV employs a small-bore injector or narrow cannula where gas is delivered in short pulses under high pressure into a specifically designed ETT.
      b. With HFJV, frequency ranges from 4 to 10 Hz, expiration is passive, and positive-pressure breaths are delivered.
      c. Relative contraindications to HFJV treatment include obstructive lung diseases such as asthma.
      d. The initial set-up for high-frequency ventilation includes the following:
         (1) Obtain chest radiograph after placing the infant on HFV. Obtain frequent chest radiographs the first few hours after initiating HFV.
         (2) The appropriate expansion of chest is to have the diaphragm at the level of the 9th to 10th ribs (counting down from the first rib).
         (3) Monitor transcutaneous oxygen and carbon dioxide, oxygen saturation, and arterial blood gases frequently.
         (4) The patient's chest should be wiggling or vibrating between the umbilicus and clavicles.
         (5) The initial jet ventilator rate is set at 5 to 10 Hz. Conventional mechanical ventilator rate is set at 5–10 bpm to maintain lung expansion.
         (6) Jet ventilator PIP is set 10 to 30% lower than conventional ventilation. The conventional ventilation PIP is then set 10 cm $H_2O$ above the HFJV pressure and the IMV is decreased and PEEP is increased to maintain the same mean airway pressure as conventional mechanical ventilation.
      e. To improve oxygenation, increase $FIO_2$, PEEP, and respiratory rate on conventional mechanical ventilation (15–20 bpm). Overexpansion can cause poor oxygenation, which requires a reduction in mean airway pressure.
      f. Hypercarbia is treated by widening the pressure gradient between PIP and PEEP. If increasing PIP or decreasing PEEP does not affect the $CO_2$, the frequency is increased.
      g. Hypocarbia is treated by decreasing PIP, increasing PEEP, and decreasing jet ventilation rate.
      h. Weaning starts with reducing PIP and $FIO_2$ to less than or equal to 0.60. PEEP is then reduced, and PIP is reduced so that both the conventional ventilator PIP and the HFJV PIP are below 15 cm $H_2O$. At this point PEEP may be increased 1–2 cm $H_2O$ to prevent atelectasis. The HFJV peak inspi-

ratory pressure is reduced, and extubation can occur with rates at approximately 5 Hz.

4. High-frequency oscillation (HFO)
   a. A piston or bellows is used to generate positive and negative pressures at the airway through a regular ETT. This can be a stand-alone ventilator.
   b. Gas exchange occurs from tidal volumes that are smaller than dead space.
   c. Oxygen is supplied by a continuous flow of gas through the circuit, which removes carbon dioxide and creates mean airway pressure. The oscillations are superimposed on this flow.
   d. Because of the piston or bellows device, both inspiration and expiration are active.
   e. Consider HFO with acute lung disease when an $FIO_2$ of 0.60 or greater and a mean airway pressure approaching 15 cm $H_2O$ is required to maintain an oxygen saturation of greater than 90%.
      (1) Initiate HFO with a mean airway pressure between 5 to 8 cm $H_2O$ or 1 to 2 cm $H_2O$ greater than when the patient was on mechanical ventilation. Increase mean airway pressure until the $FIO_2$ can be reduced to 0.60 or less while maintaining an oxygen saturation of greater than 90%. Chest radiograph shows lung expansion to 8th–9th rib.
      (2) Rates for newborns begin at 10 to 15 Hz. Pediatric patients start at 5 to 10 Hz. Set inspiratory time at 33%.
      (3) Amplitude is set to achieve chest vibration between the clavicles and umbilicus. An incremental change of 2 to 5 cm $H_2O$ is accomplished to achieve an acceptable $PaCO_2$ or transcutaneous $CO_2$. Increased carbon dioxide levels or reduced vibrational quality may be caused by secretions in the airway, dislodged ETT, or pneumothorax. Suctioning should only be done when absolutely necessary. After suctioning the mean airway pressure, $FIO_2$ and rate may need to be increased to stabilize the patient again.
      (4) To improve oxygenation, adjust mean airway pressure and $FIO_2$.
      (5) To reduce carbon dioxide, adjust amplitude and rate.
      (6) Reducing the frequency by 1 to 2 Hz can help increase effective alveolar ventilation. Increasing frequency can reduce hyperventilation. Increasing inspiratory time may help, but there is a potential for gas trapping with this maneuver.
   f. Once the infant has stabilized and lung ventilation improves, weaning may begin by reducing $FIO_2$ first, then reducing the mean airway pressure by 1 to 2 cm $H_2O$. Monitor chest radiograph, oxygenation, and transcutaneous $CO_2$.
      (1) With continual improvement, the amplitude is reduced by incremental changes of 2 to 5 cm $H_2O$ until chest wall vibrations are no longer visible.
      (2) Incorporate conventional ventilation when the mean airway pressure has been reduced to 8 to 10 cm $H_2O$, $FIO_2$ is less than or equal to 0.60, and there is an improved chest radiograph or resolution of pathology such as a pulmonary air leak.

## XIII. Transporting the mechanically ventilated infant and child within the hospital

A. Patient transport includes preparation, movement to and from, and time spent at the destination. During movement, oxygenation, ventilation, and monitoring remain constant.

B. Contraindications to movement
   1. Unable to provide continuous monitoring, oxygenation, or ventilation by either manual ventilation or portable ventilator
   2. Unable to monitor the hemodynamic status of the patient
   3. Airway control cannot be monitored and effectively maintained.
   4. Less than an adequate number of health care team members are able to assist in the transportation.

C. Hazards and complications
   1. Respiratory alkalosis, hypotension, and cardiac dysrhythmias resulting from hyperventilation from manual ventilation
   2. Hypoxemia from loss of PEEP/CPAP
   3. Loss of monitoring capabilities due to failure of equipment
   4. Loss of airway from accidental extubation from equipment pulling on the ETT
   5. Loss of IV site, preventing administration of pharmacologic agents

6. Loss of oxygen from portable tank, causing hypoxemia

D. Equipment
   1. Emergency airway equipment, including laryngoscope blade and handle, appropriate size ETT, suction equipment, suction catheters, stylet, resuscitation bag, and appropriate size mask
   2. Portable oxygen source with adequate pressure
   3. Transport ventilator if possible.
   4. Portable pulse oximeter; cardiac monitor displaying ECG and respiratory rate
   5. Stethoscope

E. Personnel
   1. The transport team must possess considerable pediatric and neonatal critical care experience.
   2. Transporting mechanically ventilated patients requires the presence of a respiratory care practitioner and registered nurse.
   3. At least one team member should be proficient in ETT intubation, and both team members should be trained in neonatal resuscitation or pediatric advanced life support.
   4. At least one team member should be able to troubleshoot equipment problems.

F. Monitoring during transport
   1. The following should be monitored during transport of the patient:
      a. ECG and heart rate
      b. Respiratory rate and blood pressure
      c. Airway pressures, tidal volume, and $FIO_2$ (neonates) if a transport ventilator is used
      d. Continuous $SpO_2$
      e. Breath sounds to ensure placement of ETT or continuous end-tidal $CO_2$

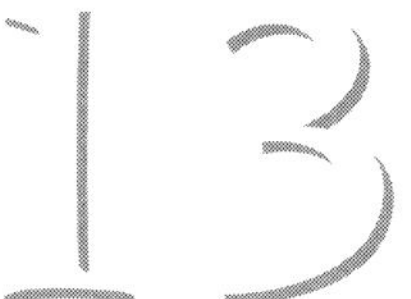

# REVIEW QUESTIONS

1. What is the tidal volume delivered to a patient receiving 6 L/min with an inspiratory time of 0.5 s?

2. When the patient is receiving either pressure-targeted or volume-targeted ventilation, how would a respiratory care practitioner know when lung compliance decreases?

3. Describe two methods that could be used to determine the level of pressure support ventilation to initiate for a patient receiving mechanical ventilation.

   a.

   b.

4. What is the difference between pressure control ventilation and pressure support ventilation?

5. List three indications for mechanical ventilation.

   a.

   b.

   c.

6. A patient on an $FIO_2$ of 0.50 has a $PaO_2$ of 50 mm Hg. What $FIO_2$ is required to achieve a $PaO_2$ of 70 mm Hg?

7. What two factors make up a time constant?

   a.

   b.

8. What concern is associated with administering surfactant to an infant who is receiving pressure-targeted ventilation?

9. An infant has the following ventilator settings:

   Rate = 20 bpm
   $T_I$ = 0.5 s
   Flowrate = 10 L/min

   Determine the following:

   a. Total cycle time

   b. I:E ratio

   c. Tidal volume

10. In the accompanying table, fill in the values needed to determine the need for mechanical ventilation.

| Physiologic Measurement | Normal Value | Abnormal Value |
|---|---|---|
| Maximum inspiratory pressure (MIP) | | |
| Vital capacity | | |
| Tidal volume | | |
| Forced expiratory volume in 1 s | | |
| Respiratory rate | | |
| $P(A\text{-}a)O_2$ difference | | |
| Arterial/alveolar $PO_2$ | | |
| Oxygenation index | | |
| Pulmonary shunt | | |

11. Fill in the accompanying table concerning the use of different levels of PIP with pressure-cycled ventilation.

| Level of PIP | Rationale for Use | Problems Associated with This Level of PIP |
|---|---|---|
| $\leq$ 25 cm $H_2O$ | | |
| $\geq$ 25 cm $H_2O$ | | |

12. List the factors that cause changes in mean airway pressure.

13. When is PEEP indicated for a patient receiving mechanical ventilation?

14. A patient receiving mechanical ventilation with pressure-targeted ventilation has a PIP of 20 cm $H_2O$ and no PEEP. Over the next few hours, PEEP is increased to (+) 10 cm $H_2O$ with a PIP of 20 cm $H_2O$. A blood gas shows the $PaCO_2$ has increased from 46 mm Hg to 58 mm Hg. What could be the reason for the development of the hypercarbic situation with the addition of PEEP?

15. List the factors that affect pressure-targeted ventilation.

16. Fill in the accompanying chart concerning ranges of ventilator rate setting with pressure-targeted ventilation.

| Rate Setting | Rationale | Problems Associated with This Level of Rate |
|---|---|---|
| ≥ 40 bpm | | |
| ≤ 40 bpm | | |

17. When is volume-targeted ventilation indicated over pressure-targeted ventilation?

18. A patient receiving volume-targeted ventilation has the following settings:

    $V_T$ = 350 mL
    Machine rate = 20 bpm (patient is not assisting)
    Mode = assist/control
    $FIO_2$ = 0.50
    Peep = 5 cm $H_2O$

    ABG returns when pH is 7.30, $PaCO_2$ is 50 mm Hg, and $PaO_2$ is 60 mm Hg. What should the desired $V_T$ be to produce a $PaCO_2$ of 40 mm Hg?

19. An asthmatic patient is receiving volume-targeted ventilation and has a PIP of 30 cm $H_2O$ and a plateau pressure of 20 mm Hg. Over the next few hours, the PIP rises to 40 cm $H_2O$ but the plateau pressure is still 20 cm $H_2O$. Based on this information, what changes have occurred in the lungs?

20. Twelve hours later, the PIP is 40 cm $H_2O$ and the plateau pressure is 33 cm $H_2O$. What changes have occurred with the lungs?

21. In the accompanying table, fill in the ventilator settings at which to begin pressure-targeted ventilation with both compliant and noncompliant lungs.

| Ventilator Setting | Value for Noncompliant Lung | Value for Compliant Lung |
|---|---|---|
| PIP (cm $H_2O$) | | |
| Respiratory rate (bpm) | | |
| PEEP (cm $H_2O$) | | |
| Inspiratory time (s) | | |
| Flowrate | | |
| I:E ratio | | |
| $FIO_2$ | | |

22. Fill in the accompanying table indicating the initial setting for volume-targeted ventilation.

| Ventilator Setting | Value |
|---|---|
| Tidal volume (mL/kg) | |
| Respiratory rate (bpm) | |
| PEEP (cm $H_2O$) | |
| $FIO_2$ | |
| Pressure support ventilation | |
| I:E ratio | |

23. Given the medications in the accompanying table, give a reason for the medicine's use for patients receiving mechanical ventilation.

| Medications | Reason for Use |
|---|---|
| SEDATIVES | |
| Benzodiazepines: | |
| Diazepam (Valium) | |
| Lorazepam (Ativan) | |
| Midazolam (Versed) | |
| Barbiturates: | |
| Thiopental | |
| Mexohexital | |
| Phenobarbital | |
| OTHER AGENTS | |
| Propofol (Diprivan) | |
| Ketamine | |
| Chloral hydrate (Noctec, Somnos) | |
| ANALGESICS | |
| Morphine sulfate | |
| Meperidine (Demerol) | |
| Fentanyl (Sublimaze) | |
| NEUROMUSCULAR BLOCKING AGENTS | |
| D-Tubocurarine (Curare) | |
| Pancuronium (Pavulon) | |
| Doxacurium (Nuromax) | |
| Atracurium (Tracium) | |
| Vecuronium (Norcuron) | |
| Rocuronium (Zemuron) | |

24. Fill in the accompanying table indicating the ventilator setting changes to make in pressure-targeted and volume-targeted ventilation with the given $PaO_2$ values.

| $PaO_2$ (mm Hg) | Ventilator Changes during Pressure-Targeted Ventilation | Ventilator Changes during Volume-Targeted Ventilation |
|---|---|---|
| <50 | | |
| 50–70 | | |
| >70 | | |

25. Fill in the accompanying table indicating the ventilator setting changes to make in pressure-targeted and volume-targeted ventilation with the given $PaCO_2$ values.

| $PaCO_2$ (mm Hg) | Ventilator Changes during Pressure-Targeted Ventilation | Ventilator Changes during Volume-Targeted Ventilation |
|---|---|---|
| >50 | | |
| 40–50 | | |
| <50 | | |

26. Give a brief description of the following high-frequency ventilations:
    a. High-frequency positive pressure ventilation
    b. High-frequency flow interrupter
    c. High-frequency jet ventilation
    d. High-frequency oscillation

27. Describe how oxygenation can be improved with HFJV.

28. Describe how hypercarbia is treated with HFJV.

29. Fill in the accompanying table for HFJV.

| | Values or Setting Adjustment |
|---|---|
| Starting rate | |
| PIP | |
| Setting changes to improve oxygenation | |
| Setting changes to reduce carbon dioxide | |
| Where should chest vibration occur to indicate appropriate pressure? | |
| On chest radiograph, level of diaphragm indicating good chest expansion | |
| On chest radiograph, level of diaphragm indicating overexpansion of the chest | |
| Settings at which to start weaning | |

30. Fill in the accompanying table for HFO.

| | Values or Setting Adjustment |
|---|---|
| Indication for initiation of HFO | |
| Starting rate: | |
| Newborn | |
| Pediatric | |
| Starting amplitude | |
| Where should chest vibration occur to indicate appropriate amplitude? | |
| What setting(s) should be adjusted to improve oxygenation? | |
| What setting(s) should be adjusted to reduce carbon dioxide? | |
| On chest radiograph, level of diaphragm indicating normal expansion | |
| On chest radiograph, level of diaphragm indicating overexpansion | |

31. List the equipment that should be available to ensure a safe transport of an intubated patient.

32. Describe the ventilator controls, alarms, and volume capabilities used to transport a patient.

33. List what should be monitored during transport of an intubated, mechanically ventilated patient.

## BIBLIOGRAPHY


Adams, J. A., Zabaleta, I. A., and Sackner, M. A. (1994). Comparison of supine and prone noninvasive measurements of breathing patterns in full-term newborns. *Pediatric Pulmonology* 18:8.

American Association for Respiratory Care Clinical Practice Guidelines. (1994). Neonatal time-triggered, pressure-limited, time-cycled mechanical ventilation. *Respiratory Care 39,* 8, 808.

American Association for Respiratory Care Clinical Practice Guidelines. (1992). Humidification during mechanical ventilation. *Respiratory Care 37,* 887.

American Association for Respiratory Care Clinical Practice Guidelines. (1992). Patient-ventilator system checks. *Respiratory Care 37,* 882.

American Association for Respiratory Care Clinical Practice Guidelines. (1993). Transport of the mechanically ventilated patient. *Respiratory Care 38,* 1169.

Bernstein, G. (1995). Synchronous and patient-triggered ventilation in newborns. *Neonatal Respiratory Diseases 3,* 2, 1.

Brochard, L. (1996). Pressure-limited ventilation. *Respiratory Care 41,* 5, 447.

Carlo, W. A., and Martin, R. J. (1986). Principles of assisted ventilation. *Pediatric Clinics of North America 33,* 221.

Chatburn, R. L. (1991). Principles and practice of neonatal and pediatric mechanical ventilation. *Respiratory Care 36,* 6, 569.

Coghill, C. H., Carlo, W. A., and Martin, R. J. (1994). High-frequency jet ventilation. In Boyton, B., Carlo, W., and Jobe, A. (Eds.). *New Therapies for Neonatal Respiratory Failure.* New York: Cambridge University Press.

Coghill, C. H., Haywood, J. L., and Chatburn, R. L. (1991). Neonatal and pediatric high-frequency ventilation: Principles and practice. *Respiratory Care 36,* 6, 596.

Czervinske, M. P. (1995). Mechanical ventilation of the pediatric patient. In Barnhart, S. L., and Czervinske, M. P. (Eds.). *Perinatal and Pediatric Respiratory Care.* Philadelphia: W. B. Saunders.

Fernandez-Mortorell, P., and Boynton, B. (1994). High-frequency oscillatory ventilation and high-frequency flow interruption. In Boyton, B., Carlo, W., and Jobe, A. (Eds.). *New Therapies for Neonatal Respiratory Failure.* New York: Cambridge University Press.

Frantz, I. D. (1995). High-frequency ventilation. *Neonatal Respiratory Diseases 5*, 1, 1

Grenier, B., and Thompson, J. (1996). High-frequency oscillatory ventilation in pediatric patients. *Respiratory Care Clinics of North America 2*, 4, 545.

Hargett, K. (1995). Mechanical ventilation of the neonate. In Barnhart, S. L., and Czervinske, M. P. (Eds.) *Perinatal and Pediatric Respiratory Care.* Philadelphia: W. B. Saunders.

Heldt, G., and Bernstein, G. (1994). Patient-initiated mechanical ventilation. In Boyton, B., Carlo, W., and Jobe, A. (Eds.). *New Therapies for Neonatal Respiratory Failure.* New York: Cambridge University Press.

Herridge, M. S., and Slutsky, A. S. (1996). High-frequency ventilation: A ventilatory technique that merits revisiting. *Respiratory Care 41*, 5, 385.

Keenan, J. P., and Salyer, J. W. (1996). Pediatric mechanical ventilation terminology. *Respiratory Care Clinics of North America 2*, 4, 487.

MacDonald, K., and Johnson, S. R. (1996). Volume and pressure modes of mechanical ventilation in pediatric patients. *Respiratory Care Clinics of North America 2*, 4, 607.

Mammel, M. C., and Boros, S. J. (1996). High-frequency ventilation. In Goldsmith J. P., and Karotkin, E. H. (Eds.). *Assisted Ventilation of the Neonate*, ed. 3. Philadelphia: W. B. Saunders.

Merideth, K. (1995). High-frequency ventilation. In Barnhart, S. L., and Czervinske, M. P. (Eds.). *Perinatal and Pediatric Respiratory Care.* Philadelphia: W. B. Saunders.

Movius, A. J., and Martin, L. D. (1996). Sedation, analgesia, and neuromuscular blockade during pediatric mechanical ventilation. *Respiratory Care Clinics of North America 2*, 4, 509.

Patterson, C., and Chatburn, R. (1992). Initiating resuscitation and respiratory support in newborn and pediatric patients. In Pilbeam, S. (Ed.). *Mechanical Ventilation.* St. Louis: Mosby–Year Book.

Salyer, J.W. Respiratory care in the transport of critically ill and injured infants and children. *Respiratory Care 36*, 7, 720–734.

Servant, G. M., et al. (1992). Feasibility of applying flow-synchronization ventilation to very low birthweight infants. *Respiratory Care 37*, 3, 252.

Smith-Wenning, K., et al. (1995). Neonatal and pediatric respiratory care. In Scanlon, C. L., Spearman, C. B., and Sheldon, R. L. (Eds.). *Egan's Fundamentals of Respiratory Care*, ed. 6. St. Louis: Mosby–Year Book.

Spitzer, A., and Fox, W. (1996). Positive-pressure ventilation: Pressure-limited and time-cycled ventilators. In Goldsmith, J. P., and Karotkin, E. H. (Eds.). *Assisted Ventilation of the Neonate*, ed. 3. Philadelphia: W. B. Saunders.

Spitzer, A. (1996). Mechanical ventilation. In Spitzer, A. (Ed.). *Intensive Care of the Neonate.* St. Louis: Mosby–Year Book.

Spitzer, A. (1996). High-frequency jet ventilation. In Spitzer, A. (Ed.). *Intensive Care of the Neonate.* St. Louis: Mosby–Year Book.

Truog, W. E. (1996). High-frequency oscillatory ventilation. In Spitzer, A. (Ed.). *Intensive Care of the Neonate.* St. Louis: Mosby–Year Book.

Vernon, D., Lynch, J. M., and Salyer J. W. (1996). High-frequency jet ventilation in the pediatric intensive care unit. *Respiratory Care Clinics of North America 2*, 4, 559.

Venkataraman, S. T., et al. (1995). Pediatric respiratory care. In Dantzker, D. R., MacIntyre, N. R., and Bakow, E. D. (Eds.). *Comprehensive Respiratory Care.* Philadelphia: W. B. Saunders.

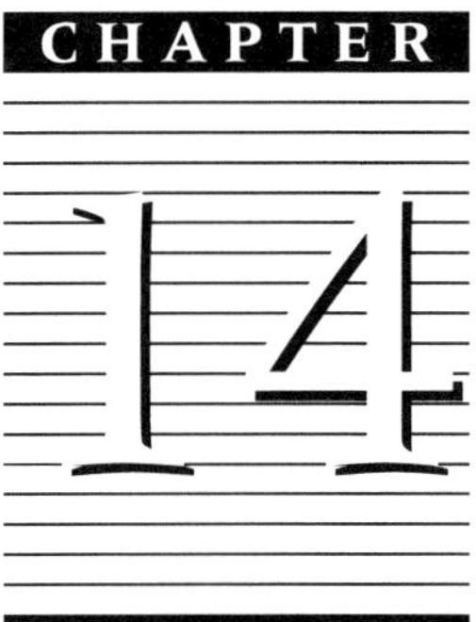

# Pulmonary Function Testing

## I. Indications for pulmonary function testing

A. To aid in the diagnosis of lung disorders such as reactive airway disease
B. To follow the natural history of lung growth or diseases presenting in infancy such as cystic fibrosis
C. To evaluate response to therapy
D. Used to make preoperative assessments in patients with compromised lung function when the surgical procedure is known to affect lung function
E. To allow for the prediction of risk of subsequent pulmonary dysfunction based on initial testing

## II. Measurement of flow and pressure

A. Pneumotachometer
   1. The pneumotachometer measures gas flow.
   2. A differential pneumotach, either variable orifice and fixed orifice, detects flow by measuring the difference in pressure between two points.
      a. A variable-orifice pneumotach uses a variable orifice to generate a pressure drop in response to flow. Changes in flow cause changes in the variable orifice, which alters the resistance to the flow.
      b. The fixed-orifice differential pressure pneumotach uses baffles to interfere with flow to create a pressure drop. A wire mesh screen acts as a baffle to alter flow. This type of pneumotach may be nondisposable or disposable.
   3. Hot wire anemometry detects flow by using the thermal properties of the gas being delivered. The pneumotach contains heated wires. As gas flows into the pneumotach and comes into contact with the heated wires, they cool. Flow is determined by the change in current needed to maintain the temperature of the heated wires.

B. Pressure transducer
   1. A typical pressure transducer has two pressure ports, one for measuring airway pressure and the other as a reference pressure port. The reference pressure port measures barometric pressure, allowing the pressure transducer to be used at any altitude.

## III. Spirometric pulmonary function measurement in children

A. Pulmonary function testing is performed in such common diseases as cystic fibrosis, asthma, and chest deformity. The tests used in these diseases are the same as those used for the adult who has obstructive or restrictive disease.
B. Lung volume and capacities (Table 14–1)
   1. Volume-measuring devices include the water-sealed spirometer, bellows spirometer, and dry-rolling spirometer. The accuracy of a volume-measuring device is determined with a 3-L syringe.
   2. Static lung volumes are determined when airflow velocity does not play a role. When two or more lung volumes are added together, a capacity is determined. Units of measurement are in liters and are at body temperature and pressure saturated with water vapor (BTPS).
      a. Tidal volume (TV) is the volume of air inhaled or exhaled with each respiratory cycle. The average volume is calculated following six breaths.
      b. Inspiratory reserve volume (IRV) is the maximal amount of air that is inhaled at the end-inspiratory tidal volume level.

TABLE 14–1. ***Volumes and Capacities of the Lung***

| Inspiratory Reserve Volume (IRV) | Inspiratory Capacity (IC) | Vital Capacity (IC) | Total Lung Capacity (TLC) |
|---|---|---|---|
| Tidal Volume (TV) | | | |
| Expiratory Reserve Volume (ERV) | Functional Residual Capacity (FRC) | | |
| Residual Volume (RV) | | Residual Volume (RV) | |

c. Expiratory reserve volume (ERV) is the maximal amount of air that is exhaled after a normal tidal exhalation. Exhalation is begun at functional residual capacity (FRC).

d. Residual volume (RV) is the volume of gas remaining in the lungs after a maximal exhalation. Calculation of RV is determined by FRC – ERV, or total lung capacity (TLC) – vital capacity (VC).

e. Inspiratory capacity (IC) is the amount of air that can be inhaled from end-expiratory tidal volume: TV + IRV = IC.

f. FRC is the amount of air left in the lungs at the end-expiratory tidal volume level. FRC is determined by helium dilution, nitrogen washout, and body plethysmography.

g. TLC is the total amount of air left in the lungs after a maximal inspiration: TLC = FRC + IC, or RV + VC. Measurements used to determine TLC include body plethysmography and gas dilution.

h. VC includes three volumes: VT, IRV, and ERV. VC is the maximal amount of air that can be inhaled and exhaled. It is appropriate to perform three VC maneuvers and to report the largest of the three VCs. The two largest VCs should agree within 5% or 100 mL of one another, whichever is largest. Predicted values can be obtained from a chart or from the following formulas:

(1) Males: $VC = 27.63 - (0.112 \times \text{age}) \times (\text{height in cm})$

(2) Females: $VC = 21.78 - (0.101 \times \text{age}) \times (\text{height in cm})$

C. Forced vital capacity (FVC)

1. FVC is the maximum volume of gas that can be expelled from the lungs during a forceful, rapid exhalation following a maximal inspiration (Fig. 14–1).
2. Predictive equation for children. Use the same equation for vital capacity.

a. For children 42 to 59 in (107 to 150 cm):

(1) Male: $(0.094 \times \text{height in cm}) - 3.04$

(2) Female: $(.077 \times \text{height in cm}) - 2.37$

b. For children 60 to 78 in (152 to 198 cm):

(1) Male: $(0.164 \times \text{height in cm}) + (0.174 \times \text{age}) - 9.43$

(2) Female: $(.0117 \times \text{height in cm}) + (0.102 \times \text{age}) - 5.87$

3. The FVC and VC should normally be within 5% of each other.
4. In general, decreased FVC is common with restrictive diseases such as pneumonia, scoliosis, and myasthenia gravis.

D. $FVC_{Timed}$

1. Timed vital capacity maneuvers can be derived from the FVC curve. These include the following:

a. Forced expiratory volume in 0.5 s ($FEV_{0.5}$)

b. Forced expiratory volume in 1 second ($FEV_1$)

c. Forced expiratory volume in 2 s ($FEV_2$)

d. Forced expiratory volume in 3 s ($FEV_3$)

2. Forced expiratory volume curve (Fig. 14–2)
3. Predictive equation for $FEV_1$

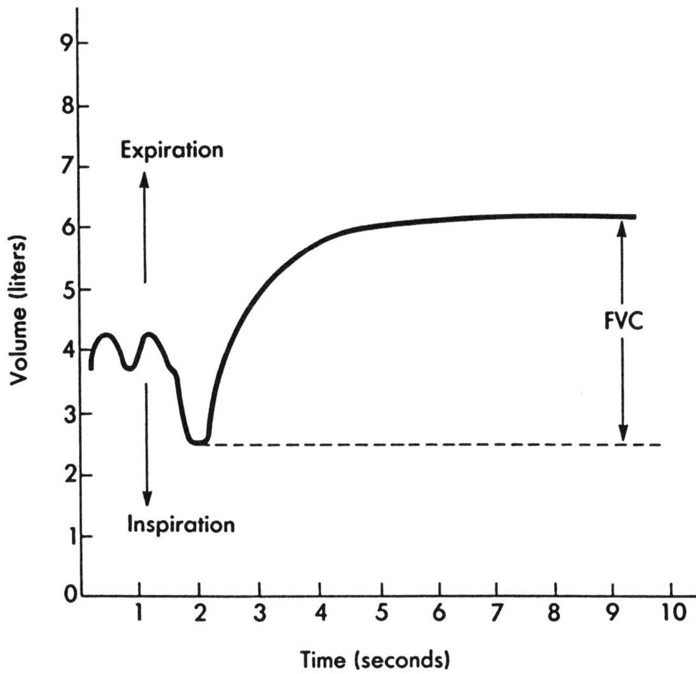


**FIGURE 14–1** Forced vital capacity. After exhaling normally, the patient is instructed to take a deep breath and blow out as hard and as fast as possible. (Ruppel, G. [1994]. *Manual of Pulmonary Function Testing*, ed. 6. St. Louis: Mosby–Year Book, p. 44, with permission.)

a. In children 42 to 59 in (107 to 150 cm) tall:
   (1) Male: (0.085 × height in cm) – 2.86
   (2) Female: (0.074 × height in cm) – 2.48
b. In children 60 to 78 in (152 to 198 cm) tall:
   (1) Male: (0.143 × height in cm) + (0.126 × age) – 7.86
   (2) Female: (0.100 × height in cm) + (0.085 × age) – 4.94

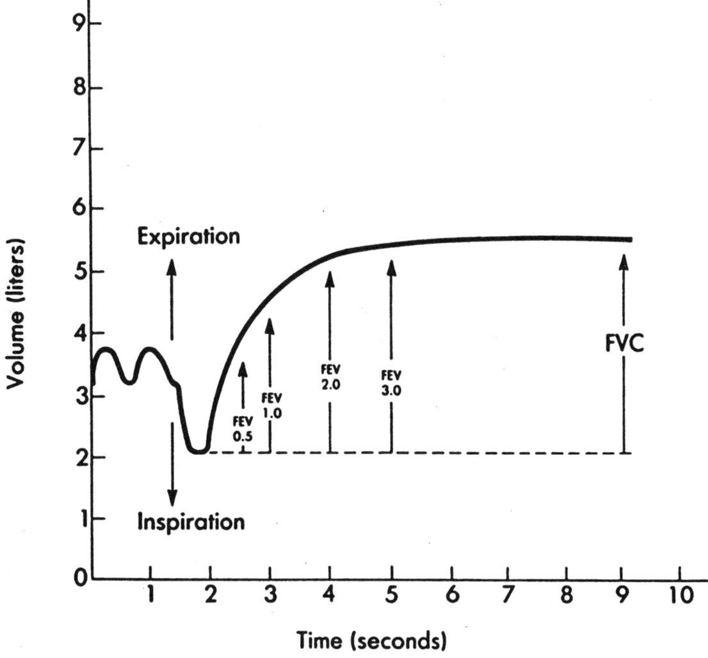


**FIGURE 14–2** Forced vital capacity maneuver showing FEV intervals of 0.5, 1.0, 2.0, and 3.0 seconds. (Ruppel, G. [1994]. *Manual of Pulmonary Function Testing*, ed. 6. St. Louis: Mosby–Year Book, p. 47, with permission.)

4. $FEV_1$ may be decreased with an obstruction in the airways, which is present with asthma, bronchitis, or bronchospasm.

E. Ratio of forced expiratory volume in 1 s to forced vital capacity ($FEV_1/FVC$, or $FEV_{T\%}$)
   1. The $FEV_1$ and the $FEV_1/FVC$ are the most widely used measurements to determine obstructive disease. They determine the percentage of vital capacity that is expelled in 1 s. Normally, $FEV_{1\%}$ is equal to 75 to 85% of the FVC, $FEV_{2\%}$ is 94% of the FVC, and $FEV_{3\%}$ is 97% of the FVC.
   2. Equations follow:
      a. $$FEV_{1\%} = \frac{FEV_1}{FVC} \times 100$$
      b. $$FEV_{2\%} = \frac{FEV_3}{FVC} \times 100$$
      c. $$FEV_{3\%} = \frac{FEV_3}{FVC} \times 100$$
   3. Obstructive disease reduces the $FEV_{T\%}$ ratio for a particular timed interval.
   4. The primary spirometry tests used to determine obstructive disease include FVC, $FEV_1$, and $FEV_1/FVC$.

F. Forced expiratory flow, 25 to 75% ($FEF_{25-75\%}$)
   1. The $FEF_{25-75\%}$ is measured from the FVC maneuver. This flow is from the medium and small airways.
   2. Reduced flows are common in early obstructive disease.
   3. Predictive equations follow:
      a. For children 42 to 59 in (107 to 152 cm) tall:
         (1) Males: (0.094 × height in cm) – 2.61
         (2) Females: (0.087 × height in cm) – 2.39
      b. For children 60 to 78 in (152 to 198 cm ) tall:
         (1) Males: (0.135 × height in cm) – (0.126 × Age) – 6.50
         (2) Females: (0.093 × height in cm) + (0.083 × Age) – 3.50

G. Peak expiratory flowrate (PEF)
   1. PEF is the amount of air that is expelled in a FVC maneuver (Fig. 14–3).
   2. PEF is effort-dependent and may be limited.
   3. When performed well, PEF correlates with FVC.

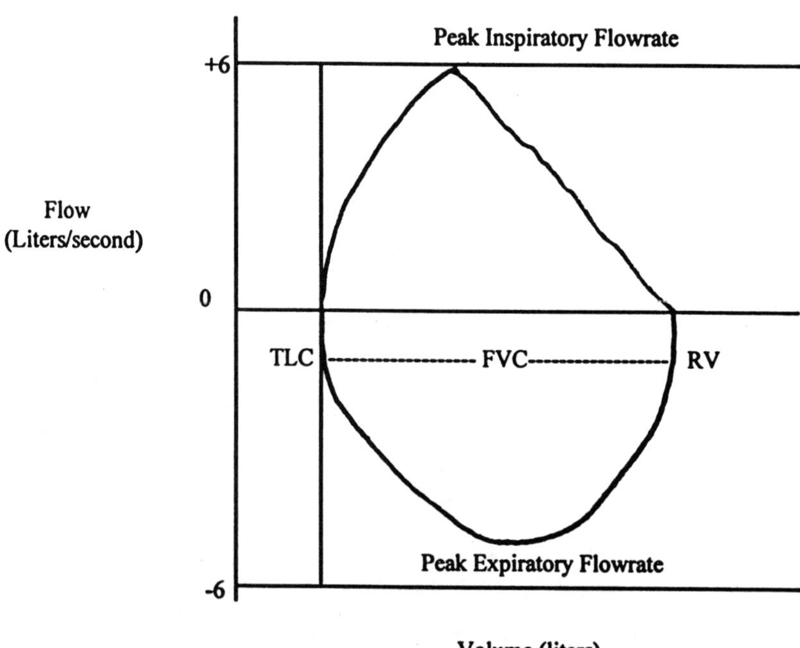


**FIGURE 14–3** Flow-volume loop.

4. In general, reduced PEF is associated with large airway obstructions. Using flow-volume loops will help determine the site and severity of the obstruction.
5. Predictive equations follow:
   a. For children 42 to 59 in (107 to 150 cm) tall:
      (1) Males: $(0.161 \times \text{height in cm}) - 5.88$
      (2) Females: $(0.131 \times \text{height in cm}) - 4.51$
   b. For children 60 to 78 in (152 to 198 cm) tall:
      (1) Males: $(0.181 \times \text{height in cm}) + (0.205 \times \text{age}) - 9.54$
      (2) Females: $(0.100 \times \text{height in cm}) + (0.139 \times \text{age}) - 4.12$

H. Prebronchodilator and postbronchodilator study
1. After performing a baseline PFT study, a sympathomimetic is administered with either a small-volume nebulizer (SVN) or a metered-dose inhaler (MDI) with a spacer device. Small children, who may be uncoordinated with the MDI, may require a SVN.
2. Proper breathing pattern is important. With a SVN, a breath-hold of 3 to 5 s should be performed by the patient. With a MDI, the breath-hold should be for 5 to 10 s and there should be a delay of 5 to 10 min between puffs.
3. Five to 10 min after administration of the bronchodilator, the patient performs the postbronchodilator study.
4. Equations follow:
   a. $$\% \text{ change} = \frac{\text{postdrug test} - \text{predrug test}}{\text{predrug test}}$$
   b. If the test used to calculate the percentage change is the $FEV_1$, then the calculation is as follows:
      (1) $$\% \text{ change} = \frac{\text{post–}FEV_1 \text{ value} - \text{pre–}FEV_1 \text{ value}}{\text{pre–}FEV_1 \text{ value}}$$
   c. A significant response is an increase in $FEV_1$ of 12 to 15%.

## IV. Methods for determining FRC

A. Nitrogen washout (open-circuit method)
1. The patient breathes 100%, and the tidal volume is collected over a period of 7 min or until the nitrogen expired is less than 1%. Breathing begins and ends at FRC.
2. Once FRC is determined, RV can be determined by the following equation:
   a. RV = FRC – ERV.

B. Helium dilution (closed-circuit method)
1. The patient breathes a certain percentage of helium through a circuit and bellows system. Breathing continues until a constant helium percentage occurs. Breathing begins and ends at FRC. This takes approximately 7 min.
2. Although helium is inert, a small amount of helium will be lost to the blood.
3. A carbon dioxide soda lime absorber is placed in line to remove carbon dioxide, and oxygen is titrated into the circuit to meet the patient's needs. Changes in the patient's rate and volume will occur if the carbon dioxide absorber is not in line or the soda lime absorber has expired (as indicated by a change in color).
4. Leaks in the circuit or in the patient (such as a punctured eardrum) will result in an increase in volume determination and give an erroneous FRC. Questionable values should be compared to the patient's clinical state.

C. Body plethysmography
1. The most common volume measured is thoracic gas volume. Thoracic gas volume, which is expressed in liters (BTPS), is the volume of gas in the lungs when the mouth shutter is closed. This gas volume is used to represent FRC.
2. Indications for using body plethysmography include evaluating for obstructive lung diseases and cystic fibrosis, for children unable to perform multi-breath tests, for determining bronchodilator response, and for following the course of a disease's response to treatment.
3. The patient is enclosed in a chamber to measure pressure, volume, and flow changes. Small children may need a parent to sit in the chamber with them. The child can sit on the parent's lap and be coached in the maneuvers. Gas-displacement corrections must take the total volumes in the cabinet into account. Oxygen should not be discontinued during the test.
4. Relative contraindications include the following:
   a. The presence of devices that must be continued while inside the chamber, such as IV pumps or other equipment that will not fit in the chamber
   b. Equipment or conditions that interfere with pressure changes, such as chest tubes or a ruptured eardrum

5. During the test, the patient breathes through a mouthpiece with a pressure transducer and a valve (shutter) that closes, obstructing the mouthpiece.
6. As the patient breathes through the mouthpiece and when FRC is reached, the shutter valve is closed and the patient pants at a rate between 20 to 40 breaths per minute (bpm). If a parent is in the chamber with a child, the parent is instructed to breath-hold during the child's panting. Nonpanting maneuvers can be used in situations where the child cannot perform the panting maneuver. Proximal airway pressure and pressure within the body plethysmograph are measured simultaneously. Because the mouth is obstructed, new volumes and pressure are generated. Mouth pressure reflects alveoli pressure, and chamber pressure reflects a change in lung volume. With intubated newborns and children, esophageal balloons are used to measure alveoli pressure changes instead of proximal airway pressure (see Airway Graphic Monitoring in this chapter).
7. Boyle's law, $P_1V_1 = P_2V_2$, is used to determine the final volume in the body plethysmograph, where:
   a. $P_1$ is the original barometric pressure in the body plethysmograph.
   b. $V_2$ is the original volume of the body plethysmograph minus the volume occupied by the patient (if the parent is in the body plethysmograph with the child, this also is taken into account).
   c. $P_2$ is the increased pressure within the body plethysmograph that results from the expansion of the thorax.
   d. $V_2$ is the final volume in the body plethysmograph.
8. Infant plethysmography is not commonly used. The infant lies supine within the small chamber or cabinet with the head, mouth, and nose positioned against a padded, cuffed opening. Measurements of pressure and flow are made through a mask placed over the infant's mouth. The infant may be sleeping or may be given a sedative during the procedure.

## V. Single-breath carbon monoxide diffusing capacity ($D_{LCO}$)

A. This test is used for evaluating and following up children with cystic fibrosis.
B. The predictive equation for males and females is 0.693 × height – 20.13.
C. Steady state and single breath are the two basic methods of determining diffusing capacity using carbon monoxide (CO).
   1. Steady-state method
      a. The subject breathes in a known concentration of CO until a steady state occurs, usually about 5 to 6 min.
      b. The $D_{LCO}$ is calculated from the difference between inhaled and exhaled CO.
   2. Single-breath method
      a. A maximal inhalation (vital capacity maneuver) of a mixture of CO, helium, and oxygen is followed by a 10-s breath hold.
D. $D_{LCO}$ is reduced in restrictive and obstructive disorders, where there is a loss of lung volume, alveolar surface area, and/or capillary bed.

## VI. Infection control

A. The possibility of cross-contamination from patient to patient or patient to therapist exists.
B. The hands should be washed whenever the mouthpiece is handled. If contaminants such as blood or mucus are present on the mouthpiece, gloves should be used. If the test has the potential for causing the patient to cough, then a surgical mask should be worn.
C. The room in which pulmonary functions are performed should be well ventilated. A specific area should be designated for patients in isolation. If a room is not available, bedside testing should be performed, if possible.
D. The tubing, mouthpiece, and any part of the equipment that comes in contact with the patient should be disposed of or a high-level disinfection should be performed. Bacterial filters that allow rebreathing should be handled with gloves and disposed of properly. Because of the possibility of added resistance, bacterial filters are not recommended.
E. A water-sealed spirometer should be drained and allowed to dry weekly.
F. The body plethysmograph should be cleaned thoroughly between patients.

## VII. Specific pulmonary function tests for diseases

A. Normal values for children are determined by height, sex, and age. Spirometric values increase in males up to the age of 18, in females up to the age of 16.
B. Chest deformity (restrictive)

1. $FEV_1$
2. Flow studies
3. Lung volumes, including VC, TLC, FRC, and RV/TLC ratio
4. $D_{LCO}$

C. Cystic fibrosis (obstructive)
1. Lung volumes, including VC, TLC, FRC, and RV/TLC ratio
2. PEF
3. $FEV_T$
4. $FEV_{T\%}$
5. $FEV_{25-75\%}$

D. Asthma
1. Lung volumes, including VC, TLC, FRC, and RV/TLC ratio
2. PEF is very useful for performing a day-to-day evaluation of therapy (see Chapter 10).
3. Flow measurements, including $FEV_T$, $FEV_{T\%}$, and $FEV_{25-75\%}$
4. Blood gas studies to monitor for hypercapnia and the need for ventilation

**VIII. Infant airway graphic monitoring**

A. Airway graphic monitoring is helpful for the following:
1. To study the characteristics and timing of mechanical ventilator breaths
2. To assess and identify lung changes
3. To assess patient-ventilator synchrony
4. To identify changes in the patient's work of breathing
5. To identify changes in compliance and other mechanical parameters
6. To evaluate the effects of therapy

B. Normal pressure, volume, and flow scalar record inspiration as positive values or above the baseline and expiration as negative values or below the baseline. These scalars are useful in determining adverse ventilator effects, such as patient-ventilator dyssynchrony, alveolar overdistention, air leak, and gas trapping (auto-PEEP).

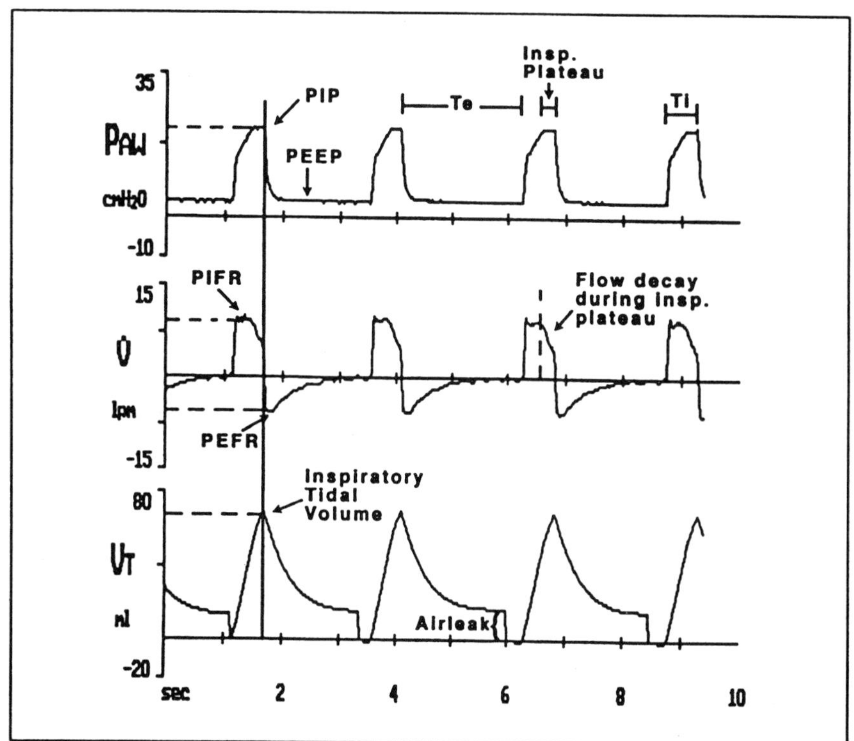


**FIGURE 14–4** Illustration of normal pressure, flow, and volume scalar from a pressure-limited, time-cycled, constant-flow ventilator. Important points in each scalar are labeled. Note the presence of an air leak identified by the volume scalar staying above baseline until the next breath is taken. This is common with infants who are intubated with cuffless endotracheal tubes. (Wilson, B. G., Cheifetz, K. M., and Meliones, J. N. [1995]. *Optimizing Mechanical Ventilation in Infants and Children With the Use of Airway Graphics*. Palm Springs, CA: Bird Corp., p. 2–1, with permission.)

1. Normal scalar from constant-flow, pressure-limited, time-cycled ventilation (Fig. 14–4).
2. Normal scalar developed from volume-limited, constant flow ventilation (Fig. 14–5).

C. Flow-volume loops record inspiration above the baseline and expiration below baseline. Pressure-volume loops record a positive-pressure breath to the right of baseline and a negative-pressure effort, such as is seen when triggering the ventilator. These loops are helpful in determining alterations in compliance, work of breathing, alterations in peak flow, overdistention of the lung, and premature termination of inspiration.
   1. Constant-flow, pressure-limited, time-cycled ventilation (Fig. 14–6)
   2. Volume-limited, constant-flow ventilation (Fig. 14–7)

D. Spontaneous and mechanical ventilation (Fig. 14–8)

E. Pressure support and SIMV (Fig. 14–9)

F. Volume-pressure loops (Table 14–2)

G. Common flow-volume loops (Table 14–3)
   1. For reference in the following Table inspiration is above baseline and exhalation is below baseline. The loop develops in a clockwise manner as indicated by arrows.

H. Identification of intrinsic PEEP (Fig. 14–10)
   1. Intrinsic PEEP can be identified but not quantified on scalars and flow-volume loops.
   2. Clinical consideration for treatment for intrinsic PEEP includes:
      a. Shorten inspiratory time
      b. Increase flowrate
      c. Optimal extrinsic PEEP
      d. Bronchodilator therapy

I. Excessive trigger work (Fig. 14–11)
   1. Clinical consideration for excessive patient triggering
      a. Adjust the sensitivity setting to make the ventilator more sensitive to the patient's inspiratory effort.

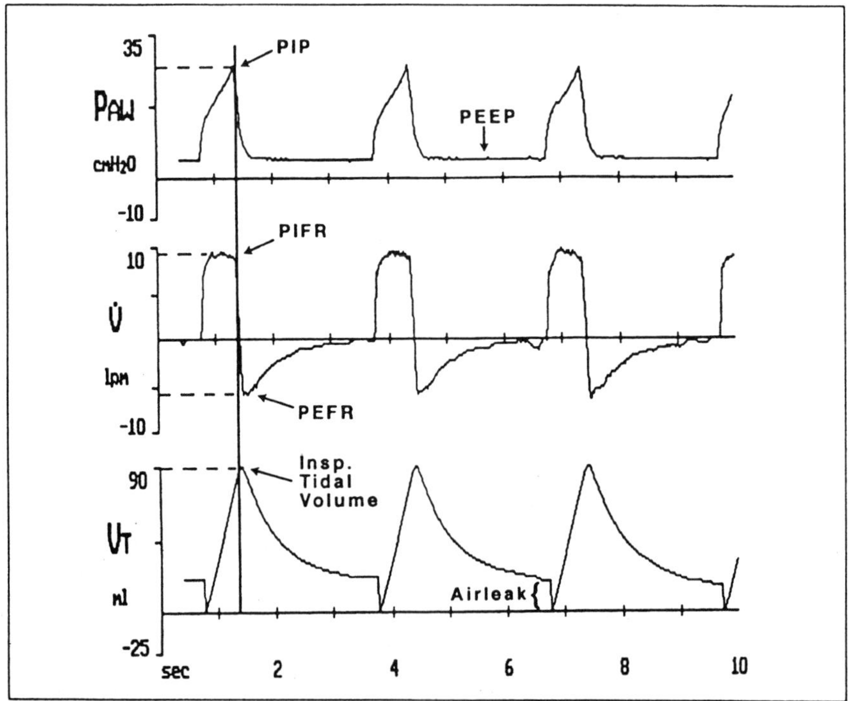


**FIGURE 14–5** Pressure, flow, and volume scalar identifying PIP, PEEP, PIFR, PEFR, and inspiratory tidal volume during volume-limited, constant-flow ventilation. Note the air leak that is present as identified by the volume scalar not returning to baseline. Measurements were taken on SIMV, rate 20/min, VT 90 mL, flow rate 8 L/min, PEEP (+) 4 cm $H_2O$ and sensitivity of (–) 1 cm $H_2O$. (Wilson, B. G., Cheifetz, K. M., and Meliones, J. N. [1995]. *Optimizing Mechanical Ventilation in Infants and Children With the Use of Airway Graphics.* Palm Springs, CA: Bird Corp., p. 2–6, with permission.)

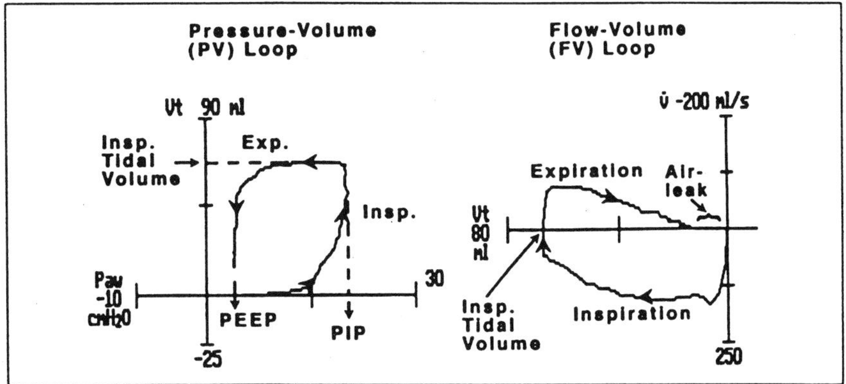


**FIGURE 14–6** Pressure-volume curve on the left illustrating PIP, PEEP, and inspiratory tidal volume. The arrows indicate development of the loop during inspiration and expiration. Dynamic compliance can be calculated by dividing the tidal volume by pressure (PIP delivered – PEEP). The flow-volume curve on the right illustrates tidal volume and the curve not returning to baseline. This may be due to an endotracheal tube leak. The arrows indicate how the curve develops during inspiration and expiration. Both curves developed from constant-flow, pressure-limited, time-cycled ventilation in normal lungs. (Wilson, B. G., Cheifetz, K. M., and Meliones, J. N. [1995]. *Optimizing Mechanical Ventilation in Infants and Children With the Use of Airway Graphics.* Palm Springs, CA: Bird Corp., p. 2–4, with permission.)

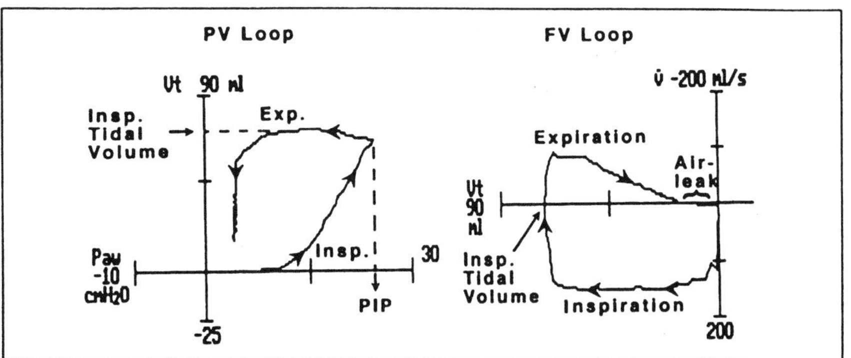


**FIGURE 14–7** The pressure-volume loop on the left illustrates PIP, inspiratory tidal volume, inspiration, and expiration. The arrows indicate the development of the loop during inspiration and expiration. The volume-pressure loop on the right illustrates inspiration, expiration, and inspiratory tidal volume. The curve does not return to baseline because of an air leak. Both curves developed from volume-limited, constant-flow ventilation in normal lungs. (Wilson, B. G., Cheifetz, K. M., and Meliones, J. N. [1995]. *Optimizing Mechanical Ventilation in Infants and Children With the Use of Airway Graphics.* Palm Springs, CA: Bird Corp., p. 2–8, with permission.)

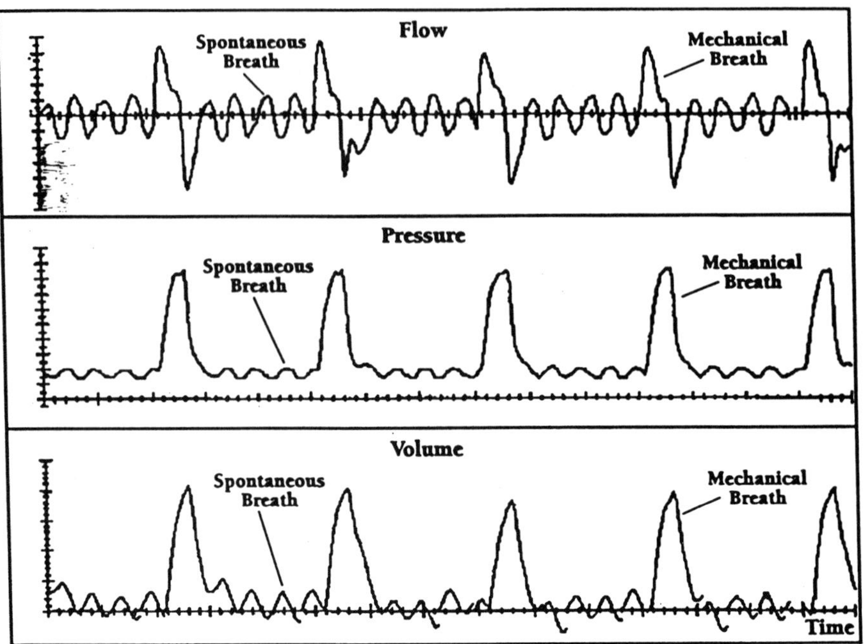


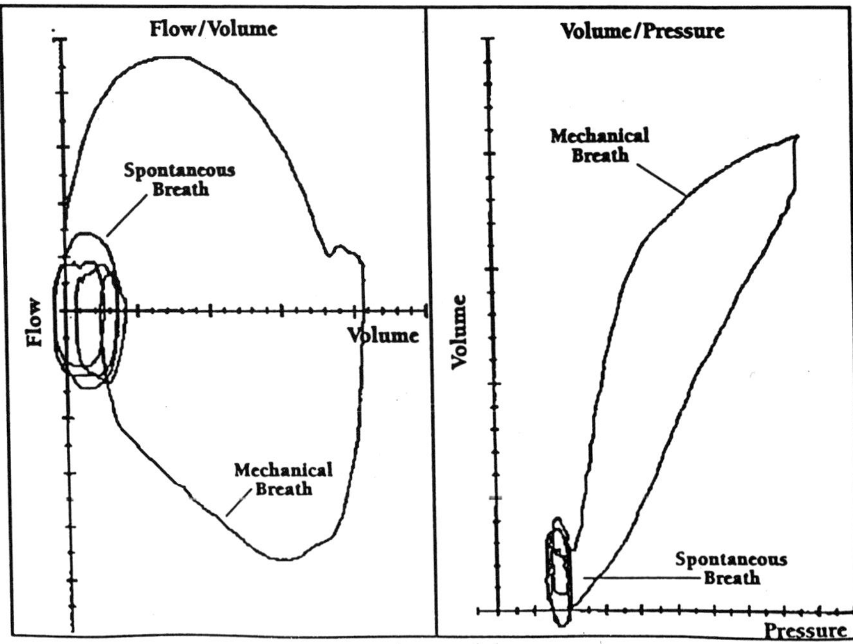


**FIGURE 14–8** Both spontaneous and mechanical ventilation breaths are identified on scalars, flow-volume loop, and volume-pressure loop. (Novametrix Medical Systems. [1995]. *Respiratory Mechanics: A Reference Handbook.* Wallingford, CT: Author, p. 5, with permission.)

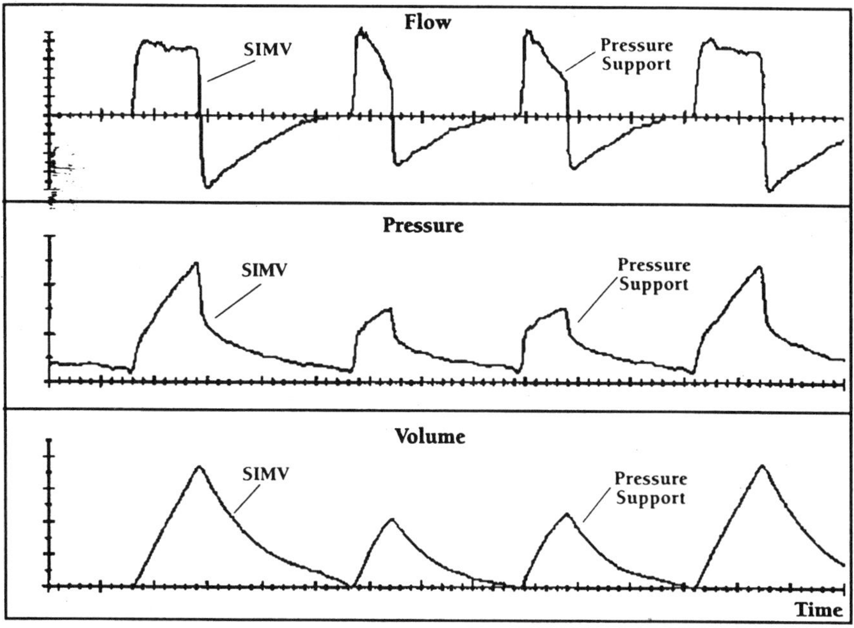


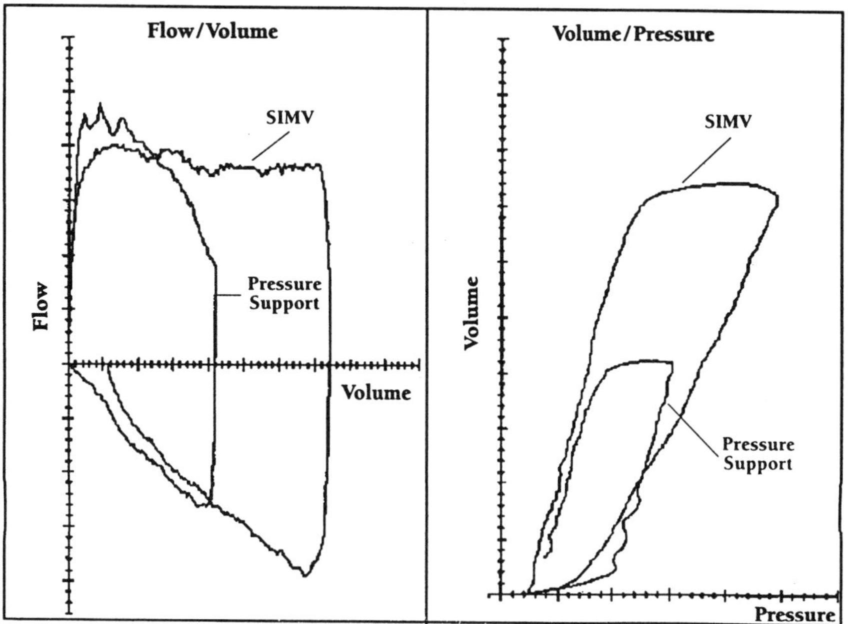


**FIGURE 14–9** Pressure, volume-flow scalars, flow-volume and pressure-volume loops show pressure-support breaths and SIMV breaths. (Novametrix Medical Systems. [1995]. *Respiratory Mechanics: A Reference Handbook.* Wallingford, CT: Author, p. 6, with permission.)

TABLE 14–2. ***Common Volume-Pressure Loops, Problems, and Suggestions***

| Volume-Pressure Loop | Description | Suggestions |
|---|---|---|
| 1. 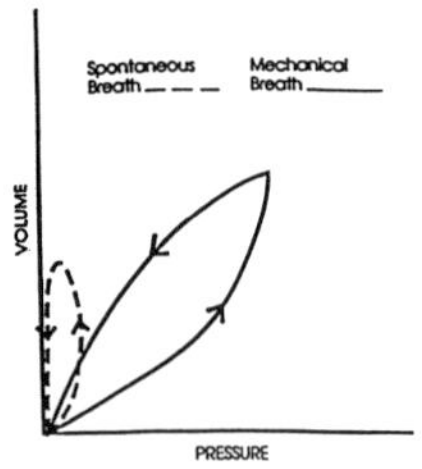 | Normal loop. Arrows indicate formation of loop in a counterclockwise fashion. The pressure begins at zero baseline and ends at zero baseline. Good compliance indicated by this curve. Dynamic compliance is calculated by: $\frac{\text{Change in volume}}{\text{PIP–PEEP}}$ | No suggestion required. |
| 2. 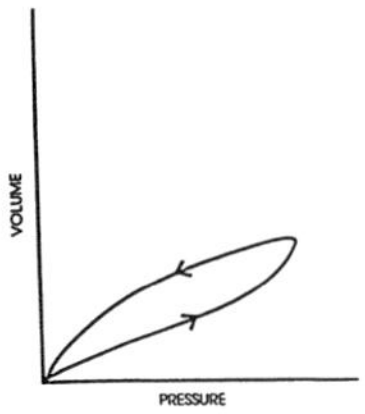 | Low compliance curve as indicated by the curve shifting to right and the curve becoming compressed. Greater pressure is required to produce a volume change. Low compliance results from restrictive problems such as atelectasis, diaphragmatic hernia, RDS. | For immature lungs, surfactant replacement therapy. Placing the infant in the prone position or placing the diseased lung up and diseased lung down. Diaphragmatic hernia requires surgery. |
| 3. 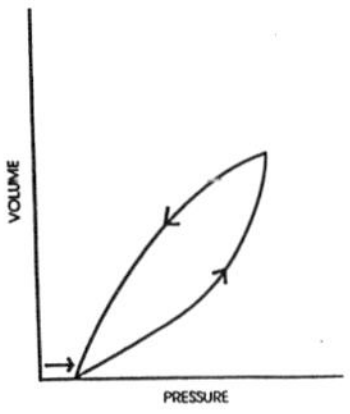 | Loop originates at the PEEP level set on the ventilator. | This is a normal position for the loop when PEEP is added. |
| 4. 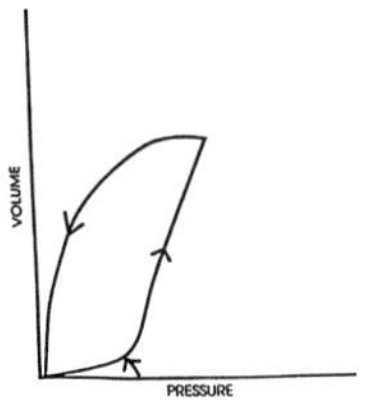 | PEEP is below critical opening pressure. The loop flattens out at the beginning of inspiration. This represents the amount of pressure required before signficant volume change occurs. The inflection point is identified by the arrow. | The PEEP level should be set above the inflection point.<br>When properly set, the loop shape rounds out. |
| 5. 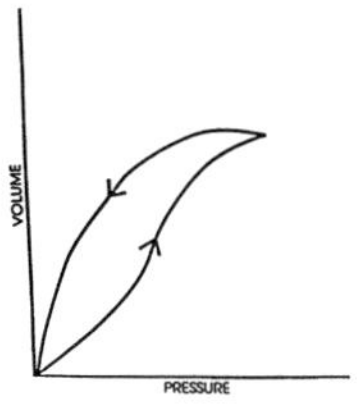 | Lung overdistention. Flattening out at the end of inspiration, causing a "penguin beak." Pressure increases with little to no volume change. This can lead to volutrauma from overdistension and can cause pneumothorax, pneumomediastinum, PIE. | Adjust PIP to reduce "beak effect." |
| 6. 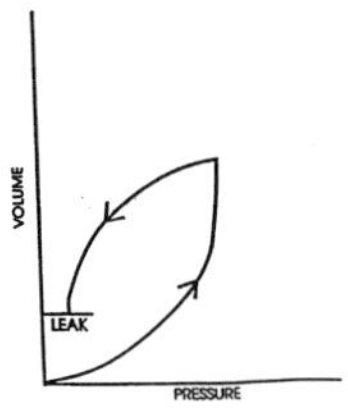 | Endotracheal tube leak. Exhale portion of the loop terminates before reaching baseline, resulting in an open-ended loop. The difference between the baseline and the termination point of the loop is the volume lost due to the leak. A leak >20% is excessive when using a cuffless tube. | Consider using a larger cuffless endotracheal tube.<br>A leak using a cuffed endotracheal tube requires immediate attention (see Chapter 11). |

Pressure-volume loops from Novametrix, Wallingford, CT, with permission.

TABLE 14–3. *Common Flow-Volume Loops, Problems, and Suggestions*

| Flow-Volume Loop | Description | Suggestions |
|---|---|---|
| 1. 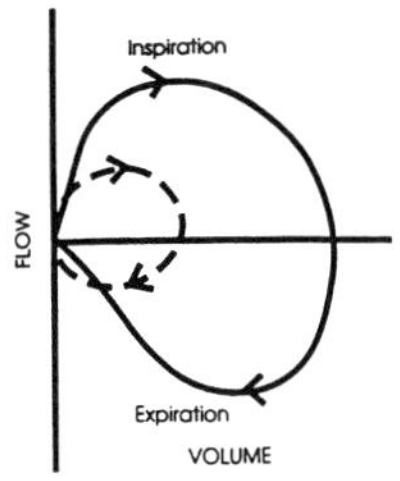 | This is a normal loop showing a rounded, symmetrical appearance. The dotted line indicates a spontaneous breath, and the solid line indicates a mechanical breath. Each breath returns to baseline and zero flow. The flow and volume are larger with the mechanical breath as compared to the spontaneous breath. | No change or alteration in the mechanical settings or therapy required. |
| 2. 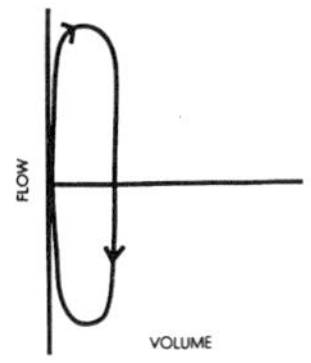 | Low-compliance, restrictive disease or high respiratory rate. The loop is compact, vertically shaped. There is low volume and high flow. Meconium aspiration, RDS, and diaphragmatic hernia present with this loop. | Surfactant therapy for RDS.<br>Surgical repair for diaphragmatic hernia.<br>Optimal PEEP for meconium aspiration and good bronchial hygiene. |
| 3. 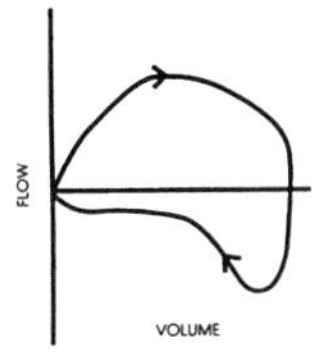 | Obstructive airway disease. The loop presents with a long, flat expiratory phase indicative of the obstruction from airways closing during exhalation. Asthma, bronchopulmonary dysplasia, and cystic fibrosis present with this shaped loop. | Bronchodilator therapy.<br>PEP therapy (see Chapter 10). |
| 4. 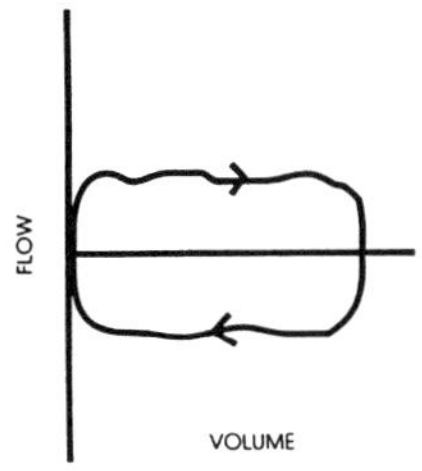 | Fixed upper airway obstruction develops a square-shaped loop. Kinked or plugged endotracheal tube, undersized endotracheal tube, and tracheal stenosis present with this shaped loop. | Assure the tube is not kinked.<br>Reposition the head, neck extension.<br>Suction the tube if plugging is suspected.<br>An undersized tube should be replaced.<br>Tracheal stenosis may require surgical repair. |
| 5. 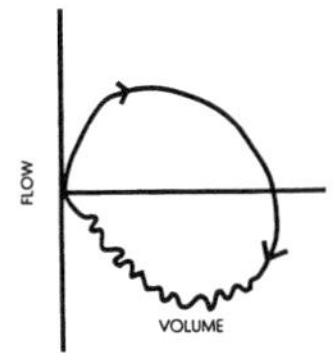 | Water in ventilator tubing or secretions in the airway. The expiratory phase of the loop is rough with indentations in the loop. | Drain the water from the tubing.<br>Suction the airway. |
| 6. 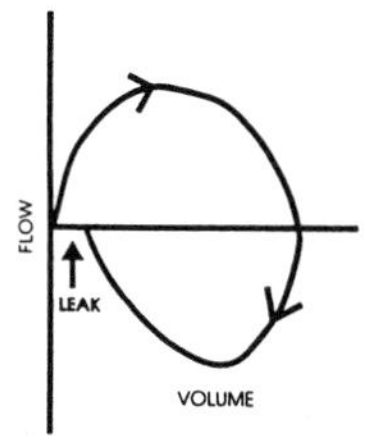 | Endotracheal tube leak. Open-ended loop on expiratory phase. The difference between the baseline and where the loop ended on the volume axis indicates the amount of volume lost. | <20% loss of volume is considered normal for a cuffless endotracheal tube. A larger volume loss requires replacement with a larger tube.<br>A cuffed endotracheal tube with a leak requires immediate attention (see Chapter 11). |

Flow-volume loops from Novametrix, Wallingford, CT, with permission.

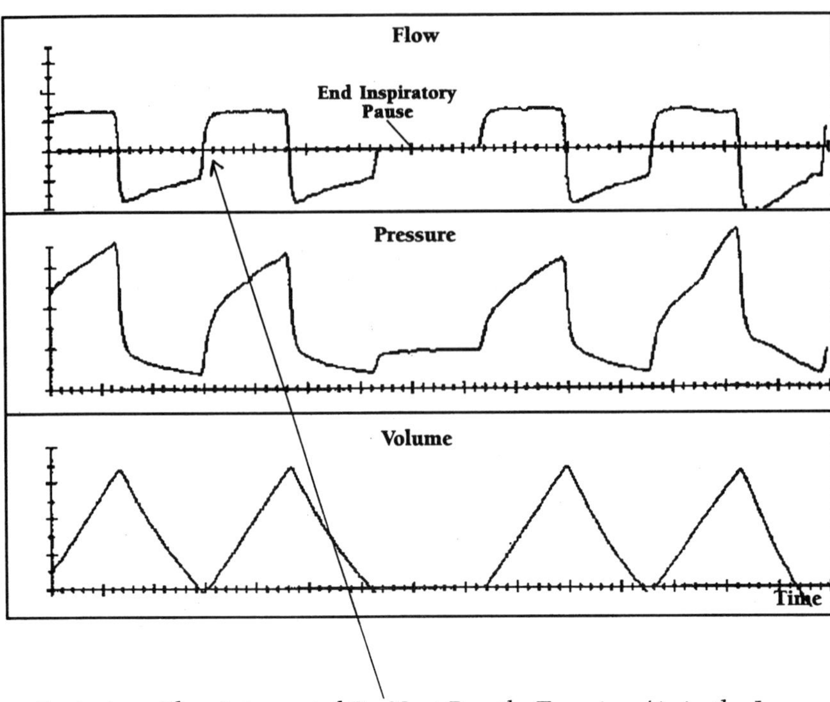


Expiratory Flow Interrupted By Next Breath, Trapping Air in the Lungs

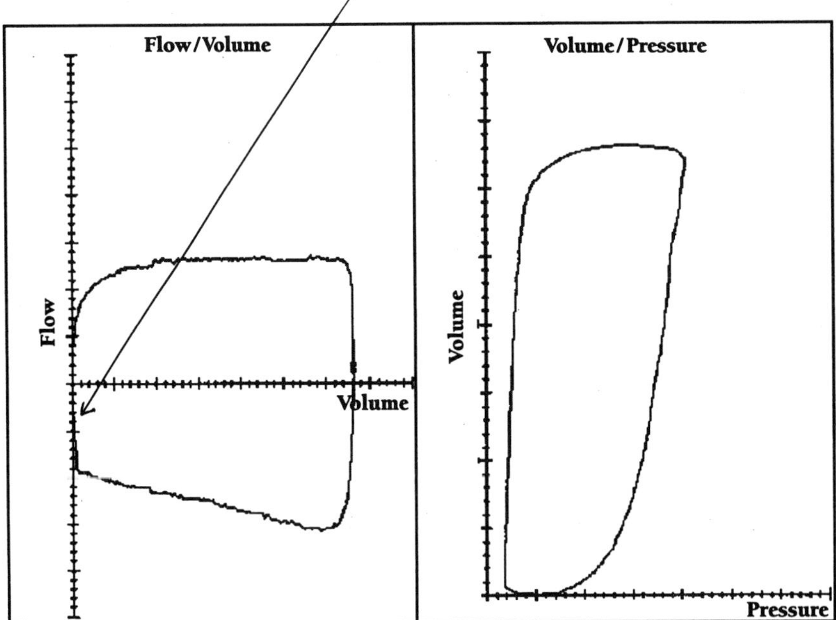


**FIGURE 14–10** Identification of intrinsic PEEP with mechanical ventilation. Flow does not reach zero before the next machine breath and pressure remains above baseline. The flow-volume loop shows the expiratory volume greater than inspiratory volume, and flow does not return to zero. (Novametrix Medical Systems. [1995]. *Respiratory Mechanics: A Reference Handbook.* Wallingford, CT: Author, p. 10, with permission.)

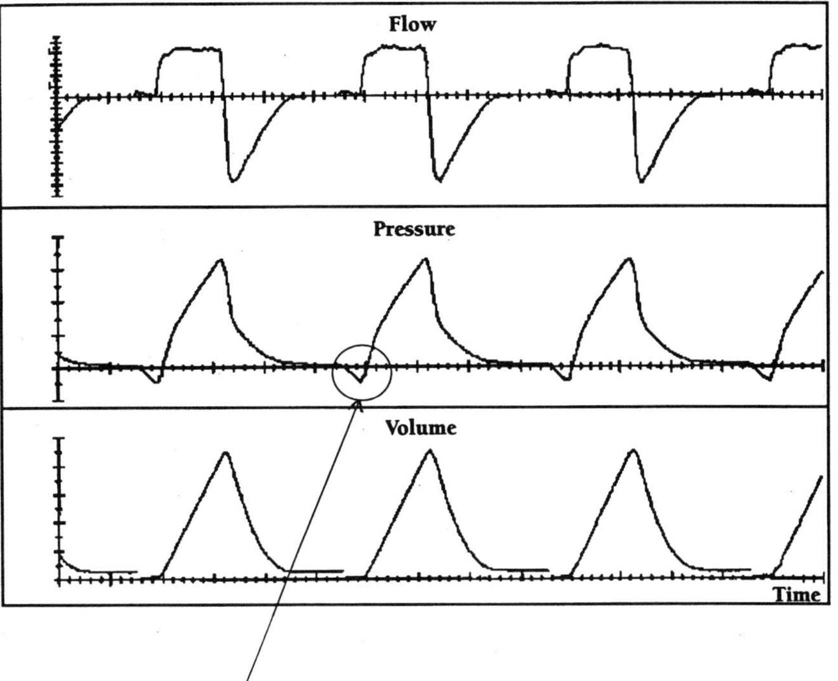


Start of Inspiration Goes Well Below Baseline Pressure

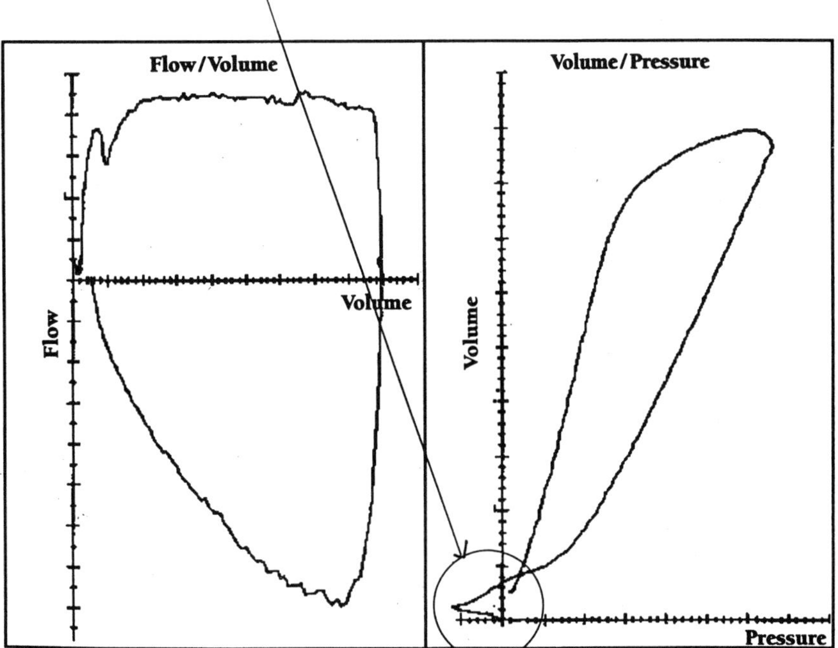


**FIGURE 14–11.** Illustration shows excessive trigger work as indicated by the pressure scalar and the volume-pressure loop. Note on the volume-pressure loop the level of negative pressure required before the machine breath is triggered. (Novametrix Medical Systems. [1995]. *Respiratory Mechanics: A Reference Handbook.* Wallingford, CT: Author, p. 12, with permission.)

TABLE 14–4. ***Pulmonary Functions in Normal-Term, RDS, and BPD Infants***

| | Units | Normal Term | RDS | BPD |
|---|---|---|---|---|
| Tidal volume | mL/kg | 5–7 | 4–6 | 4–7 |
| Respiratory rate | bpm | 30–40 | 50–80 | 45–80 |
| Minute ventilation | mL/kg/min | 200–300 | 250–400 | 200–400 |
| Functional residual capacity | mL/kg | 20–30 | 15–25 | 20–30 |
| Static compliance | mL/cm $H_2O$/kg | 1–4 | 0.1–0.6 | 0.2–0.8 |
| Dynamic compliance | mL/cm $H_2O$/kg | 1–2 | 0.3–0.5 | 0.2–0.8 |
| Resistance | cm $H_2O$/mL/s | 25–50 | 60–150 | 30–150 |
| Work of breathing | gm/cm/min/kg | 500–1000 | 800–3000 | 1800–6500 |
| VD/VT ratio | percent | 22–38 | 60–80 | 35–60 |
| Physiologic dead space | mL/kg | 1.0–2.0 | 3.0–4.5 | 3.0–4.5 |
| Alveolar ventilation | mL/kg/min | 110–160 | 55–90 | 90–170 |
| $CO_2$ production | mL/kg/min | 5–6 | | |
| Oxygen consumption | mL/kg/min | 6–8 | | |
| Respiratory quotient | | 0.75–0.83 | | |
| Calories | kcal/kg/day | 105–133 | | |

From SensorMedics Corp., Yorba Linda, California, with permission.

b. Switch from pressure triggering to flow triggering.
c. Check for the presence of auto-PEEP.

J. Low-flow setting (Fig. 14–12)
1. Low flow as indicated by the pressure scalar and volume-pressure loop
2. Clinical consideration to treat low flow
a. Increase flowrate on mechanical ventilation.

K. Patient-ventilator asynchrony
1. Clinical considerations (Fig. 14–13) for patient-ventilator asynchrony
a. Increase flowrate.
b. Increase respiratory rate.
c. Sedate, paralyze patient.

L. Severe obstruction (Fig. 14–14)
1. Clinical considerations for severe obstruction
a. Reduce inspiratory flowrate.
b. Check for proper exhalation valve functioning. A patient receiving MDI or aerosolized medications in-line may have drug buildup on the valve, causing obstruction to flow. Place a filter proximal to the exhalation valve during the treatment and remove it upon completion of the treatment.

M. Esophageal pressure
1. Clinically, esophageal pressure monitoring is used to quantify the work of breathing, lung compliance, patient-ventilator synchrony, as well as evaluating intrinsic PEEP and determining the amount of extrinsic PEEP to add to counterbalance intrinsic PEEP.
2. A catheter with a large air-filled balloon is placed in the esophagus. Proper placement is determined by equal airway pressure and esophageal pressure changes against an occluded airway in the spontaneously breathing patient. Proper placement is attained when atrial contractions are seen on the esophageal tracing in the mechanically ventilated patient. In general the catheter should be placed in the lower third of the esophagus.
3. Patient-ventilator synchrony is assessed with esophageal pressure (Fig. 14–15).

N. Lung mechanics improve when an infant is placed in the prone position as compared to the supine position.
1. In infants that are mechanically ventilated, tidal volume, minute ventilation, dynamic compliance total pulmonary resistance, and work of breathing improve.
2. In infants that are spontaneously breathing, compliance, total pulmonary resistance, and total work of breathing improve.

O. Overview of pulmonary function values in infants (Table 14–4)

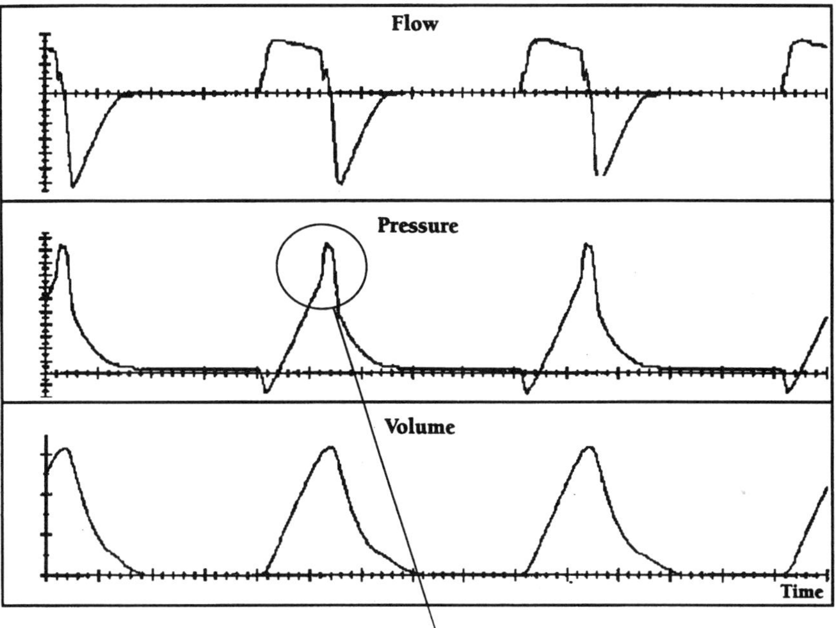


*Inspiratory Slope of Pressure Tracing Caves In*

*Inspiratory Slope of Volume/Pressure Curve Loses its Convex Shape*

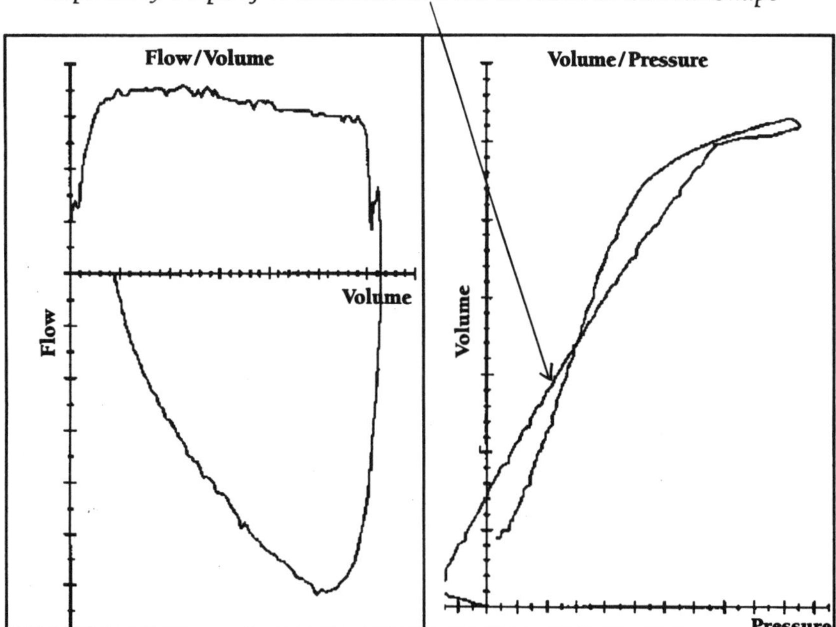


**FIGURE 14–12** Illustration of low-flow setting on mechanical ventilation. (Novametrix Medical Systems. [1995]. *Respiratory Mechanics: A Reference Handbook.* Wallingford, CT: Author, p. 13, with permission.)

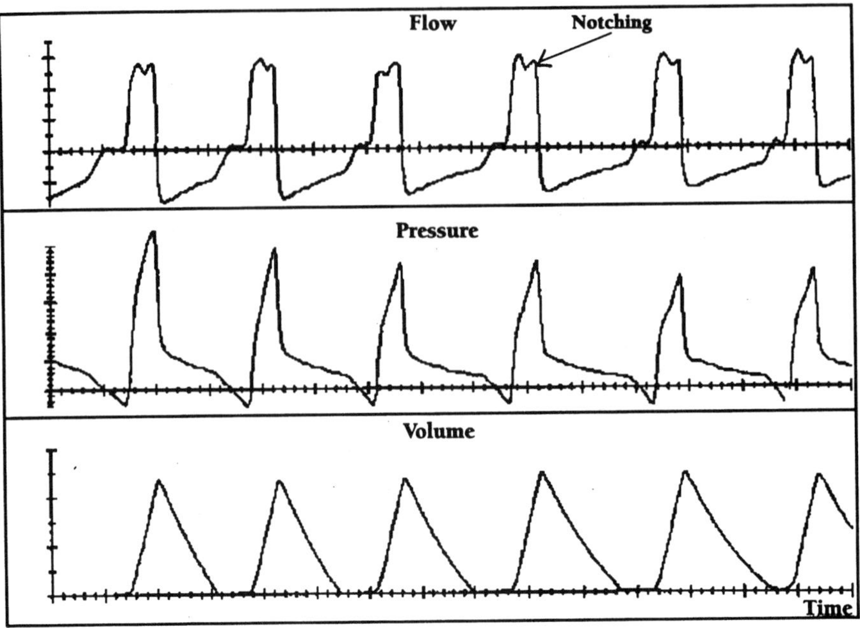


*Patient's Effort Exceeds Mechanically Delivered Breath Flow*

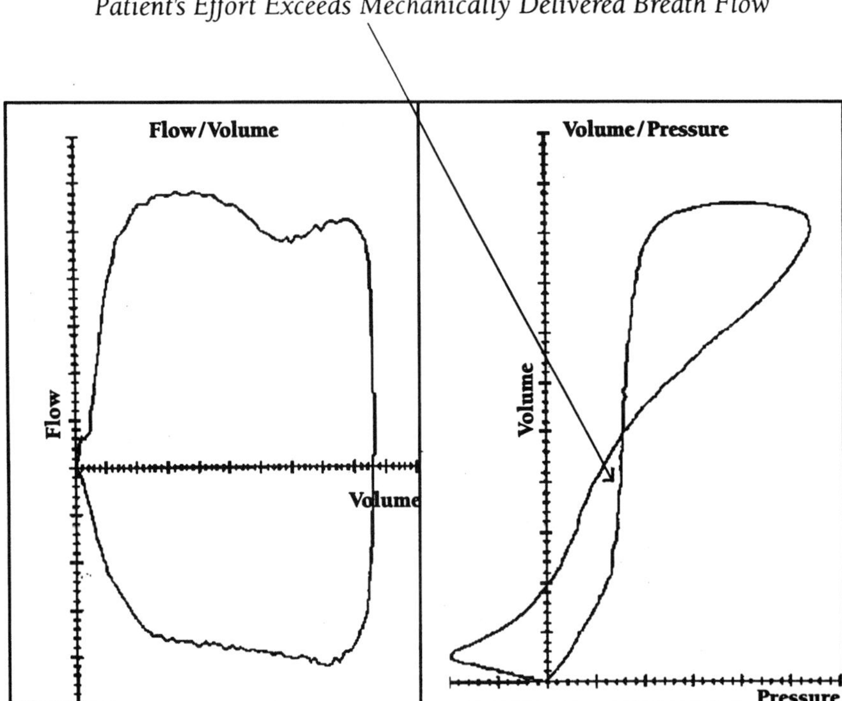


**FIGURE 14–13** Illustration of patient-ventilator asynchrony indicated by the flow scalar and volume-pressure loop. (Novametrix Medical Systems. [1995]. *Respiratory Mechanics: A Reference Handbook.* Wallingford, CT: Author, p. 11, with permission.)

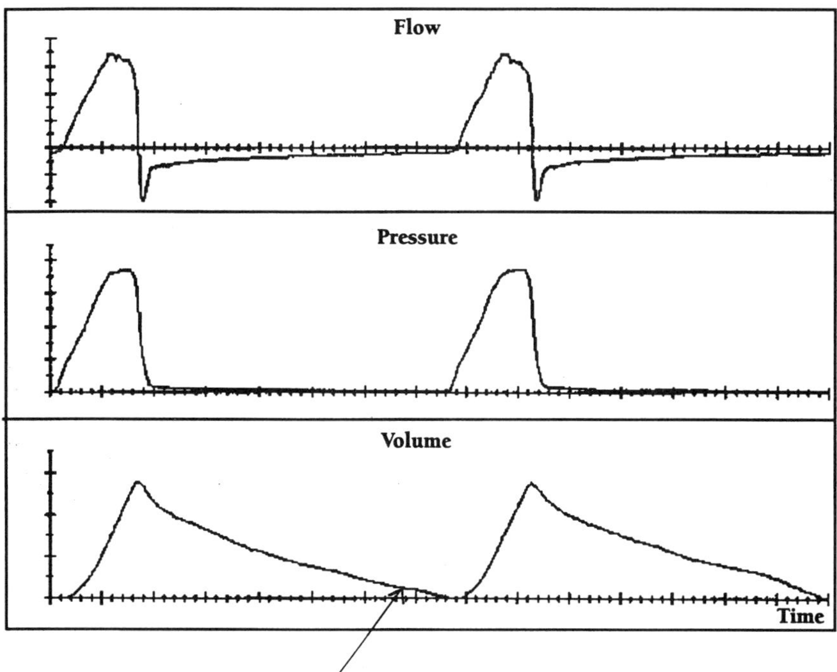


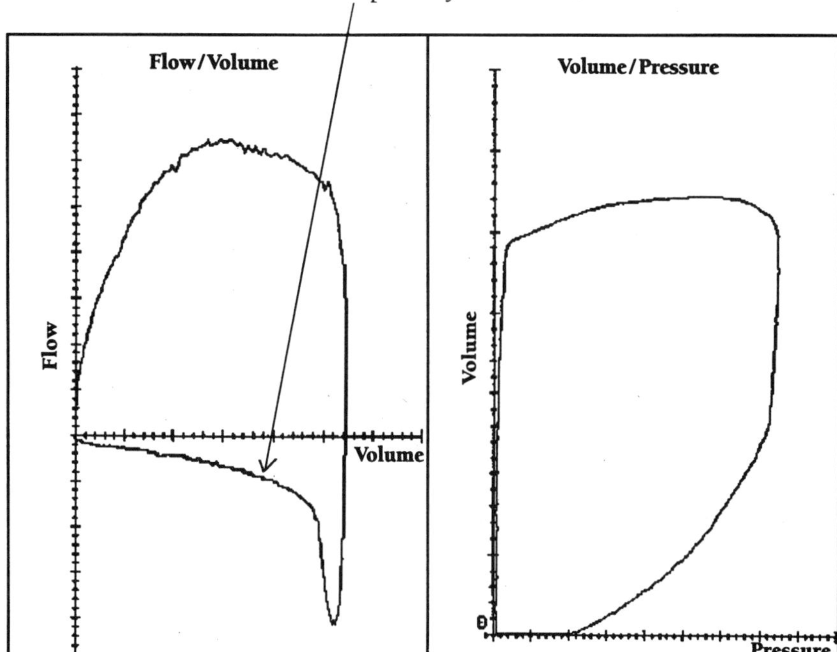


**FIGURE 14–14** Illustration shows severe obstruction to exhalation as indicated by the volume scalar and the flow-volume loop. (Novametrix Medical Systems. [1995]. *Respiratory Mechanics: A Reference Handbook.* Wallingford, CT: Author, p. 12, with permission.)

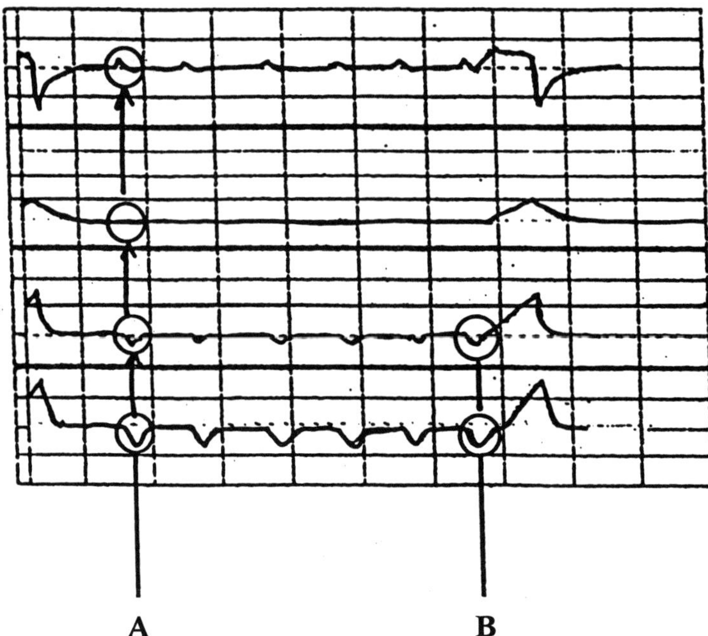


**FIGURE 14–15** Illustration of patient-ventilator synchrony (*A*). At point 1 the patient takes a breath and the airway pressure (PAW) and esophageal pressure (PES) scalars deflect. The ventilator senses the patient response and a breath is delivered as indicated by the pressure, flow, and tidal volume curves. Patient-ventilator asynchrony is illustrated in (*B*). Both the PES and PAW deflect but there is no change in the volume and flow scalars. Following point 1 there is still deflection of the PES and PAW but no response by the ventilator. Point 2 identifies patient-ventilator synchrony.

# 14 REVIEW QUESTIONS

1. Give two indications for performing pulmonary function testing on infants and children.

   a.

   b.

2. What does a pneumotachometer measure?

3. What devices measure volume and capacities during a pulmonary function test?

4. Give a brief definition of the following volumes and capacities:

   a. Tidal volume

   b. Inspiratory reserve volume

   c. Expiratory reserve volume

   d. Residual volume

   e. Inspiratory capacity

   f. Functional residual capacity

   g. Total lung capacity

   h. Vital capacity

5. Describe the difference between a forced vital capacity maneuver and a vital capacity maneuver.

6. What are the primary tests used to determine obstructive disease?

7. How is $FEV_{1\%}$ calculated?

8. What is the peak expiratory flow used to make a diagnosis?

9. On the flow-volume loop on page 265 (see Fig. 14–3), identify the peak expiratory flowrate, peak inspiratory flowrate, total lung capacity, forced vital capacity, and residual volume.

10. A 10-year-old has a prebronchodilator $FEV_1$ of 1.3 L and a postbronchodilator $FEV_1$ of 1.8 L. What is the percentage change between these two values? Is this considered a significant response?

11. During a closed-circuit helium dilution test, the patient begins to breathe fast and deep. What could be the cause of this type of breathing in your patient?

12. During a body plethysmography, what adjustments must be made if a parent has a child sitting in his or her lap?

13. What causes a reduction in the $D_{LCO}$ in both restrictive and obstructive diseases?

14. List the tests performed that diagnose cystic fibrosis, asthma, and chest deformity.

| **Asthma** | **Cystic fibrosis** | **Chest deformity** |
|---|---|---|

15. Referring to Figure 14–4 on page 267, describe the difference between the pressure, flow, and volume scalar graphics.

16. Referring to Figure 14–6 on page 269, identify the following on pressure-volume (P-V) and flow-volume (F-V) loop:

    a. Inspiration

    b. Expiration

    c. PIP

    d. Inspiratory tidal volume

    e. Air leak

17. Referring to page 272, give one clinical suggestion to correct the abnormal V-P loop numbered 4, 5, and 6 in Table 14–2.

18. Referring to page 273, give one clinical suggestion to correct the abnormal F-V loop numbered 2, 3, and 6 in Table 14–3.

19. Describe why the scalar graphics and V-P and F-V loops on page 274 (refer to Fig. 14–10) indicate intrinsic PEEP.

20. Referring to the scalar graphics and V-P and F-V loops on page 274 (see Fig. 14–10), what should be done for a patient on mechanical ventilation?

21. Referring to the scalar graphics and V-P and F-V loops on page 278 (see Fig. 14–13), list one clinical change that could correct this problem.

22. Referring to Figure 14–14 on page 279, what type of pediatric disease would cause this alteration in the scalar graphics and V-P and F-V loops? Give one clinical change that could help reverse this problem. List one change that could correct this problem.

23. How could patient-ventilator asynchrony be determined using esophageal pressure monitoring?

## BIBLIOGRAPHY


American Association for Respiratory Care, Clinical Practice Guideline. (1994). Static lung volumes. *Respiratory Care 39*, 8, 830.

American Association for Respiratory Care, Clinical Practice Guideline. (1995). Infant/toddler pulmonary function test. *Respiratory Care 40*, 7, 761.

American Association for Respiratory Care, Clinical Practice Guideline. (1991). Spirometry. *Respiratory Care 36*, 1414.

American Association for Respiratory Care, Clinical Practice Guideline. (1994). Body plethysmography. *Respiratory Care 39*, 12, 1184.

American Association for Respiratory Care, Clinical Practice Guideline. (1993). Single-breath carbon monoxide diffusing capacity. *Respiratory Care 38*, 511.

American Thoracic Society/European Respiratory Society. (1995). Respiratory function measurements in infants: Measurement conditions. *American Journal of Respiratory Critical Care Medicine 151*, 2058.

Antunes, M. J., and Greenspan, J. S. (1996). Pulmonary function testing. In Spitzer, A. (Ed.). *Intensive Care of the Newborn*. St. Louis: Mosby–Year Book.

Cullen, J. A., et al. (1994). Pulmonary function testing in the critically ill neonate. Part II: Methodology. *Neonatal Network 13*, 7.

Davis, M. G., and Coates, A. L. (1990). Pulmonary function testing in infants and neonates. *Seminars in Respiratory Medicine 11*, 2, 185.

Greenspan, J. S., et al. (1994). Pulmonary function testing in the critically ill neonate. Part I: An Overview. *Neonatal Network 13*, 1, 9.

Kacmarek, R. M., and Hess, D. R. (1993). Airway pressure, flow and volume waveforms, and lung mechanics during mechanical ventilation. In Kacmarek, R. M., Hess, D. R., and Stoller, J. K. (Eds.). *Monitoring in Respiratory Care*. St. Louis: Mosby–Year Book.

Kacmarek, R. M., Mack, C. W., and Dimas, S. (1990). *The Essentials of Respiratory Care,* ed. 3. St. Louis: Mosby–Year Book.

Lodrup-Carlsen, K. C., and Carlsen, K. H. (1993). Lung function in awake healthy infants: The first five days of life. *European Respiratory Journal 6,* 1496.

Madama, V. C. (1993). *Pulmonary Function Testing and Cardiopulmonary Stress Testing.* Albany: Delmar Publishers.

Marini, J. J. (1990). Lung mechanics determinations at the bedside: Instrumentation and clinical application. *Respiratory Care 35,* 7, 669.

McAnn, E., et al. (1987). Pulmonary function in the sick newborn infant. *Pediatric Research 21,* 313.

McIntyre, N. R. (1991). *Graphical Analysis of Flow, Pressure and Volume during Mechanical Ventilation,* ed. 3. Riverside, CA: Bear Medical Systems.

Mendoza, J. C., Roberts, J.L., and Cook, L. N. (1991). Postural effects on pulmonary function and heart rate of preterm infants and lung disease. *Journal of Pediatrics 118,* 445.

Novametrix Medical Systems, Inc. (1995). *Respiratory Mechanics: A Reference Handbook.* Wallingford, CT: Novametrix Medical Systems.

Ruppel, G. (1994). *Manual of Pulmonary Function Testing,* ed. 6. St. Louis: Mosby–Year Book.

SensorMedics Corporation. (1990). *Pulmonary and Metabolic Function in Infants.* Yorba Linda, CA: SensorMedics Corp.

Wilson, B. G. (1996). Optimizing mechanical ventilation using airway graphics. *NBRC Horizons 22,* 4, 1.

Wilson, B. G., Cheifetz, I. M., and Meliones, J. N. (1995). *Optimizing Mechanical Ventilation in Infants & Children with the Use of Airway Graphics.* Palm Springs, CA: Bird Corporation.

Yuksel, B., Greenough, A., and Green, S. (1991). Lung function abnormalities at 6 months of age after neonatal intensive care. *Archives of Disease in Childhood 66,* 472.

Zukowsky, K., et al. (1994). Pulmonary function testing in the critically ill neonate. Part III: Case studies. *Neonatal Network 13,* 4, 31.

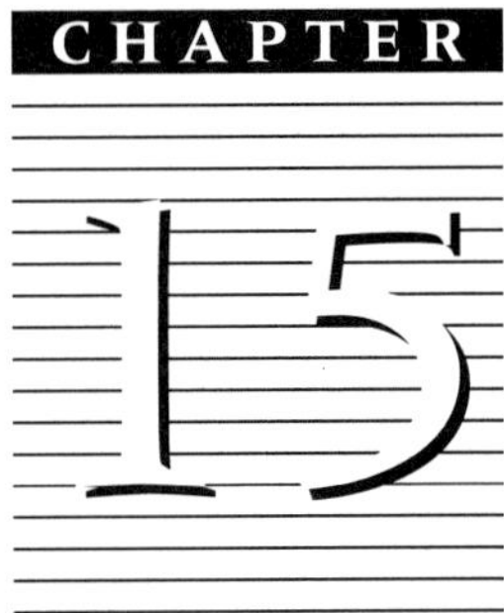

# Special Procedures

**I. Tube thoracostomy (chest tube)**

A. Indications
   1. Spontaneous pneumothorax (large, symptomatic, or presence of underlying lung disease)
   2. Presence of tension pneumothorax
   3. Progressive iatrogenic pneumothorax
   4. Penetrating chest injuries
   5. Hemopneumothorax in acute trauma
   6. Complicated empyema
   7. Bronchopleural fistula
   8. After thoracic surgery
   9. Chylothorax

B. In patients with transient symptoms, as evidenced by the pneumothorax not increasing over several hours, a chest tube is not indicated for a pneumothorax of less than 25%. If the patient exhibits respiratory distress, moderate to severe pain, or evidence of continual air leak, a chest tube is inserted.

C. Chest tube placement
   1. To drain air, a chest tube should be inserted into the anterior chest (between the second and third interspace) at the midclavicular line. The tube is directed anteroapically.
   2. For fluid drainage, a chest tube is placed in the sixth interspace at the midaxillary line. The tube is directed inferiorly and posteriorly. A free-flowing pleural effusion requires that a chest tube be inserted in this area, whereas with loculated fluid, a tube must be placed directly into the specific area of the loculation.

D. Concept of drainage unit
   1. A traditional three-bottle chest drainage system is incorporated in the plastic disposable chest drainage unit (Fig. 15–1).
   2. The collection chamber or bottle, the one closest to the patient, collects drainage from the chest drainage tubing through the open connection port. This compartment is marked in graduated increments monitoring rate and volume of drainage.
   3. The water sealed compartment or bottle is compartment 2. To prevent air from entering the chest through the chest tube, the end of a straw or tubing is placed beneath 2 to 3 cm of water within the bottle. In the disposable compartmental unit, the "U" shape at the bottom of this chamber forms a seal. When 2 to 3 cm of water is added to this chamber, it acts the same as the tubing beneath the water in the bottle system. This one-way valve system allows air to exit the chest, but prevents air from entering the chest during inspiration. During spontaneous inspiration, water draws up into the tube, or the water level rises in the water sealed chamber. During spontaneous expiration, air will move out through the tube through the water and the water level returns to the preinspiration level at end expiration. With positive pressure, the fluctuation will be the opposite. Disappearance of the fluctuation may indicate that there is no more air leak or that the chest tube or connecting tube is kinked. If the chest tube is disconnected from the water seal, atmospheric air will enter the lung during inspiration.
   4. The third bottle or compartment is for suction control. Suction is applied to the drainage system when large amounts of fluid or air are present or when small chest tubes are used. The amount of water in the suction controlled bottle regulates the amount of suction through the system, regardless of the amount of suction applied at the wall suction control. Therefore, to change

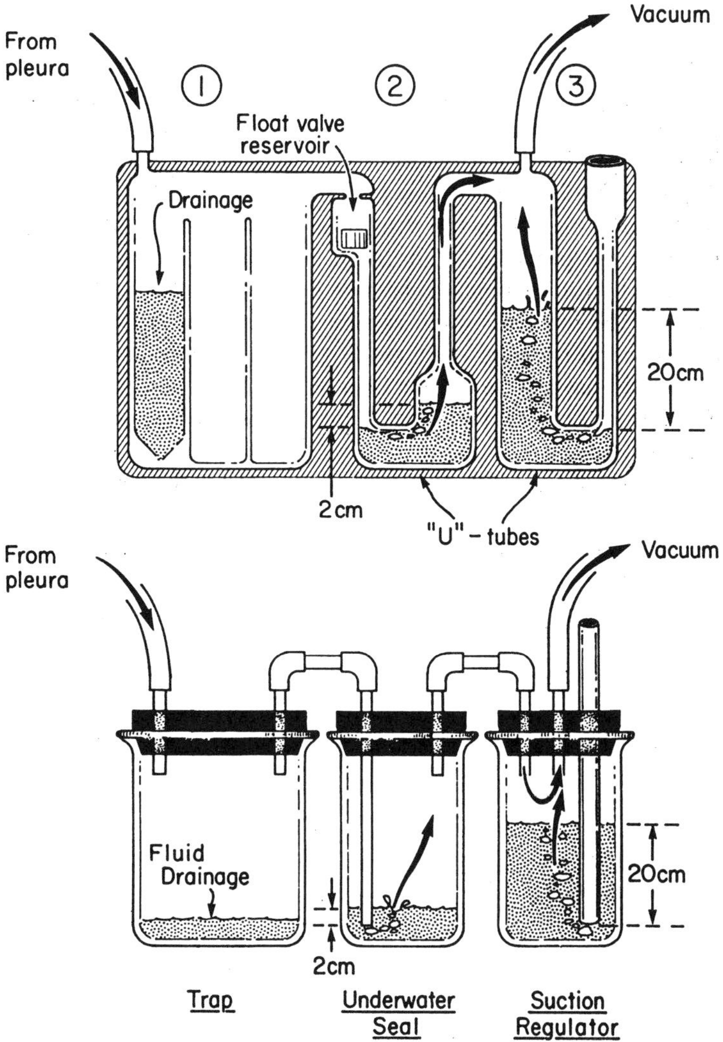


**FIGURE 15–1** Disposable compartmental chest drainage unit and a three-bottle chest tube system. Compartment 1 is the drainage compartment. Compartment 2 is the water seal compartment. Compartment 3 is the suction control compartment. (Fishman, N.H. [1983]. *Thoracic Drainage: A Manual of Procedures.* St. Louis: Mosby–Year Book, p. 84, with permission.)

the amount of suction, water will have to be added to or drawn off from this compartment. Increasing the suction pressure on the wall regulator will not increase the suction but will increase the flow through the system. With massive pleural air leaks, this may be required in order to evacuate the pleural cavity before the next breath.

E. Troubleshooting (Table 15–1)

F. Removing the chest tube

1. Removing the tube is indicated if the tube is nonfunctional or is no longer indicated (bubbling has stopped in the water sealed chamber, or on chest radiograph no air is seen in the pleural cavity).
2. To assess whether air is still in the pleural cavity, before removing the tube, it is clamped off for 12 to 24 h.
3. The patient is observed for any respiratory distress (air may still be in the pleural space or may reaccumulate).
4. A chest radiograph is taken.
5. If there is any sign of respiratory distress or if the chest radiograph indicates the presence of pneumothorax, the tubes are unclamped.
6. Just before removing the tube, if the patient can understand, a deep breath is taken and a Valsalva maneuver is performed. This reduces the possibility of air entry as tube is removed.
7. The tube is pulled and a gauze with petroleum is placed over the opening.
8. Another chest radiograph is taken following removal.

TABLE 15–1. ***Troubleshooting Chest Tube Drainage System with Suction***

| Problem | What Should be Done? |
|---|---|
| In a short period of time, an unusually large volume of blood has collected. | Check the patient for problems associated with loss of blood; assess blood pressure, pulse (peripherals), ECG, and color. Report findings. Ensure that the drainage compartment does not get filled. |
| There is no bubbling in the suction control bottle. The patient has been ordered for (–) 20 cm $H_2O$ suction. | 1. Turn the wall suction up to at least 20 cm $H_2O$.<br>2. Check the water level in the suction control compartment. It may be above 20 cm. |
| The drainage unit is level with the patient's chest-tube insertion site. | Place the drainage unit several feet below the patient's chest (recommended, 3 ft). |
| The water sealed compartment has excessive bubbling. | Check all connections in the system.<br>1. If bubbling continues, clamp the drainage tube momentarily where it enters the drainage unit. If bubbling continues, the leak is in the drainage unit.<br>2. If bubbling stops the leak is in the patient or in the chest drainage tubing. To identify where the leak is, advance toward the chest tube insertion site clamping the tube every few inches.<br>3. If, after clamping the drainage tubing closest to the insertion site of the chest tube, bubbling continues, check for air leak around the chest tube insertion site. This can be done by compressing the skin around the tube. Bubbling will stop, if the leak is here. The site needs to be sealed.<br>4. If, after compressing the skin, bubbling is still present, this indicates the leak is from the pleural space. A bronchopleural fistula could be present. |

## II. Flexible bronchoscopy

A. Definition and description
1. Flexible bronchoscopy (FB) directly visualizes the upper and lower respiratory tract for the diagnosis and management of various inflammatory, infectious, and malignant diseases of the chest.
2. Uses of FB includes the following:
    a. Removal of secretions
    b. Foreign bodies
    c. Pathological diagnostics (bronchial brushing, forceps, or needle biopsy)
    d. Removal of tissue by laser
    e. Intubation

B. Indications
1. Presence of lesions of unknown etiology on chest radiograph
2. Need to evaluate the presence of recurrent or persistent atelectasis or pulmonary infiltrates
3. To assess the patency of mechanical properties in the upper airway
4. To assess the patient exhibiting hemoptysis, persistent unexplained cough, localized wheeze, or stridor
5. Suspicious or positive sputum cytology results
6. To obtain lower respiratory tract secretions, cell washings, and biopsies for cytology, histology, and microbiological samples
7. To determine the location and extent of injury from burns or toxic inhalation
8. To assess and evaluate problems with endotracheal and tracheostomy tubes
9. To remove mucus plugs that may have caused segmental or lobar atelectasis
10. To remove foreign bodies (this is done more commonly with rigid bronchoscopy)

C. Contraindications
1. Inability to adequately oxygenate, monitor, and provide health care personnel to assist
2. Serious complications in patients with disorders including the following:
    a. Bleeding or coagulopathy disorder that cannot be corrected
    b. Severe obstructive airway disease
    c. Unstable cardiovascular status including dysrhythmias
3. Relative contraindications include the following:
    a. Lack of cooperation by the patient
    b. Partial obstruction of the trachea

c. Moderate to severe hypoxia or any degree of hypercarbia
d. Respiratory failure requiring mechanical ventilation

4. Asthma does not preclude the use of FB, but greater monitoring may be required.

D. Complications
1. Epistaxis
2. Air leak
3. Fever
4. Drug reaction
5. Heart rhythm disturbance
6. Hypoxemia
7. Hypercarbia
8. Wheezing
9. Hypotension
10. Laryngospasm
11. Hemoptysis
12. Cross-contamination of specimens and bronchoscope
13. Increased airway resistance
14. Bradycardia

E. Equipment for procedure
1. Bronchoscopic devices
a. Bronchoscope, light source, video or photographic equipment
b. Cytology brushes, flexible forceps, aspiration needle and basket, and specimen collecting devices
c. Syringes for bronchoalveolar lavage, needle aspiration, and drug administration
d. Bite block, laryngoscope, various sizes of endotracheal tubes, and resuscitation bag and mask
2. Monitoring devices, including pulse oximeter, ECG, and blood pressure device
3. Equipment in procedure room including the following:
a. Oxygen and various equipment for delivery of oxygen
b. Suction systems
c. Protease enzyme agent (Protozyme) for cleaning and removing blood and protein before disinfection or sterilization; any other detergent capable of removing this debris is acceptable.

F. Preparing the patient
1. Specific protocol for patient preparation should be established.
a. Empty the stomach to prevent vomiting and aspiration.
b. Blood studies should be done to establish any coagulation problems that could cause bleeding following lung biopsy.
c. Establish intravenous line for administration of medication (if needed).
d. Administer medication to prevent coughing, bronchospasm, anxiety, bradycardia, and dysrhythmias.
2. Apply medications prior to bronchoscopy.
a. Anesthesia may be given via aerosol, direct gargle, or injection (spray) into the posterior pharyngeal wall. Lidocaine (1%, 2%, or 4%) can accomplish topical anesthesia. Anesthetics are administered with the patient in a semi-Fowler's position. The respiratory therapist can test the degree of anesthesia by lightly touching the pharynx with a tongue depressor. Further anesthesia will be needed if a gag reflex is still present or the patient is still sensitive in this area. Watch for side effects, such as tremors, nervousness, blurred vision, talkativeness, dizziness, hypotension, and bradycardia, that may be caused by the topical anesthetic agent.
b. If the bronchoscope is inserted transnasally, 0.5% phenylephrine hydrochloride or dilute epinephrine (1:10,000) may also be used for vasoconstriction to reduce epistaxis or control bleeding following lung biopsy.
c. Patients may require administration of an antianxiety drug (codeine, meperidine, midazolam, morphine, or hydroxyzine) before any topical anesthetics are administered. To relieve anxiety, reduce secretions, and minimize vasovagal reflexes, the patient should receive an antianxiety drug and an anticholinergic agent (atropine or glycopyrrolate). Antianxiety drugs will sedate the patient mildly and suppress the cough reflex. Anticholinesterase drugs will inhibit vagal stimulation, reducing the potential for bradycardia, arrhythmia, and hypotension.
d. IV medications such as diazepam, meperidine, and fentanyl
e. Inhaled beta 2 agonists, including albuterol and metaproterenol

f. Water-soluble lubricant or combined lubricant-anesthetic (viscous lidocaine)
g. Sedative antagonist medication, including physostigmine (Antilirium), used as an antidote for CNS effects (delirium, coma), and naloxone (Narcan), a narcotic antagonist

G. Insertion of the bronchoscope
1. Insertion may be accomplished transnasally with or without a nasal airway, transorally through a bite block, or through a tracheostomy or endotracheal tube.
2. Transnasal insertion allows viewing of the nasal fossa, pharynx, and larynx.
3. When passing the bronchoscope transorally in a nonintubated patient, having a bite block in place is preferred. This will prevent the bronchoscope from being damaged by biting.
4. Patients receiving mechanical ventilation will need a special adapter for advancement of the bronchoscope. The adapter should allow a fit tight enough to prevent loss of ventilating pressure, loss of PEEP, and loss of volume. Further precautions that should be taken for patients receiving mechanical ventilation include the following:
a. Prior to insertion of the bronchoscope, a topical anesthetic should be administered down the endotracheal tube or tracheostomy tube.
b. Increase the $FIO_2$ (may require 100% oxygen).
c. Monitor the exhaled volume and any leaks that may occur. This can be compensated for by turning up the tidal volume until the desired volume is achieved.

H. Treatment of side effects and complications
1. Bronchospasm and laryngospasm may occur if the patient's airway has not been adequately anesthetized. Administration of intravenous aminophylline or an aerosol containing beta 2-adrenergic effects will prevent any further episode. If the patient is receiving positive-pressure ventilation, a muscle relaxant with a sedative may be used.
2. Hemorrhage is not uncommon but varies in the degree to which it occurs. In most cases, bleeds can be controlled by saline lavage and time. If a major bleed occurs, then one or more of the following can be implemented to reduce and stop it.
a. Instillation of epinephrine: Epinephrine is a vasopressor and can be injected into the lungs through the biopsy channel.
b. Compression with the bronchoscope: The distal tip is wedged against the bleed site, which compresses the site and allows clotting.

I. Patient monitoring during bronchoscopy
1. Heart and ECG
2. Pulse oximeter
3. BP, respiration rate
4. Level of consciousness
5. Subjective response to procedure such as pain, discomfort, and dyspnea
6. $SpO_2$ and $FIO_2$
7. Ventilatory parameters including tidal volume, rate, peak airway pressure, inspiratory flow, PEEP, and exhaled volume
8. Monitoring after the procedure for the first 24 to 48 h: Assess the patient and identify problems such dyspnea, fever, chest pain, wheezing, hemoptysis, or any new findings after the procedure was performed.
9. Chest radiograph, especially if tissue samples are obtained

J. Collecting samples
1. Wash hands.
2. Wear gloves when touching body substances, mucous membranes, or nonintact skin.
3. Wear gown.
4. Wear mask or eye protection.

K. Cleaning and disinfecting the equipment
1. Nosocomial infections are a major problem associated with bronchoscopy.
2. Cleaning and disinfecting agents that can be used include the following:
a. Betadine
b. Alcohol
c. Ethylene oxide
d. Alkaline glutaraldehyde
e. Protozyme
3. Immediately following the procedure, rinse saline through the biopsy channel.
4. The outside of the scope and entire biopsy channel should be exposed to disinfecting solution. Rinse with sterile distilled water.

5. The bronchoscope is then cleaned with a disinfecting agent, and the biopsy channel is rinsed with sterile water.
6. The outside of the bronchoscope is dried with a sterile gauze pad, and oxygen is applied to the biopsy channel for drying or allowed to air dry.
7. The bronchoscope is wrapped to prevent any dust from accumulating and stored.

## III. Thoracentesis

A. Indications
   1. Removing air and fluid from the pleural cavity to relieve symptoms
   2. Obtaining a sample of fluid for laboratory examination

B. Pleural disease
   1. Pleural effusion is an excess fluid that accumulates between the visceral and parietal pleura in relationship to the amount that is reabsorbed.
   2. Pleural effusion has a number of etiological factors such as *Mycoplasma* pneumonia, streptococcal pneumonia, and congestive heart failure.
   3. Other factors are not as evident and require an analysis of the fluid in the pleural cavity.
   4. The presence of pleural effusion may be established by the following:
      a. Lateral decubitus chest radiograph or CT scan
      b. Physical examination with flatness to percussion and diminished breath sounds; blunting of costophrenic angle on chest radiograph

C. Procedure
   1. Performed through the intercostal space at the site of maximal dullness
   2. The site is marked, sterilized, and draped.
   3. Reassure the patient and inform the patient what is about to happen.
   4. Lidocaine hydrochloride is used to anesthetize the skin.
   5. After anesthetizing the area, insert the thoracentesis needle. Placing the patient in an upright or supine position provides dependent drainage of the fluid.
   6. The needle is inserted into the eighth intercostal space until fluid level is reached. This is established when fluid can be withdrawn. Inserting the needle into any area lower than this may puncture the spleen or the diaphragm.
   7. A small amount of pleural fluid is aspirated for diagnostic purposes.
   8. For therapeutic thoracentesis, tubing is connected to a large bottle, which is then attached to a vacuum source. The chest tube is then placed in the sixth intercostal space.
   9. After the thoracentesis is completed, the needle is withdrawn and the puncture hole is pinched between the fingers to prevent air entry. The puncture hole may be sutured closed or closed with adhesive tape.

D. Types of pleural fluid problems
   1. Transudate
      a. Clear, straw-colored appearance
      b. Ultra filtrate of the plasma containing protein
      c. Caused by increased pulmonary venous pressure or decreased serum protein levels
      d. Problems such as congestive heart failure or pulmonary atelectasis cause transudate fluid.
      e. Laboratory characteristics include specific gravity less than 1.016, few lymphocytes, few red blood cells, and glucose similar to serum glucose level.
   2. Exudate
      a. A cloudy, turbid fluid
      b. Problems such as bacterial infection or lymphatic problems cause exudative fluid.
      c. Laboratory characteristics include specific gravity more than 1.016, many lymphocytes, and variable red blood cells; glucose may be less than serum glucose levels.
      d. Types of exudates
         (1) Empyema is pus-filled secretions caused by pneumonitis.
         (2) Chylothorax is the result of presence of chyle from intestinal lymph vessels. It may be caused by trauma. This fluid contains products of digestion and fats.
   3. Hemothorax
      a. Bleeding into the pleural cavity because of trauma or penetrating injury
   4. Hydrothorax

a. Caused by fluid entering the pleural cavity because of a misplaced IV line or CVP line
5. Hydropneumothorax
a. Combination of air and fluid in the pleural cavity

E. Test performed for pleural fluid analysis
1. Gram stain culture and sensitivity for bacterial infection
2. Acid-fast stain and culture for tuberculosis
3. Red blood cell count for frank bleed versus bloody effusion (check hematocrit count)
4. Leukocyte count for sepsis; leukocytes are the first line of defense for fighting infection.
5. Blood clots may indicate tuberculosis or neoplasm.
6. Specific gravity of more than 1.016 may indicate infection, whereas a value less than 1.016 may indicate pleural effusion from CHF.
7. Glucose level less than the serum glucose level may indicate bacterial infection.

## IV. Extracorporeal membrane oxygenation (ECMO)

A. For infants who fail to respond to conventional ventilation because of respiratory failure from hyaline membrane disease, meconium aspiration, persistent pulmonary hypertension of the newborn, congenital diaphragmatic hernia, or sepsis, ECMO provides systemic life support, which allows the lungs to rest at low mechanical ventilator settings. Gas exchange in the form of cardiopulmonary bypass is provided.

B. ECMO circuit and cannulation
1. The most common ECMO circuit is the venoarterial bypass (Fig. 15–2). A venous drainage cannula is placed in the internal jugular vein with the distal tip in the right atrium. A second cannula is placed in the right common carotid artery with its tip in the innominate artery at the junction of the aortic arch. Gravity allows venous blood to be removed from the patient via the right atrium to a bladder. A roller device then pumps the blood to a

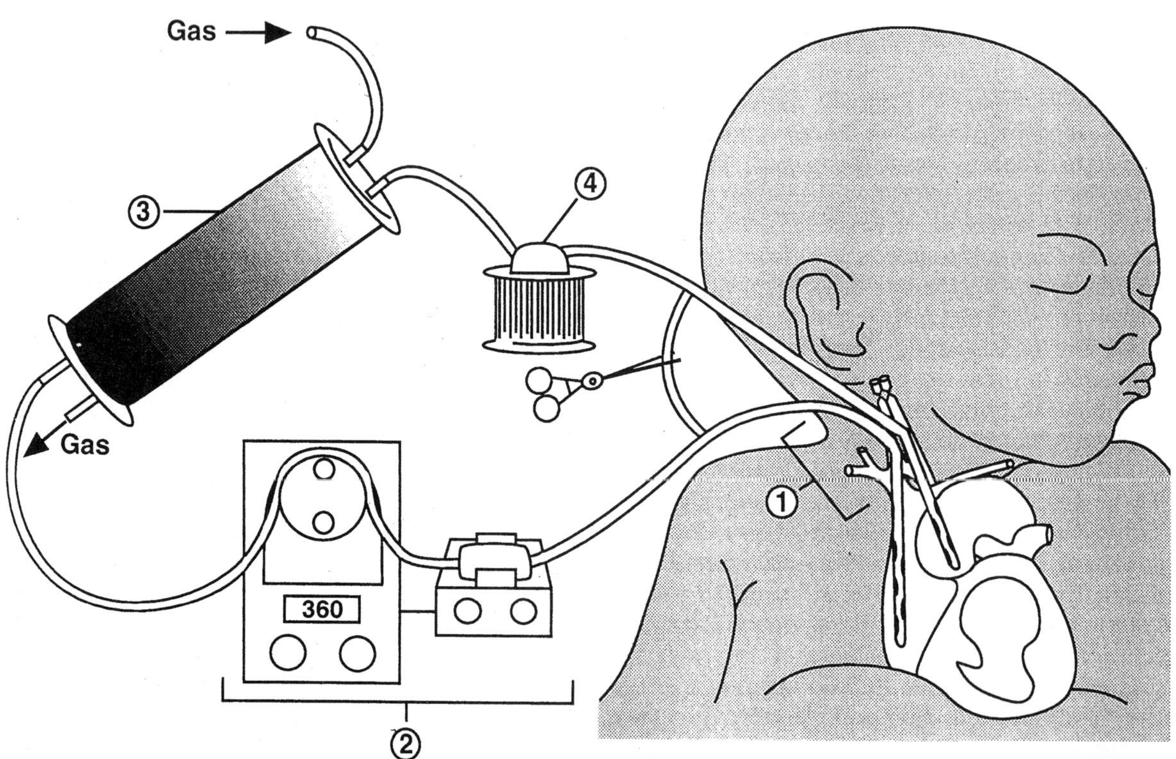


**FIGURE 15–2** Veno-arterial ECMO circuit. Major components of the circuit include 1) the venous and arterial cannulae (note clamping of the bridge to permit blood flow through the cannulae to and from the infant); 2) the servoregulated roller pump; 3) the artificial membrane lung; and 4) the heat exchanger for rewarming blood prior to recirculation to the infant. (From Spitzer, A.R. [1996]. Intensive Care of the Fetus and Neonate. St. Louis: Mosby–Year Book, p. 605, with permission.)

polyurethane membrane (artificial lung) oxygenator, through a warmer, and returns to the patient by the arterial cannula.

2. The rate of blood flow through the ECMO circuit controls the $PaO_2$. Normal flow is 100 to 120 mL/kg/min.
3. Venovenous (V-V) bypass is also used with ECMO therapy. With the V-V bypass, a catheter in the right atrium is inserted through the right jugular vein. Blood travels through the circuit, is oxygenated, and enters the infant through the femoral vein. This circuit is not used as often as the V-A circuit. In general, to use this circuit, infants must have a good cardiac output.

C. Inclusion criteria for ECMO therapy
   1. Infants on mechanical ventilation for less than 10 days on maximal therapy
   2. Infants weighing more than 2000 gm who are more than 35 weeks old (greater incidence of intracranial hemorrhage in premature infants)
   3. Reversible cardiopulmonary disease
   4. No major cardiac anomalies

D. Scoring systems that determine the need for ECMO
   1. $A\text{-}aDO_2$ gradient
      a. $PAO_2 = (Pb - PH_2O) \times FIO_2 - \frac{PaCO_2}{0.8} - PaO_2$
      b. Example: $PAO_2 = 747 - 47 \times 1.0 - \frac{48}{0.8} - 40$
         $PAO_2 = 700 - 60 - 40$
         $PAO_2 = 600$ mm Hg
      c. The gradient determines the degree of shunting taking place before entering the systemic circulation. A normal $A\text{-}aDO_2$ is less than 25 mm Hg. Infants with a gradient more than 600 for more than 8 h have a mortality rate of more than 80%. Patients that meet this criterion are considered for ECMO.
   2. Oxygenation index (OI)
      a. Mean airway pressure: $\times$ ( $FIO_2 \times 100$) $\div PaO_2$
      b. Example: $OI = 20\ (1.0 \times 100) \div 40$
         $OI = 2000 \div 40$
         $OI = 50$
      b. The OI is determined from three blood gases drawn at least 30 min apart. An OI more than 40 predicts an 80% chance of dying without ECMO.

E. Ventilator settings while on ECMO
   1. To rest the lungs and prevent barotrauma and oxygen toxicity, ventilator settings are reduced.
   2. Common settings include the following:
      a. PIP: 20 cm $H_2O$
      b. $FIO_2$: 0.25
      c. Rate: 20/min
      d. PEEP: 10 to 14 cm $H_2O$ (This level of PEEP helps reduce atelectasis and white-out and may help the lungs to recover more quickly.)

F. Weaning and decannulation
   1. In general, the average ECMO lasts for 3 to 7 days. A trial off of ECMO may be initiated during this time after lung recovery has begun. Chest radiograph shows improvement, oxygen saturation is stable, and lung compliance shows improvement. As the patient improves, less blood flow is needed through the circuit to maintain the $PaO_2$.
   2. At this point, the ventilator parameters are increased to levels to support the infant when ECMO is being weaned. Common settings include the following: PIP, 20 to 25 cm $H_2O$; rate, 30/min; PEEP, 5 cm $H_2O$; and $FIO_2$, 0.40. After the infant has been on these settings for 20 to 30 min, the ECMO is discontinued by clamping the cannula of the ECMO circuit. Blood gases are taken every 20 min. If blood gases show deterioration of the infant's condition, the infant is placed back on ECMO. Several trials may take place before the infant is permanently off ECMO.
   3. Once the infant is permanently off ECMO, the cannulae are removed.

15

# REVIEW QUESTIONS

1. List two indications for chest tube insertion.

   a.

   b.

2. Where should a chest tube be placed to drain air? To drain free-flowing fluid?

3. Describe the three chambers in the disposable chest drainage unit.

4. How would one determine by observing a disposable chest drainage unit if an air leak is still present in the lung?

5. In order to provide 20 cm $H_2O$ to a chest tube, how much water must be added to the suction control chamber?

6. Fill in the accompanying table concerning troubleshooting a chest tube drainage unit.

| **Problem** | **What Should Be Done?** |
|---|---|
| In a short period of time, an unusually large volume of blood has collected. | |
| There is no bubbling in the suction-control bottle. The patient has been ordered for (–) 20 cm $H_2O$ suction. | |
| The drainage unit is level with the patient's chest-tube insertion site. | |
| The water sealed compartment has excessive bubbling. | |

7. When should a chest tube be removed?

8. After clamping the chest tube for 12 h, the patient begins showing signs of respiratory distress. What should be done at this time?

9. What maneuver is performed to prevent air from entering the chest as the chest tube is removed?

10. List two indications for flexible bronchoscopy.

    a.

    b.

11. The following is a list of medications that should be available for use during the bronchoscopy procedure. Give a reason why this drug may be used for this procedure.
    a. Lidocaine (1%, 2%, and 4%)
    b. Epinephrine (1:10,000)
    c. Meperidine
    d. Atropine
    e. Albuterol
    f. Viscous lidocaine
    g. Naloxone

12. While bronchoscopy is being performed in a patient receiving mechanical ventilation, what should be monitored?

13. What agents are used to disinfect a bronchoscope?

14. List two indications for a thoracentesis.
    a.
    b.

15. Given the following types of pleural fluid, describe the difference between each one.
    a. Transudate
    b. Exudate
    c. Empyema
    d. Hemothorax
    e. Hydrothorax

16. In the accompanying table, give the rationale as to why each test is performed on pleural fluid.

| **Test** | **Rationale for Performing Test** |
|---|---|
| Gram stain | |
| Acid-fast stain | |
| Red blood cell count | |
| Leukocyte count | |

17. Describe the location of cannulation in a venoarterial ECMO circuit.

18. What controls the $PaO_2$ in the ECMO circuit?

19. Describe the location of cannulation in a venovenous ECMO circuit.

20. List two inclusion criteria for ECMO therapy.

    a.

    b.

21. After placing an infant on ECMO, what adjustment in ventilator settings should be made to reduce the incidence of barotrauma and oxygen toxicity?

22. What are the A-a$DO_2$ and oxygenation index (OI) of a 36-week-old infant receiving mechanical ventilation with the following settings:

    PIP: 30 cm $H_2O$; pH: 7.22

    Rate: 60/min; $PaCO_2$: 64 mm Hg

    $FIO_2$: 1.0; $PaO_2$: 40 mm Hg

    Itime: 0.4 s; mean airway pressure: 20 cm $H_2O$

    PEEP: 10 cm $H_2O$

23. What are common ventilator settings for an infant during a trial off of ECMO?

## BIBLIOGRAPHY

American Association for Respiratory Care: Clinical Practice Guideline. (1993). Fiberoptic bronchoscopy assisting. Respiratory Care 38, 1173.

Fishman, N. H. (1983). *Thoracic Drainage: A Manual of Procedures*. St. Louis: Mosby–Year Book.

Baumgart, S. (1996). Extracorporeal membrane oxygenation. In Spitzer, A. (Ed.). *Intensive Care of the Fetus and Neonate*. St. Louis: Mosby–Year Book.

Finer, N. N. (1996). Flexible fiber-optic bronchoscopy. In Spitzer, A. (Ed.). *Intensive Care of the Fetus and Neonate*. St. Louis: Mosby–Year Book.

Klein, M. D., and Whittlesey, G. C. (1994). Extracorporeal membrane oxygenation. *Pediatric Clinics of North America 41*(2), 365.

Miller, S. K., and Sahn, S. A. (1987). Chest tubes: Indications, technique, management and complications. *Chest 91*(2), 258.

O'Rourke, P. P. (1991). ECMO: Where have we been? Where are we going? *Respiratory Care 36*(7), 683.

O'Rourke, P. P. (1993). ECMO: Current status. *Neonatal Respiratory Diseases 3*(3), 1.

Ortiz, R. M., Cilley, R. E., and Bartlett, R. H. (1987). Extracorporeal membrane oxygenation in pediatric respiratory failure. *Pediatric Clinics of North America 34*(1), 39.

Steele, R. W. (1994). *The Clinical Handbook of Pediatric Infectious Disease*. New York: The Parthenon Publishing Group.

Torosian, M. B., Statter, M. B., and Arensman, R. M. (1996). Extracorporeal membrane oxygenation. In Goldsmith, J. P., and Karotkin, E. H. (Eds.). *Assisted Ventilation of the Neonate*, ed. 3. Philadelphia: W. B. Saunders.

Wong, S. J. (1997). Pulmonary system. In Seidel, H. M., Rosenstein, B. J., and Pathak, A. (Eds.). *Primary Care of the Newborn*, ed. 2. St. Louis: Mosby–Year Book.

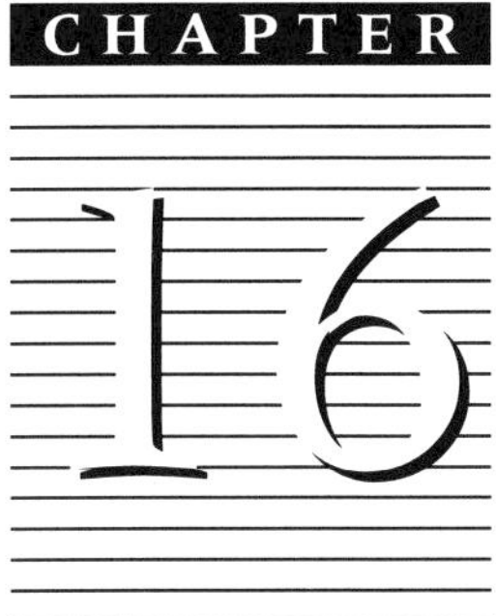


# Pediatric Home Care

I. **Goals of pediatric home care**
   A. To provide an environment in which the child can function at the highest possible level
   B. To allow the child to develop properly within a framework of a nurturing home environment
   C. To increase the independence of and participation in his or her own care
   D. To reinstate the family roles and socialization as much as possible
   E. To improve the quality of life

II. **Discharge planning**
   A. A mechanism that guides a multidisciplinary effort to successfully transfer the child from the hospital environment to a home environment
   B. The discharge plan includes the following:
      1. Patient evaluation to determine if the patient is ready for discharge
      2. Determination of the site for the infant after discharge, as well as the supplies and equipment required for continual care at the site
      3. Determine adequacy of financial resources.
   C. The discharge plan should be developed and implemented as soon as possible prior to transfer. How soon the plan is implemented is based on the severity of the patient's medical condition, supplies and equipment required, and goals.
   D. The discharge planning process includes the following:
      1. Evaluation of the patient
         a. Medical condition
         b. Equipment for oxygen therapy, bronchial hygiene, cardiovascular monitoring, sleep-disorder breathing, aerosol therapy, and airway maintenance
         c. Mechanical ventilation equipment, including negative-pressure and positive-pressure equipment
      2. The functional ability of the patient
      3. The family's and patient's psychosocial condition
      4. Evaluation of the site for continuing care
         a. The site should be capable of operating and supporting equipment used in the continual care of the patient.
         b. The site should be evaluated and determined to be free of fire, health, and safety hazards. Adequate heating, cooling, and ventilation should be available. The site should have adequate room for the equipment and storage of the supplies and should provide easy access and mobility.
      5. Development of a care plan. This plan should include the following:
         a. Patient self-care as appropriate
         b. Roles and responsibilities of team members and members who will provide daily care
         c. Documentation of training additional caregivers
         d. Emergencies and contingencies
         e. Maintenance and troubleshooting equipment
         f. Appropriately responding to changes in the patient's medical condition
         g. Types of medications administered
         h. Assessment of the patient
         i. Communication to all health care team members
      6. Evaluation of the caregivers' ability to learn and perform the required care before discharge. Discharge may be postponed because of the patient's and/or caregiver's inability to learn and adequately perform the appropriate care.

7. Outcome goals of the discharge plan include the following:
    a. Satisfactory administration of all treatments by caregivers as instructed
    b. The goals and needs of the patient are being met by the treatments and equipment.
    c. The patient and caregivers are satisfied with the care and plan.
    d. The site is optimal for the patient's needs.
    e. The caregiver is able to adequately assess the patient's needs and troubleshoot the equipment.

E. Education of the caregivers
1. Providing education and training to the caregivers is required to increase their knowledge and understanding of the patient's health status and therapy, to improve the caregivers' skills at providing safe and effective therapy, and to foster a positive attitude toward the care and compliance of therapy.
2. The respiratory care practitioner's goal in educating the caregiver is to equip him or her with the knowledge, skills, and attitudes to better understand the patient's condition.
3. To properly instruct the caregiver, resources such as written materials, audiovisual aids, anatomic models, respiratory equipment, mannequins, a computer, and software should be available.
4. The patient and caregiver should be questioned as to what they perceive is important and relevant to the care. Information obtained from questioning will help determine the capabilities of the patient and caregiver.
5. After instructing the patient and caregiver in a particular skill using the appropriate educational resources, the RCP should do the following:
    a. Require the caregiver and/or patient to demonstrate the skill and repeat any information in his or her own words without prompting.
    b. Upon completion of the skill, the RCP should then provide correction or additional instruction. Have the caregiver and/or patient repeat the skill.
    c. Complete the skill task by asking the caregiver to adapt the skill in the home environment.
6. Once in the home, documenting the caregiver's and/or patient's continuing acquisition of skills should be done on a consistent basis.

## III. Oxygen in the home

A. Indications for oxygen therapy in the home
1. Documented hypoxemia (for children and infants older than 28 days)
    a. $PaO_2$ less than or equal to 55 mm Hg, or $SaO_2$ less than or equal to 88% in subjects breathing room air, or
    b. $PaO_2$ of 56 to 59 mm Hg, or $SaO_2$ or $SpO_2$ less than or equal to 89% with specific clinical conditions such as cor pulmonale, erythrocythemia, or a hematocrit greater than 56%.
2. Subjects who do not qualify for oxygen therapy at rest but who will qualify during exercise, ambulation, or sleep.

B. Assessing the need for oxygen
1. Initially, the need for oxygen is determined by assessing arterial blood gas values and pulse oximetry values.
2. Reassessment requires additional blood gas analysis if any change in the patient's cardiopulmonary condition occurs. Within 1 to 3 months of beginning oxygen therapy, another blood gas should be assessed to determine the need for long-term oxygen therapy.

C. Steel oxygen cylinders
1. For stationary home use, cylinder size H or K is used. Cylinder sizes D and E are used for travel.
2. Primarily used for intermittent oxygen requirement because of the limited amount of oxygen depending on the flowrate and cylinder size. Also for children requiring a flowrate of less than 1 L/min.
3. One cubic ft of gas volume equals 28.316 L of gas volume.
4. Estimating duration of flow
    a. To determine cylinder factor, use the following formula:

(1) $$\text{Cylinder factor (L/psig)} = \frac{\text{cubic feet in full cylinder} \times 28.3}{\text{pressure of full cylinder in psig}}$$

(2) $$\text{Cylinder factor for an E cylinder} = \frac{22\ \text{ft}^3 \times 28.3}{2200\ \text{psig}} = 0.283 \text{ or } 0.3$$

    b. To determine flow duration:

(1) $$\text{Duration of flow (min)} = \frac{\text{pressure in cylinder (psig)} \times \text{cylinder factor}}{\text{flowrate to patient}}$$

(2) Duration of flow of a full E cylinder at a flowrate of 2 L/min. Consider the cylinder empty at 500 psig. This will ensure an uninterrupted supply of oxygen.

$$\text{Duration of flow} = \frac{2200 - 500 \text{ psig} \times 0.28}{2 \text{ L/min}} = 238 \text{ min/60 min} = 4 \text{ h}$$

5. Oxygen flowrates of less than 4 L/min do not require humidification, unless the patient complains of dryness with the oxygen administration device.
6. Table 16–1 shows liters, cubic feet, and conversion factors for cylinders commonly used in home care.

D. Aluminum and fiber-wrapped cylinders
1. Lightweight cylinders used with specific oxygen delivery devices (demand-flow oxygen device) are more portable than steel cylinders.
2. Lighter cylinders are capable of delivering appropriate liter flow in a certain amount of time. For example, Oxylite Mini weighs 4.5 lb and supplies oxygen for 10.5 h at 2 L/min.

E. Liquid oxygen
1. Liquid oxygen is the most economical way of providing stationary, portable oxygen.
2. One liter of liquid oxygen is the equivalent of 860 L of gaseous oxygen. One pound of liquid oxygen equals 342 L of gaseous oxygen.
3. To determine the duration of flow, use the following formula:
   a. $$\text{Duration of flow (min)} = \frac{\text{weight of oxygen} \times 342 \text{ L}}{\text{flowrate to patient}}$$
   b. For a patient receiving 3 L/min from a device with 60 lb of oxygen, the duration of flow is as follows:
      (1) $$\text{Duration of flow (min)} = \frac{60 \text{ lb} \times 342}{3 \text{ L/min}}$$
      (2) Duration of flow = 6840 min/60 min = 114 h/24 h = 5 days
4. A portable tank is filled from the larger stationary tank. An ambulatory tank providing a flowrate of 1 L/min lasts approximately 15 h. At 2 L/min, it will last approximately 7 to 8 h.
5. The disadvantages to this system are that the oxygen is extremely cold, requiring the patient to handle the equipment with gloves; the equipment is more costly; and there is evaporative oxygen loss.

F. Oxygen concentrator
1. Using an oxygen concentrator is the most economical way of providing oxygen but is not able to provide portable oxygen capabilities. Concentrators extract oxygen from ambient air and should deliver oxygen at concentrations of 85% or greater at liter flows up to 4 L/min.
2. Children requiring a specific oxygen concentration in order to achieve an acceptable oxygen saturation may benefit from the oxygen concentrator. The flowrate is adjusted to achieve the acceptable oxygen saturation.

G. Oxygen-conserving devices
1. Reservoir cannulas (Oxymizer Cannula)
   a. This device has a large reservoir located just beneath the nasal prongs that sit just below the nose.
   b. During inspiration, a large bolus of pure oxygen is inhaled, therefore requiring a lower flow in order to maintain appropriate oxygen saturation.
   c. This results in savings because of the decreased oxygen use.
2. Oxygen-conserving nasal cannula
   a. This device has a reservoir that is located below the nose, nasal prongs, and oxygen-supply tubing. The reservoir contains nearly pure oxygen,

TABLE 16–1. ***Liters, Cubic Feet, and Conversion Factors for D, E, H and K Cylinders***

| Cylinder Size | Cubic Feet | Liters | Conversion Factor |
|---|---|---|---|
| D | 12.6 | 356 | 0.16 |
| E | 22 | 622 | 0.28 |
| H | 186 | 5260 | 3.14 |
| K | 244 | 6900 | 3.14 |

and as the patient inspires, the reservoir collapses, delivering high $FIO_2$ to the patient.

3. Oxygen-conserving pendant
   a. This device consists of a reservoir that sits on the patient's chest and connects to a nasal cannula by wide-diameter connecting tubes. Operation is the same as with the oxygen-conserving nasal cannula.
4. Humidification is not required when flowrates are less than 4 L/min.

H. Demand-flow oxygen devices
   1. Demand-flow oxygen administration devices deliver oxygen by pressure, flow, pressure and flow, or other ways.
   2. The flow of oxygen is delivered when the device senses either early inspiration or a crossover between inspiration and exhalation. The triggering mechanism uses a solenoid valve to deliver a pulse of oxygen.
   3. Alarms, such as a low-battery alarm, are incorporated in the device.
   4. In some devices, if the inspiration is not sensed or the unit malfunctions, the device automatically switches to continuous flow. In others, a switch may be provided in order to change from demand flow to continuous flow.
   5. Some devices can be programmed to deliver an oxygen pulse for a prescribed number of breaths.
   6. Humidification is not required when flowrates are less than 4 L/min.
   7. These devices can be attached to portable and stationary liquid oxygen systems and high-pressure cylinders.

I. Troubleshooting home oxygen equipment (Table 16–2)

J. Oxygen safety (Table 16–3)

## IV. Aerosol therapy in the home (see Chapter 9)

A. Troubleshooting compressor-nebulizer systems in the home (Table 16–4)

## V. Airway care and maintenance of the tracheostomy tube

A. When infants and children go home with a tracheostomy tube, humidity is required. Humidity can be provided by a heat moisture exchanger or a heated humidifier (see Chapter 9).

B. The tracheostomy tube size should be evaluated every 2 to 4 months. With the child's growth, the tube size will need to be increased. The younger the child with a tracheostomy, the sooner will the need arise to change the tracheostomy size.

C. Pediatric tracheostomy tubes may not have inner cannulas and may require weekly changing to prevent obstruction by mucus. Observe the patient for indications of the need for suctioning.
   1. Increased gurgling, bubbling, or coughing
   2. Anxiousness, restlessness, or crying
   3. Flaring nostrils
   4. Change in color of the fingernails, mouth, or lips to pale, gray, or blue
   5. Difficulty eating
   6. Suprasternal, intercostal retractions
   7. Unable to cough out secretions
   8. Pulling in of the skin around the stomal opening

D. Suctioning procedure

TABLE 16–2. ***Common Troubleshooting Techniques for Home Oxygen Equipment***

- Set cannula in a glass of water and watch for bubbling.
- Check contents gauge on tank.
- Check flow setting on oxygen source.
- Check on-off switch if there is no flow.
- Check all tubings for kinks and connections.
- Check washable filter on concentrator for clogging.
- Check humidifier bottle for leaks at threads, cross-threading.
- Remove or replace humidifier.
- If concentrator spontaneously stops, check positioning of machine and make sure it has 18 in of space on each side (concentrator can overheat without sufficient ventilation, causing it to quit running spontaneously).
- Check circuit breaker on back of concentrator; push back in if it has popped.
- Check power cord on concentrator to be sure it is plugged in.
- Check to be sure light switch is turned on if concentrator is plugged into outlet controlled by that light switch.

(From Dunne, P.J., and McInturff, S.L., p. 59, with permission.)

TABLE 16–3. ***Home Oxygen Safety Tips***

- Always keep cylinders in carts or safety collars.
- Small cylinders should be laid on the floor if not secured in a cart.
- Avoid knocking cylinders together (this may create sparks).
- Remove and avoid combustible materials (i.e., petroleum jelly, hair oil, hair and other aerosol sprays, petroleum-based skin lotions, and grease).
- Remove and avoid sources of ignition (i.e., hair dryers, electric razors, open flames, heaters, sparking toys, and lit cigarettes).
- Place oxygen source at least 6 ft away from flames or other sources of ignition.
- Do not place oxygen tanks in the trunk of the car.
- Keep oxygen tanks in a well-ventilated area to prevent the buildup of an oxygen-enriched atmosphere.
- Use "No Smoking—Oxygen in Use" signs to alert others to the presence of oxygen in the home.
- When filling a liquid oxygen portable tank, avoid contact with the stream of liquid oxygen that is seen at the vent when the tank is full.

(From Dunne, P.J., and McInturff, S.L., p. 61, with permission.)

1. The suction catheter can be cut to the distance or 1 cm beyond the distal end of the tracheostomy tube to prevent irritation and damage to the airway.
2. Wash hands, put on glove, and attach the catheter to the suction machine (a battery-operated suction machine should be available in case of a power failure). The suction pressure is adjusted to suction the secretions adequately at the lowest suction pressure.
3. Thick secretions may require a few drops of saline down the tracheostomy tube to loosen the mucus. From insertion of the catheter to removal should take no longer than 10 s. Repeat if necessary.
4. Observe the secretions for color, consistency, and odor. Monitor the patient for signs of infection, which include the following:
   a. Localized redness, swelling
   b. Fever, generalized malaise
   c. Pain at site
   d. Increased cough
   e. Abnormal drainage at site
   f. Increased sputum production
   g. Change in sputum color to yellow or green
5. If signs of infection are present, call the physician.
6. A bulb syringe can be used to remove secretions at the top of the tracheostomy tube.

E. Tracheostomy tube
   1. Changing the cuffless tracheostomy tube
      a. A small infant will need to be held by another caregiver, or the infant will need to be swaddled in a blanket during the procedure.
      b. After obtaining the new tracheostomy tube, attach the tape ties, insert the obturator, and lubricate the end of the tube with water-based lubricant.
      c. If needed, suction the old tube, and then remove the tube (provide blow-by oxygen as needed).
      d. Gently insert the new tube and immediately remove the obturator. Secure the tube with the ties.
   2. Changing the cuffed tracheostomy tube
      a. The procedure is the same as with the cuffless tube, except that the cuff's integrity should be tested prior to inserting it into the infant. This can be

TABLE 16–4. ***Troubleshooting the Compressor-Nebulizer System in the Home***

- If the unit will not turn on, check the power cord.
- If the unit has been in a cold environment and will not turn on, rock the power switch on and off several times (this should free the compressor).
- Check the nipple adapter on the compressor to ensure that it has no leaks.
- Check the medication nebulizer to be sure it has been assembled properly.
- Check the tiny jet holes to be sure they are not clogged.
- Inspect the compressor's filter; change it if it looks gray.
- Replace the medication nebulizer.

(From Dunne, P.J., and McInturff, S.L., p. 62, with permission.)

done by taking the tracheostomy tube with the cuff inflated and inserting it into sterile water and observing for bubble formation from the cuff.
   b. After inserting the tracheostomy tube, inflate the cuff with the proper pressure (measure cuff pressure).
   c. Foam cuffs help reduce the incidence of tracheomalacia (see Chapter 11).
3. Cleaning the tracheostomy inner cannula and opening
   a. Larger tracheostomy tubes have inner cannulas that can be removed to be cleaned. A disposable or nondisposable inner cannula is used. For a child receiving mechanical ventilation, an immediate replacement of the inner cannula is required until the nondisposable inner cannula can be cleaned. For infants not on mechanical ventilation, the inner cannula can be removed and cleaned. The oxygenation and humidification device can be placed over the outer tracheostomy tube.
   b. The inner cannula is placed in a bath of half-strength hydrogen peroxide (one-half water and one-half hydrogen peroxide). Scrub the inside and outside, removing mucus, rinse with sterile water, remove excess water, and insert into tracheostomy tube. Do not use a cloth to dry the cannula because the cloth may leave lint on the cannula.
   c. The tracheostomy opening can be cleaned with a cotton swab, using half-strength hydrogen peroxide (in the case of infection) or sterile water.
4. Decannulation
   a. Progressively decrease the size of the tracheostomy tube, then capping the tracheostomy tube. If capping is tolerated, then decannulate.
   b. Use a fenestrated tracheostomy tube in place of the standard tube.
   c. Replace the standard tube with a trach button (see Chapter 11).

## VI. Apnea monitoring

A. Apnea monitoring is indicated for infants who are at high risk for sudden death.
   1. Low-birth-weight infants with apneic episodes
   2. Siblings of infants who die of sudden infant death syndrome (SIDS) after a second SIDS death in the family. SIDS is defined as the sudden death of an infant less than 1 year of age, in which the death remains unexplained in spite of a postmortem examination, investigation of the death scene, and case history review.
   3. Infants who had apparent life-threatening events (ALTEs) and required vigorous stimulation and resuscitation. An ALTE is an episode characterized by apnea, bradycardia, change in color, loss of muscle tone, and choking or gagging.

B. Types of apnea
   1. Obstructive apnea is a cessation of airflow, despite continuous chest and abdominal movement (Fig. 16–1).
   2. Central apnea is the loss of respiratory effort caused by the loss of diaphragmatic movement and other respiratory muscle function (Fig. 16–2).
   3. Mixed apnea is a combination of central and obstructive apnea (Fig. 16–3).

C. The home monitoring device monitors heart rate and apneic events. It uses impedance pneumography with use of electrodes on the abdomen. Alarms are activated if the infant's heart rate falls out of the parameters set (i.e., a low heart rate alarm is activated at rates of fewer than 100 beats/min, and a high heart rate alarm is activated at rates of more than 170 beats/min) or if apnea occurs for longer than the set apnea parameter (i.e., 20 s). Apnea events are automatically documented by a recording of the event when the alarm limits have been exceeded. The date, time, infant's breathing pattern, and heart rate are recorded.

D. Technical problems with impedance monitors
   1. False alarms caused by shallow breathing
   2. Inability to detect obstructive apnea
   3. Inappropriate placement of the lead (on the chest versus the abdomen)

E. Obstructive sleep apnea (OSA)
   1. OSA is a breathing disorder characterized by repeated collapse of the upper airway during sleep, with consequent cessation of breathing. Sleep disorder breathing is more common in rapid eye movement sleep (REM).
   2. Polysomnography is a diagnostic tool used to identify sleep disturbances. Of school-aged children, 7 to 9% snore and 1 to 3% may have OSA.
   3. Symptoms
      a. Chronic, loud snoring (not as loud as adults)
      b. Gasping or choking episodes during sleep
      c. Excessive daytime sleepiness
      d. Personality change or cognitive difficulties related to fatigue
      e. Irritability, crankiness, low frustration tolerance, and short attention span

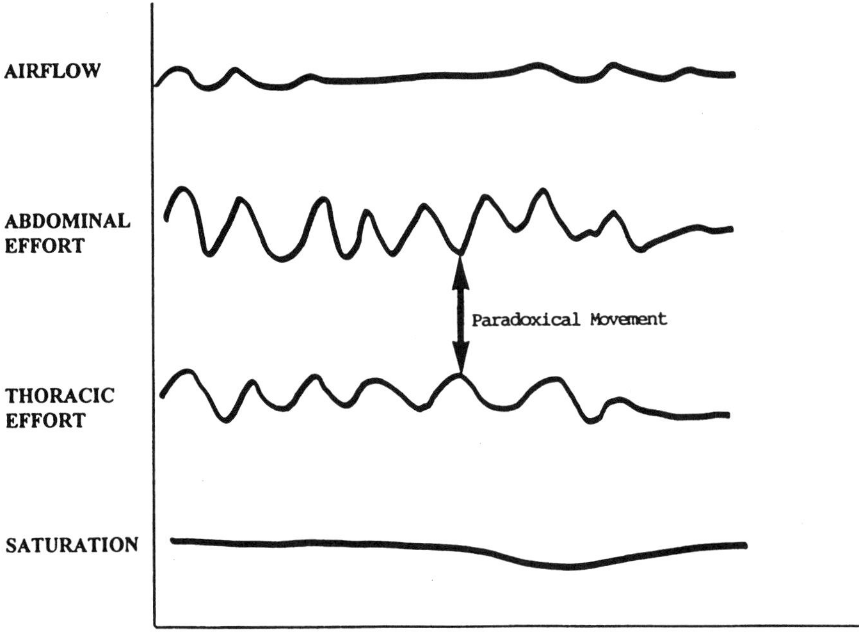


**FIGURE 16–1** Obstructive apnea tracing. Note the cessation of nasal airflow but continual abdominal and thoracic movement.

4. Signs
   a. Nasopharyngeal narrowing
   b. Obesity
   c. Small neck and micrognathia (small lower jaw) (Down syndrome and Pierre Robin syndrome)
   d. Craniofacial abnormalities
5. OSA is characterized by closure of the upper airway, resulting in cessation of airflow, despite persistent ventilatory efforts. OSA may present with nocturnal respiratory dysfunction, ranging from OSA with mild hypoxemia to prolonged episodes of obstructive hypopnea with hypercarbia.
6. The common cause of OSA is tonsils and adenoids. An adenotonsillectomy cures OSA in many children.
7. Treatment
   a. Some infants will outgrow apnea and will not require further monitoring.

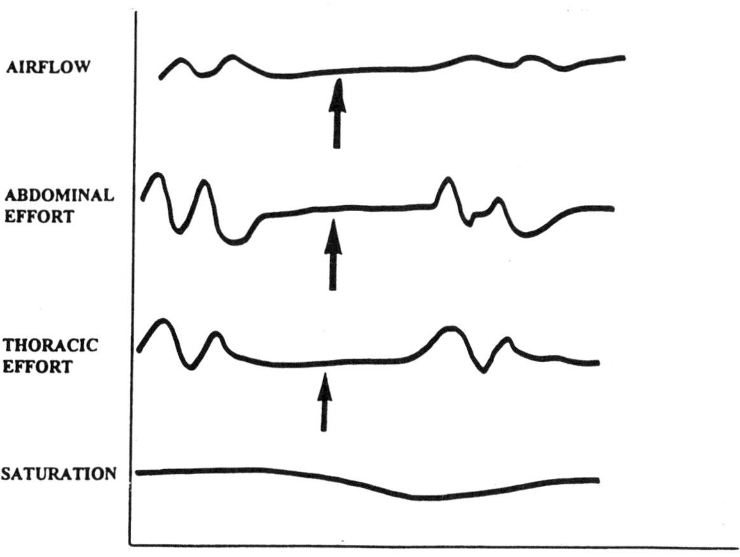


**FIGURE 16–2** Central apnea tracing. Note the airflow obstruction as well as cessation of abdominal and thoracic movement.

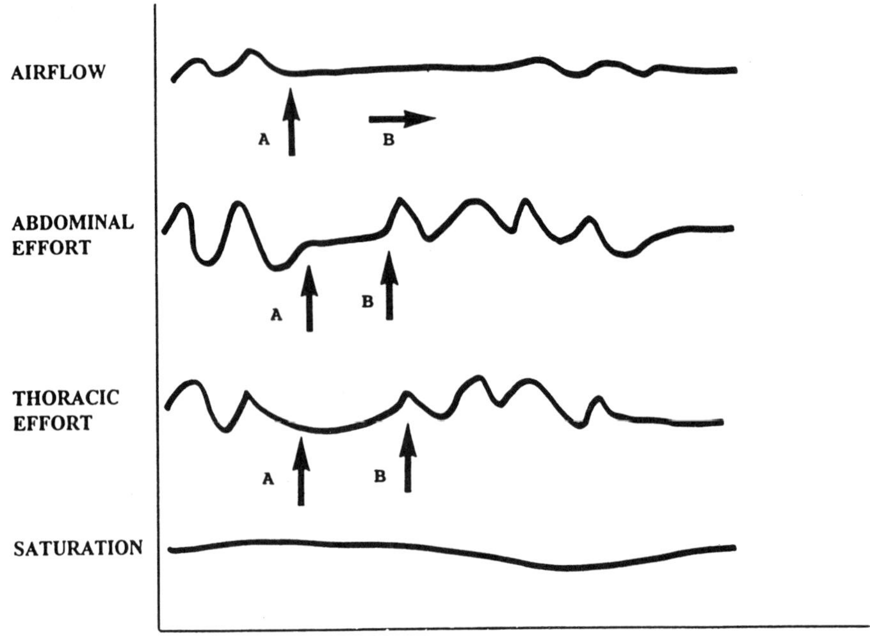


**FIGURE 16–3** Mixed apnea tracing. Mixed apnea begins with central apnea *(A)*, with cessation of airflow, abdominal movement, and thoracic effort. This is followed by continuous cessation of airflow, but there is abdominal and thoracic effort *(B)*.

b. Surgical procedures
c. Weight loss

**VII. Noninvasive ventilation**

A. CPAP and BiPAP (see Chapter 9)

B. Negative-pressure ventilation (NPV)

1. Indications
   a. NPV is seldom used in the acute care setting (other than instructing patients in the use of the equipment prior to discharge from hospital) and is mostly used for home care.
   b. Helpful in supporting chronic neuromuscular disorders and obstructive disorders, with the advantage of not requiring endotracheal intubation
   c. Symptomatic chronic respiratory failure ($PaCO_2$ greater than 45 mm Hg and compensated pH) with symptoms of morning headaches and hypersomnolence
   d. Adequate airway
   e. Intolerance of, or inability to use, noninvasive positive-pressure ventilation
2. Contraindications
   a. Same as for BiPAP
   b. Patients whose sleep apnea is caused by airway obstruction
3. Types of negative-pressure (NP) ventilators
   a. Chest cuirass
   b. Iron lung
   c. Poncho or suit type
4. Controls (All of these controls may not be on NP ventilators, but generally a combination of these.)
   a. Negative pressure
   b. Inspiratory time
   c. Expiratory time
   d. Rate

C. Settings

1. The patient should be instructed not to eat or drink during NPV.
2. Begin setting the negative pressure based on spontaneous tidal volume values of 5 to 7 mL/kg of body weight, subjective feelings from the patient, and chest rise.
3. The following modes are available:
   a. Time-triggered (control)
   b. Control with sigh
   c. Assist-control

TABLE 16–5. ***Troubleshooting Negative Pressure Ventilation***

| Patient Complaint | Clinical Consideration |
|---|---|
| Patient's tidal volume has decreased. | Check fitting of device (chest cuirass). A loose-fitting shell will not create the appropriate level of negative pressure and result in a reduction of the patient's tidal volume. Apply the appropriate size shell or other device. |
| Patient complains of shortness of breath. | Increase the applied negative pressure to increase alveolar ventilation or increase rate or decrease expiratory time. |
| Patient complains of dizziness and tingling in the fingers. | Reduce the applied negative pressure to reduce alveolar ventilation or decrease rate or increase expiratory time. |
| Patient's $SpO_2$ is < 90%. | Increase the $FIO_2$. This may require the addition of an oxygen source such as a nasal cannula or increasing the flowrate of the device currently being used. |

d. Assist-control with sigh
e. Assister (no backup rate)

4. Inspiratory-expiratory time or rate is set according to the patient's needs and is set if there is no rate control. If there is a rate control, the rate will be directly set. If the patient is spontaneously breathing, the patient will set his or her own rate, inspiratory time, and expiratory time.
5. With $FIO_2$ delivery, a separate oxygen delivery system, such as a nasal cannula, is used to supplement oxygen to the patient.
6. Some NPVs do not have alarms.

D. Troubleshooting and patient complaints (Table 16–5)

## VIII. Mechanical ventilation

A. A patient is eligible for home mechanical ventilation, if, even when a tracheostomy tube is required, the patient no longer needs intensive medical and monitoring services.

B. Goals
1. To sustain and extend life
2. To enhance the quality of life
3. To reduce morbidity
4. To improve and sustain physical and psychological function of all ventilated-assisted individuals (VAI) and to enhance growth and development
5. To provide cost-effective care

C. Indications
1. For patients unable to be completely weaned from invasive ventilatory support
2. Where there is progression of a disease requiring ventilatory support

D. Contraindications
1. Where there is a medical condition requiring high-level care or an unstable condition that requires hospital expertise and care. Indicators determining instability for home care include the following:
   a. $FIO_2$ greater than 0.40
   b. PEEP greater than 10 cm $H_2O$
   c. Lack of mature tracheostomy
   d. Inadequate resources for home care, including both financial and personal
   e. Patient's refusal to receive mechanical ventilation in the home
   f. Unsafe home environment including fire, health, and unclean conditions
   g. Lack of essential utilities

E. Criteria for discharge to home on mechanical ventilation
1. Oxygen requirements stable for 1 week and able to achieve this requirement at home. Medically stable infants weaned to maintenance levels of ventilatory support are candidates for home care.
2. Weight gain on a specific diet constant for 1 week
3. Stable drug therapy
4. Patient's siblings and patient immunized. Because of respiratory infections, half of all children discharged will require rehospitalization. Respiratory syncytial virus (RSV) is a frequent cause. Practical advice for parents to follow in order to avoid hospitalization and infection includes the following:
   a. During winter months, monitor the infant closely and avoid sibling contact if suspicious of contamination.
   b. Watch for signs of infection, including irritability, low-grade fever, nasal congestion, cough, tachypnea, and wheezing.

c. Maintain routine immunizations for patients, parents (flu shot), and siblings.

5. Education of patient's family regarding smoking, environmental inhalants, equipment, medication, and procedures. Planning for home care and education of the parents is extremely important. Knowledge of the equipment, problems that might arise, and how to respond to those situations should be reviewed prior to leaving the hospital. The parents must have confidence in the equipment and other medical personnel who will be assisting them at home. The parents must know CPR.
6. Before discharging to home, switch ventilators to the one that will be used at home. Assess settings according to chest movement, ABG, $SpO_2$, heart rate, and general work of breathing. Set alarms accordingly.

F. Establishing mechanical ventilation in the home

1. A neonatal ventilator is ideal for home use but consumes a lot of gas because of the continuous flow. These ventilators require compressed oxygen, air, and electricity. Because of this, it is recommended for short-term use (1 to 2 months).
2. Adult home ventilators require electricity, have internal batteries, and can achieve an $FIO_2$ of up to 0.50. The assist-control mode is used with the adult ventilator. If IMV is used with an adult home-care ventilator, then an add-on flow-through system should be attached to reduce the imposed work of breathing.
3. Pressure control ventilation is used. Chest excursion should be monitored to ensure adequate volume delivery. The peak pressure and inspiratory time is set directly or by setting tidal volume or tidal volume and peak flow. With ventilators that do not have pressure control capabilities, a pressure-relief valve can be added to the patient's circuit. A small leak should be present with each breath. Set the pressure limit 5 cm $H_2O$ above the pop-off pressure.
4. Some ventilators have valves that provide precise oxygenation. Others require oxygen add-on reservoirs that provide concentrations in the range of 40 to 50%. If the respiratory rate changes, the oxygen concentration will change. For example, a higher respiratory rate will decrease the concentration of oxygen available.
5. If PEEP is used, a PEEP valve is incorporated into the patient's circuit. These valves are often flow resistors that increase the work of breathing. If the ventilator is not PEEP compensated, the ventilator's sensitivity must be adjusted accordingly. Set the sensitivity 0.5 to 1.0 cm $H_2O$ below the level of PEEP. Observe the patient for signs of increased work of breathing and readjust the sensitivity as needed.
6. Heated humidifiers should be used for mechanical ventilation. Heat moisture exchangers should be for temporary use and are not recommended for subjects with small tidal volumes (less than 150 mL) or leaks around the tracheostomy tube.
7. Monitoring mechanical ventilation
   a. High- and low-pressure alarm or low-exhaled volume alarm
   b. $FIO_2$ (intermittent assessment)
   c. Apnea (if on the ventilator, no need for a separate monitoring device)
   d. Pulse oximetry (for use with high $FIO_2$ requirements, even then they may not be required)
8. Other equipment should be available for the patient on mechanical ventilation.
   a. A self-inflating resuscitation bag and mask
   b. A second ventilator should be available if needed within 2 h.
   c. Suction equipment
   d. Replacement tracheostomy tube with obturator and inner cannula, plus one size smaller
   e. Ventilator circuits
   f. Adequate means of communicating
9. A plan of care should be provided for each patient. In this care plan, include ventilator settings, equipment function, patient's physical condition, and emergency equipment that is available and functional. At each home-care visit, each of these should be consistently assessed by the respiratory care practitioner and the caregiver. Interventions by the respiratory care practitioner should be documented as to the type of intervention and results of the intervention.
10. Weaning
    a. Prior to weaning, a complete weaning schedule should be developed and communicated with the physician. Contingency plans should be available in case of problems.

b. Monitor for intolerance and cardiovascular changes.
c. Weaning may be initiated by using a T piece, varying the time the patient is off ventilation.
d. Because of neurological and/or neuromuscular problems, some infants may not be able to be weaned.

## IX. Infection control

A. Limit visitors who have an acute infection.
B. Wash hands before cleaning the equipment.
C. Nebulizers
  1. To clean the nebulizer, place the unassembled parts in hot water and detergent and rinse them thoroughly with tap water every 48 h.
  2. To disinfect the nebulizer after cleaning the nebulizer parts, place the parts in a solution of 1 part white vinegar and 3 parts tap water and allow to soak for 30 min. Rinse the parts thoroughly in tap water and dry.
D. Humidifiers
  1. Empty and refill the humidifier daily with distilled water or boiled tap water.
  2. Cleaning and disinfecting is the same as for nebulizers.
  3. Oxygen administration devices such as cannulas are replaced every week and the oxygen connecting tube once a month.
E. BiPAP mask
  1. Wash the mask with mild detergent, rinse with tap water, and dry.
  2. The headgear is hand-washed weekly and air-dried.
  3. The hose should be washed with mild detergent and hot water and hung up to air dry.
F. Suction machine
  1. Empty the contents into the toilet at least once per day and more often with more frequent suctioning.
  2. To remove debris in the suction connecting tube, suction hydrogen peroxide and water through the tube, tonsil tip, and suction catheter.
  3. Wearing gloves, wash the collection bottle in detergent and hot water every other day. Rinse with tap water and dry.
  4. Replace the suction connecting tube and tonsil tip once per week or as often as needed. Replace the suction catheter once per day.
G. Mechanical ventilator
  1. Change patient-ventilator tubing no more than once per week, unless otherwise indicated. While it is connected to the patient, enter the circuit as little as possible.
  2. Dispose of medical waste appropriately.

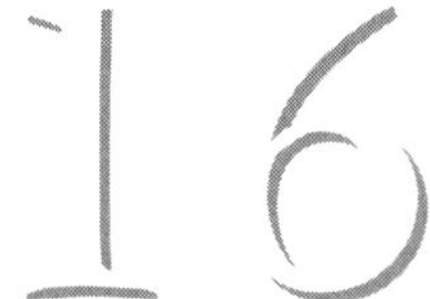

# REVIEW QUESTIONS

1. What should be included in a discharge plan for an infant who is being discharged to home on oxygen?

2. The parents of an infant are to be instructed in suctioning their child's airway through a tracheostomy tube. Explain how you would assess the parents to be certain they understand the procedure and are able to perform the procedure correctly.

3. For infants more than 28 days of age and children, what is the indication for oxygen therapy in the home?

4. An infant is receiving 1 L/min by nasal cannula from an H cylinder with 2000 psig. What is the duration of flow in hours?

5. A patient is receiving 2 L/min from a nasal cannula attached to a liquid oxygen system. There is 50 lb of oxygen in the system. What is the duration of flow in days?

6. Give a brief description of the following oxygen-conserving devices:

   a. Reservoir cannula

   b. Oxygen-conserving nasal cannula

   c. Oxygen-conserving pendant

7. What is a demand-flow oxygen device? What are the alarms and safety features that may be part of the demand-flow system?

8. A parent complains over the phone that she does not feel oxygen coming from her child's nasal cannula that is running at 5 L/min. You instruct the parent to place the cannula in water, and she tells you that there is no bubbling. Give three troubleshooting tips that may solve this problem.

   a.

   b.

   c.

9. List two oxygen safety tips you would tell a patient who has an H cylinder in the home for the first time.

   a.

   b.

10. A parent at home calls the pulmonary clinic and complains that the small-volume nebulizer being powered by an air compressor is not nebulizing. What would you tell this parent to check to troubleshoot this problem?

11. List two indications that an infant with a tracheostomy needs suctioning.

    a.

    b.

12. What are two signs that an infant with a tracheostomy has an infection?

    a.

    b.

13. To reduce the incidence of tracheomalacia, what type of cuffed tracheostomy tube would you suggest?

14. What are two indications for home apnea monitoring?

    a.

    b.

15. Describe the difference between the following types of apnea:

    a. Obstructive

    b. Central

    c. Mixed

16. What type of test is used to diagnose obstructive sleep apnea (OSA)?

17. What are two symptoms of OSA?

    a.

    b.

18. What are two common causes of OSA in children?

    a.

    b.

19. List two indications for negative-pressure ventilation (NPV).

    a.

    b.

20. How would a patient be assessed for appropriate volume delivery when receiving NPV?

21. Fill in the accompanying table for troubleshooting NPV.

| **Patient Complaint** | **Clinical Consideration** |
|---|---|
| Patient's tidal volume has decreased. | |
| Patient complains of shortness of breath. | |
| Patient complains of dizziness and tingling in the fingers. | |
| Patient's $SpO_2$ is < 90%. | |

22. List two contraindications for home mechanical ventilation.
    a.
    b.

23. What are three criteria that are used to determine if an infant is ready to be discharged to home on mechanical ventilation?
    a.
    b.
    c.

24. Fill in the information for capabilities that should be on an adult home mechanical ventilator used for a child.
    a. Power source
    b. $FIO_2$
    c. Mode
    d. Set pressure on pressure relief valve.
    e. Sensitivity with and without PEEP
    f. Humidity device
    g. Alarms

25. Describe the cleaning and disinfecting procedure for each piece of equipment.
    a. Nebulizer
    b. Humidifier
    c. Suction machine
    d. Patient-ventilator circuit

## BIBLIOGRAPHY

American Association for Respiratory Care, Clinical Practice Guideline. (1992). Long-term invasive mechanical ventilation in the home. *Respiratory Care 40*(12), 1313.

American Association for Respiratory Care, Clinical Practice Guideline. (1992). Oxygen therapy in the home or extended care facility. *Respiratory Care 37*, 918.

American Association for Respiratory Care, Clinical Practice Guideline. (1996). Providing patient and care giver training. *Respiratory Care 41*(7), 658.

American Association for Respiratory Care, Clinical Practice Guideline. (1996). Training the health-care professional for the role of patient and caregiver educator. *Respiratory Care 41*(7), 654.

American Association for Respiratory Care, Clinical Practice Guideline. (1995). Discharge planning for the respiratory care patient. *Respiratory Care 40*(12), 1308.

American Association for Respiratory Care, Association of Polysomnography Technologists Clinical Practice Guideline. (1995). Polysomnography. *Respiratory Care 40*(12), 1336.

Downy, R., et al. (1997). Sleep-disordered breathing. *Respiratory Therapy 10*(4), 53.

Hill, N. S. (1994). Use of negative pressure ventilation, rocking beds and Pneumobelts. *Respiratory Care 39*(5), 532.

Leger, P. (1994). Noninvasive positive pressure ventilation in the home. *Respiratory Care 39*(5), 501.

Kacmarek, R. M. (1994). Home mechanical ventilatory assistance for infants. *Respiratory Care 39*(5), 550.

Kacmarek, R. M., and Spearman, C. B. (1986). Equipment used for ventilatory support in the home. *Respiratory Care 31*(4), 311.

McDonald, M., McInturff, S. L., and McIntyre, C. (1998). Pediatric respiratory home care. In Dunne, P. J., and McInturff, S, L. (Eds.). *Respiratory Home Care: The Essentials*. Philadelphia: F. A. Davis.

Mallinckrodt Medical. (1996). *A Parent's Guide to Tracheostomy Home Care for Your Child*. St. Louis: Mallinckrodt Medical.

McInturff, S. L., and Dunne, P. J. (1998). Infection control. In Dunne, P. J., and McInturff, S. L. (Eds.). *Respiratory Home Care: The Essentials*. Philadelphia: F. A. Davis.

McInturff, S. L., and Dunne, P. J. (1998). Home care equipment. In Dunne, P. J., and McInturff, S. L. (Eds.). *Respiratory Home Care: The Essentials*. Philadelphia: F. A. Davis.

National Heart, Lung, and Blood Institute Working Group on Sleep Apnea: Chaska, B., et al. (Eds.). (1995). Sleep apnea: Is your patient at risk? *Respiratory Care 40* (12), 1287.

Pierson, D. J., and George, R. B. (1986). Mechanical ventilation in the home. *Respiratory Care 31*(4), 266.

Spinner, S., et al. (1995). Recent advances in home infant apnea monitoring. *Neonatal Network 14*(8), 39.
Teague, W. G. (1997). Pediatric application of noninvasive ventilation. *Respiratory Care 42*(4), 414.
Zahr, L. K., and Montijo, J. (1993). The benefits of home care for sick premature infants. *Neonatal Network 12*(1), 33.

# Post-Test

1. A patient admitted for exacerbation of asthma has been intubated and placed on volume-targeted ventilation. Upon examination of the patient and ventilator, it is determined that 10 cm $H_2O$ auto-PEEP has developed. The physician would like the auto-PEEP reduced. The perinatal/pediatric specialist should suggest to:

   A. Increase flowrate

   B. Increase respiratory rate

   C. Increase tidal volume

   D. Reduce sensitivity

2. In hospitalized infants under 2 years of age, the most common agent that causes bronchiolitis is:

   A. Parainfluenza type I

   B. Adenovirus

   C. Respiratory syncytial virus

   D. Mycoplasma pneumonia

3. After suctioning the oral endotracheal tube of a 7-year-old receiving volume-targeted ventilation, assessment reveals that breath sounds are clear, $SpO_2$ has increased from 85 to 94%, and peak inspiratory pressure has decreased. What would these findings indicate?

   A. Further suctioning is required.

   B. The child requires saline instillation prior to suctioning.

   C. Greater suction pressure is required.

   D. Suctioning was successful in clearing the lungs.

4. While monitoring the fetal heart rate, it is noticed that during a contraction, the heart decreases to 110 beats/min from 138 beats/min. At the end of the contraction, the heart rate returns to 140 beats/min. This type of fetal heart rate deceleration is called:

   A. Variable

   B. Late

   C. Early

   D. Intermediate

5. A 1-min Apgar score assessed on a newborn infant reveals the following:
   Breathing effort is good with a good cry.
   Well-flexed extremities
   Infant has a good cough.

Pulse is 142 beats/min.

Body is pink, extremities are blue.

Based on these results, which of the following should be done?

A. Begin blow-by 100% oxygen at 5 to 8 L/min.

B. Administer bag-mask ventilation with 100% oxygen.

C. Intubate and mechanically ventilate.

D. Continue to monitor and at 5 min repeat the Apgar score.

6. A chest radiograph of an 850-gm infant on mechanical ventilation for the past 14 days reveals a bubble appearance with cyst formation. This would indicate the presence of:

A. Pulmonary interstitial emphysema

B. Loculated pleural effusion

C. Lung hypoplasia

D. Pneumopericardium

7. A newborn infant delivered by vaginal delivery presents with thick meconium staining covering the face and body. The infant is taken to the radiant warmer immediately following delivery. At this time the perinatal/pediatric specialist should:

A. Perform a 1-min Apgar score.

B. Administer oxygen by blow-by at 5 to 8 L/min.

C. Suction the airway.

D. Begin bag-mask ventilation with 100% oxygen.

8. A perinatal/pediatric specialist assessing a newborn infant notices weak peripheral pulses and a systolic pressure that is higher in the upper extremities than in the lower extremities. These findings indicate:

A. Tricuspid atresia

B. Coarctation of the aorta

C. Ventricular septal defect

D. Patent ductus arteriosus

9. A 1200-gm male infant has been on mechanical ventilation for 36 days with an $FIO_2$ of 0.50. A chest radiograph shows hyperinflation, interstitial fibrosis, and cor pulmonale. These findings are consistent with:

A. Pulmonary interstitial emphysema

B. Bronchopulmonary dysplasia

C. Diaphragmatic hernia

D. Tension pneumothorax

10. A 14-year-old with cystic fibrosis is performing PEP therapy. The patient is achieving an expiratory pressure of 10 cm $H_2O$ at a set expiratory resistance. The patient complains that it is difficult to exhale and requires a forceful expiration. The perinatal/pediatric practitioner should:

A. Reduce the number of sessions the patient performs PEP therapy.

B. Instruct the patient to take a deeper breath prior to the expiratory maneuver.

C. Reduce the expiratory resistance.

D. Add a bronchodilator treatment to the PEP therapy session.

11. A newborn infant taken to a preheated radiant warmer should be dried and covered with a blanket in order to prevent heat loss by which of the following methods?

    A. Conduction

    B. Evaporation

    C. Convection

    D. Radiation

12. In a report a perinatal/pediatric specialist informs you that a just-admitted newborn infant has increased inspiratory effort. Which of the following is NOT a sign of increased inspiratory effort?

    A. Tachycardia

    B. Retractions

    C. Grunting

    D. Nasal flaring

13. Which of the following instructions are most correct to teach a child with cystic fibrosis in the use of a flutter device?

    A. Head tilted slightly back, take in a deep breath, hold for 2 to 3 s, and exhale as much as possible.

    B. Head tilted slightly back, take in a deep breath, and exhale as much as possible.

    C. Head tilted slightly back, take in a deep breath, hold for 2 to 3 s, and exhale one fast blast.

    D. Head tilted slightly back, take in a deep breath, hold for 2 to 3 s, and exhale as much as possible while bending over.

14. Following intubation of a 2500-gm infant with a 3.5-mm ID oral endotracheal tube, findings include that no air is heard entering the stomach, right lung breath sounds are greater than the left, and there is no gastric distention. Based on this information, the perinatal/pediatric specialist should:

    A. Extubate and bag-mask ventilate

    B. Insert the endotracheal tube 1 cm.

    C. Pull the tube back until bilateral breath sounds are heard.

    D. Extubate and reintubate with a 3.0-mm ID endotracheal tube.

15. A 12-year-old is intubated and mechanically ventilated with volume-targeted ventilation. The following data have been obtained:

    Tidal volume: 5 mL/kg of body weight — pH: 7.24
    Mode: Assist-control — $PaCO_2$: 58 mm Hg
    Rate: 12 breaths/min — $PaO_2$: 46 mm Hg
    $FIO_2$: 1.0

    An optimal PEEP study is performed by the perinatal/pediatric specialist with the following results:

| Peep (cm $H_2O$) | Static Effective Compliance (L/cm $H_2O$) | Cardiac Output (L/min) | % Shunt | $PaO_2$ (mm Hg) | a-v$DO_2$ (Vol %) |
|---|---|---|---|---|---|
| 5 | 0.30 | 5.6 | 32 | 50 | 4.6 |
| 7 | 0.41 | 5.8 | 24 | 58 | 4.5 |
| 10 | 0.48 | 5.8 | 22 | 69 | 4.5 |
| 15 | 0.34 | 4.8 | 24 | 75 | 6.1 |

Which of the following PEEP levels is the optimal level of PEEP?

A. 5 cm $H_2O$

B. 7 cm $H_2O$

C. 10 cm $H_2O$

D. 15 cm $H_2O$

16. Which of the following medications is recommended for a newborn who is being resuscitated and whose heart rate has been below 80 beats/min for the last 45 s while receiving positive-pressure ventilation with 100% oxygen and chest compressions?

A. Epinephrine

B. Sodium bicarbonate

C. Naloxone hydrochloride

D. Dopamine

17. An L/S ratio test showing a ratio of greater than 2:1 would indicate:

A. Increased incidence of respiratory distress syndrome from an immature lung

B. Decreased incidence of respiratory distress syndrome

C. Increased incidence of premature rupture of membranes

D. Birth weight less than 2500 gm

18. A chest radiograph of a newborn infant returns and shows a "snowman"-shaped heart. This would indicate the presence of:

A. Coarctation of the aorta

B. Tetralogy of Fallot

C. Ventricular septal defect

D. Total anomalous pulmonary venous return

19. A flow-inflated resuscitation bag is attached to an oxygen flowmeter set at 10 L/min. During manual ventilation with the resuscitation bag of an intubated infant, it is noticed that the infant's chest does not rise adequately. Action to take at this time would be to:

A. Adjust the pressure-relief valve.

B. Increase the bagging rate.

C. Decrease the oxygen flowrate.

D. Extubate the infant and apply bag-mask ventilation.

20. A 14-year-old has called the pulmonary clinic and informs the perinatal/pediatric specialist that she is having symptoms that are consistent with exacerbation of her asthma condition. She further explains that her peak expiratory flowrate has decreased to 60% from 82%. Based on this information she should:

A. Go to the emergency department immediately.

B. Take a short-acting beta$_2$-agonist and consult her physician

C. Take a corticosteroid and a short-acting beta$_2$-agonist and come to the emergency department.

D. Continue her medication regimen as usual and consult her physician

21. Which of the following reduces pulmonary artery pressure and pulmonary vascular resistance by vasodilating the pulmonary artery vasculature?

    I. Alkalotic pH by hyperventilation

    II. Nitric oxide

    III. Tolazoline

    IV. Oxygen

    A. I and II only

    B. II and III only

    C. I, II and III only

    D. I, II, III, and IV

22. Which of the following is NOT a symptom of foreign-body enlodgement in the larynx?

    A. Aphonia

    B. Hoarseness

    C. Stridor

    D. Pain radiating to the back

23. What size oral endotracheal tube would be appropriate for a 2000-gm infant?

    A. 2.5 mm

    B. 3.5 mm

    C. 4.0 mm

    D. 3.0 mm

24. Upon assessment of a newborn infant, it is noticed that there is a pattern of alternating breaths and pauses lasting 10 to 15 s. The infant's oxygen saturation and heart rate remain stable. Based on these findings, the perinatal/pediatric specialist should:

    A. Apply a nasal cannula at 0.5 L/min at 21% oxygen. Monitor oxygen saturation.

    B. Apply a nasal cannula at 1 L/min at 21% oxygen. Monitor oxygen saturation and heart rate.

    C. Apply bag and mask ventilation with 100% oxygen.

    D. Continue monitoring the infant. No other therapy is required at this time.

25. A 4-year-old has been admitted to general floor care for upper respiratory tract infection. A sweat chloride test performed on the child earlier is found to be 100 mEq/L. This finding is consistent with a diagnosis of:

    A. Allergic asthma

    B. Bronchiolitis

    C. Cystic fibrosis

    D. Pneumonitis

26. A 3-day-old newborn infant delivered vaginally has developed respiratory distress, periods of apnea, vomiting, and diarrhea. A chest radiograph shows the infant to have pneumonia. The most common organism to cause the pneumonia is:

    A. Group B streptococcus

    B. Pseudomonas

C. Klebsiella

D. *Staphylococcus epidermidis*

27. A 10-year-old patient is orally intubated and receiving mechanical ventilation. The patient communicates to his parents that he is having pain. Appropriate medication to administer to relieve pain would be:

A. Morphine sulfate

B. Diazepam (Valium)

C. Lorazepam (Ativan)

D. Chloral hydrate

28. Which of the following is NOT an acyanotic congenital heart defect with increased pulmonary blood flow?

A. Patent ductus arteriosus

B. Ventricular septal defect

C. Coarctation of the aorta

D. Atrial septal defect

29. A newborn has been on nasal prong CPAP of 5 cm $H_2O$ and $FIO_2$ 0.30 for the past 2 days. Over the last 1 hour it is noticed that the infant has periods of desaturation below 90%. The infant's heart rate and blood pressure remain stable and there is no apnea present. Upon inspection of the infant the nasal prongs are positioned properly in the nares. Based on this finding the perinatal/pediatric practitioner should:

A. Increase the $FIO_2$ to 0.40.

B. Increase the CPAP to 7 cm $H_2O$.

C. Suction the nares.

D. Obtain an arterial blood gas.

30. A perinatal/pediatric specialist is reading the chart of a 9-year-old admitted for exacerbation of asthma. The history reveals that the patient has symptoms more than 2 times per week, activity is limited, nighttime symptoms occur more than 2 times per month, and the PEF varies by 20 to 30%. These findings would indicate the patient to have which severity of asthma?

A. Mild intermittent

B. Mild persistent

C. Moderate persistent

D. Severe persistent

31. An ultrasound examination has determined the presence of polyhydramnios. This would indicate:

A. Multiple gestation

B. Increased fetal heart tones

C. An excessive amount of amniotic fluid

D. Increased size of the fetal head

32. A 14-year-old motor vehicle accident victim is intubated and receiving mechanical ventilation. The following data are obtained from the patient:

Tidal volume: 400 mL
Peak pressure: 30 cm H2O
Plateau pressure: 20 cm H2O

Peak flow: 40 L/min
Mode: SIMV

The patient has been ordered for pressure-support ventilation. To overcome airway resistance, what level of pressure support should be added initially?

A. 8 cm $H_2O$

B. 10 cm $H_2O$

C. 15 cm $H_2O$

D. 25 cm $H_2O$

33. Which of the following instructions are most correct when teaching a 10-year-old diagnosed with asthma in the use of a peak expiratory flowrate meter?

A. "While sitting, take a deep breath, filling the lungs completely; then give one fast blast of air."

B. "While sitting, take a deep breath, filling the lungs completely; then give one slow expiratory push of air."

C. "While standing, take a deep breath, filling the lungs completely, then give one fast blast of air."

D. "While sitting, take a deep breath, filling the lungs completely; then give one fast blast of air while bending over during exhalation."

34. On an A-P chest radiograph of a term newborn infant, there is a "sail-like" appearance extending into the right hemithorax. This appearance is consistent with:

A. Tension pneumothorax

B. Thymus gland

C. Complete atelectasis of the right lung

D. An enlarged right heart

35. A 5-year-old is presented to the ED with difficulty swallowing, dyspnea, and excessive oral secretions and in respiratory distress. Radiographic analysis shows hyperpharyngeal swelling. These findings are consistent with:

A. Bronchiolitis

B. Epiglottitis

C. Foreign-body aspiration

D. Laryngotracheobronchitis

36. Which of the following medications is/are used as "relievers" when treating exacerbation of asthma?

I. Ipratropium bromide

II. Methylprednisolone

III. Albuterol

A. III only

B. II and III only

C. I and III only

D. I, II, and III

37. A newborn infant is receiving tactile stimulation because of apnea and desaturation. Initially, the heart rate is 110 beats/min. Thirty seconds later, the heart rate is 46 beats/min and blood pressure decreases. At this time, the perinatal/pediatric specialist should:

A. Provide more vigorous stimulation.

B. Administer free-flowing oxygen at 5 to 8 L/min.

C. Administer epinephrine subcutaneously.

D. Begin bag-mask resuscitation with 100% oxygen.

38. Before being discharged from the hospital, an 11-year-old with asthma requires instruction in establishing the best peak expiratory flowrate (PEF) at home. Which of the following sets of instructions is most correct?

A. Measure the PEF in the morning and afternoon before taking a bronchodilator.

B. Measure the PEF in the morning and afternoon after taking a bronchodilator.

C. Measure the PEF in the morning after taking a bronchodilator and in the afternoon following a bronchodilator treatment.

D. Measure the PEF after taking a bronchodilator once in the morning only.

39. Appropriate placement of an oral endotracheal tube is determined by:

I. $SpO_2$

II. Bilateral breath sounds

III. Skin color

A. I only

B. II only

C. II and III only

D. I, II, and III

40. A 1200-gm premature infant is on mechanical ventilation. Over the last 30 min the infant has developed tachycardia, hypotension, and increased respiratory efforts. Further assessment reveals decreased breath sounds on the right and cardiac impulse shifted to the left. Based on these findings the perinatal/pediatric specialist should suggest:

A. To obtain an arterial blood gas

B. To obtain a glucose level

C. To perform a thoracentesis to the right lung

D. To perform a transillumination

41. Which of the following is the primary predictor of infant survival?

A. Infection

B. Birth weight

C. Ethnic origin

D. Maternal smoking

42. A 1500-gm infant who is receiving mechanical ventilation is experiencing respiratory distress. A chest radiograph returns and shows anterior air and the thymus is pushed upward and away from the heart. This would indicate the presence of:

A. Pneumomediastinum

B. Pneumopericardium

C. Pulmonary interstitial emphysema

D. Subcutaneous emphysema

43. A term newborn infant receiving 40% oxygen by head hood is found to have irregular respirations, apnea, jitteriness, and a weak cry. The following information has been obtained:

    pH: 7.26
    $PaCO_2$: 37 mm Hg
    $SpO_2$: 94%
    Glucose: 18 mg/dL

    Appropriate treatment for this infant would be to:

    A. Increase the oxygen to 60%.

    B. Administer glucose.

    C. Begin phototherapy.

    D. Apply CPAP at 5 cm $H_2O$.

44. A premature newborn infant has been diagnosed with hyaline membrane disease and is receiving CPAP at 7 cm $H_2O$ and a $FIO_2$ of 0.45. An A-P chest radiograph shows dark lateral projections extending to the lung periphery, surrounded by a fluffy white appearance consistent with atelectasis. The chest radiograph is consistent with:

    A. Air bronchograms

    B. Subcutaneous emphysema

    C. Spontaneous pneumothorax

    D. Pulmonary interstitial emphysema

45. A 6-year-old is intubated and is being mechanically ventilated following an automobile accident in which head trauma occurred. An intracranial pressure-monitoring device is in place and the intracranial pressure is 40 mm Hg. To treat the intracranial pressure, the perinatal/pediatric specialist should do which of the following on the mechanical ventilator?

    I. Increase minute ventilation.

    II. Decrease $FIO_2$.

    III. Add PEEP.

    A. I only

    B. II and III only

    C. I and III only

    D. I, II, and III

46. The parents of a 2-year-old are being instructed in the proper use of a suction machine and suctioning procedure for use at home. To assess whether the parents understand this information, the perinatal/pediatric specialist should:

    A. Have the parents take a written examination before discharge.

    B. Allow the parents to practice several times on other patients in the hospital.

    C. Allow the parents to demonstrate their skill at home on their child.

    D. Require the parents to demonstrate their skill and repeat any information in their own words.

47. A 12-year-old is intubated and receiving mechanical ventilation. The following are data obtained from the patient:

    Tidal volume: 400 mL
    Peak inspiratory pressure: 30 cm $H_2O$
    Plateau pressure: 25 cm $H_2O$
    PEEP: 5 cm $H_2O$

$FIO_2$: 0.60
What is the static lung compliance?

A. 40 mL/cm $H_2O$

B. 33 mL/cm $H_2O$

C. 20 mL/cm $H_2O$

D. 18 mL/cm $H_2O$

48. An 8-year-old female has been admitted to general floor care. During her interview it is found that she has weakness in her arms and legs, has trouble focusing, and has dysphagia. You notice she is tachypneic and does complain of being short of breath. These findings are most consistent with:

A. Myasthenia gravis

B. Guillain-Barrè syndrome

C. Orthostatic hypertension

D. Bacterial pneumonia

49. Which of the following is the correct position for draining the superior segment of the lower lobes?

A. Head of bed down, child lies on abdomen

B. Head of bed down, child lies on back

C. Head of bed flat, child lies on abdomen

D. Head of bed down, child lies with right or left side down

50. A term newborn has been placed on extracorporeal membrane oxygenation following 2 weeks of mechanical ventilation for meconium aspiration. The mean airway pressure is 20 cm $H_2O$, $FIO_2$ is 1.0, and $PaO_2$ is 40 mm Hg. What is the oxygenation index?

A. 50

B. 30

C. 20

D. 10

51. Which of the following differentiates complete upper airway obstruction from partial airway obstruction?

A. Stridor with weak cough

B. Sternal and clavicular retractions

C. Marked inspiratory effort with no air movement

D. Unconsciousness

52. Which of the following spirometry tests is/are used to determine obstructive diseases?

I. FVC

II. $FEV_1$

III. $FEV_1$/FVC

A. I only

B. II only

C. I and II only

D. I, II, and III

53. Which of the following is an indication for home oxygen therapy for infants and children older than 28 days?

A. $PaO_2$ less than or equal to 55 mm Hg, or $SaO_2$ less than or equal to 88% breathing room air

B. $PaO_2$ less than or equal to 50 mm Hg, or $SaO_2$ less than or equal to 88% breathing room air

C. $PaO_2$ less than or equal to 50 mm Hg, or $SaO_2$ less than or equal to 83% breathing room air

D. $PaO_2$ less than or equal to 50 mm Hg, or $SaO_2$ less than or equal to 83% breathing $FIO_2 < 0.28$

54. The quickest maneuver to establish a patent airway from soft tissue obstruction in a child is by:

A. Jaw thrust

B. Head tilt–chin lift

C. Chin lift

D. Mandibular displacement

55. A newborn infant is on pressure-limited, time-cycled ventilation with the following settings:

PIP: 20 cm $H_2O$
Rate: 30 breaths/min
$FIO_2$: 0.80
PEEP: 7 cm $H_2O$
Itime: 0.3 s

Umbilical artery blood gases results are:

pH: 7.34
$PaCO_2$: 42 mm Hg
$PaO_2$: 56 mm Hg

The perinatal/pediatric specialist should recommend which ventilator setting change?

A. Decrease PEEP.

B. Decrease rate.

C. Decrease PIP.

D. Decrease $FIO_2$.

56. A patient is receiving 2 L/min from a liquid oxygen device that contains 60 lb of oxygen. What is the duration of flow from this device?

A. 4 days

B. 7 days

C. 8 days

D. 2 days

57. Which of the following is an indication for placement of a chest tube?

I. Presence of a tension pneumothorax

II. Presence of a hemopneumothorax

III. Presence of a bronchopleural fistula

A. I only

B. II and III only

C. I and III only

D. I, II, and III

58. Upon entering a patient's room, the perinatal/pediatric specialist finds the patient slumped over in the chair. At this time it would be appropriate to:

A. Open the airway.

B. Call for help.

C. Give two rescue breaths.

D. Determine unresponsiveness.

59. A newborn infant has been intubated and placed on pressure-limited, time-cycled ventilation with the following settings:

PIP: 25 cm $H_2O$
Itime: 0.4 second
PEEP: 5 cm $H_2O$
Rate: 25 breaths/min
$FIO_2$: 0.60

Umbilical artery blood gas reveals:

pH: 7.24
$PaCO_2$: 60 mm Hg
$PaO_2$: 50 mm Hg
$HCO_3$: 21 mEq/L

Based on the umbilical artery blood gas, which ventilator adjustment is recommended?

A. Increase PIP.

B. Increase rate.

C. Increase $FIO_2$.

D. Increase PEEP.

60. A 39-week-gestational-age infant weighing 5700 gm is intubated with a 3.0-mm ID oral endotracheal tube and is placed on pressure-limited, time-cycled ventilator. After the infant is placed on mechanical ventilation, the perinatal/pediatric specialist notices the volume-pressure loop indicates a 30% leak around the endotracheal tube.

Based on this information, it would be recommended to:

A. Increase the PIP by 5 cm $H_2O$.

B. Add 5 cm $H_2O$ PEEP.

C. Extubate and reintubate the infant with a 4.0-mm ID endotracheal tube.

D. Reduce expiratory time.

61. Which of the following types of high-frequency ventilation has both positive- and negative-pressure ventilation?

A. High-frequency oscillation

B. High-frequency flow interrupter

C. High-frequency jet ventilation

D. High-frequency positive-pressure ventilation

62. An oropharyngeal airway has been inserted into an unconscious infant. Assessment following insertion reveals no air movement. The perinatal/pediatric specialist should:

A. Suction the airway.

B. Insert a nasopharyngeal airway.

C. Remove the oropharyngeal airway.

D. Perform nasotracheal intubation.

63. A 5-year-old in respiratory arrest is orally intubated and being manually ventilated with a resuscitation bag connected to oxygen. An end-tidal $CO_2$ monitor has been connected to the endotracheal tube. The following end-tidal $CO_2$ waveform appears during manual ventilation.

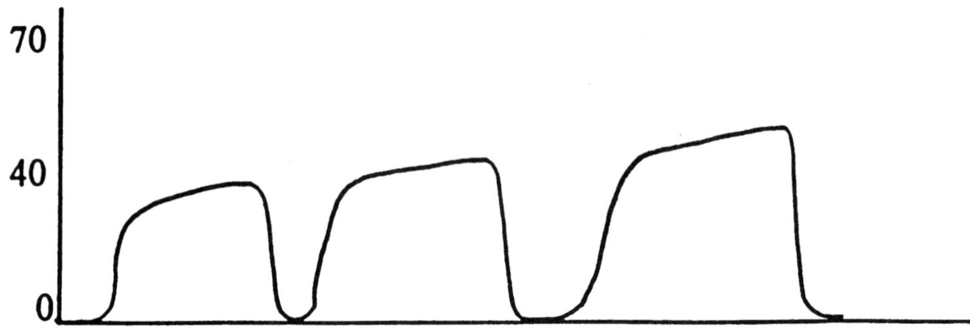


Based on this waveform the perinatal/pediatric specialist should:

A. Reintubate the patient.

B. Suction the endotracheal tube.

C. Increase minute ventilation.

D. Remove dead space between the endotracheal tube and resuscitation bag.

64. A 16-year-old is on pressure-controlled ventilation with the following settings:

PIP: 25 cm $H_2O$
$FIO_2$: 0.60
I:E ratio: 1:3
Exhaled tidal volume: 500 mL

Arterial blood gas sample obtained while on the preceding settings are:

pH: 7.34
$PaCO_2$: 42 mm Hg
$PaO_2$: 46 mm Hg
$HCO_3$: 21 mEq/L

The physician orders 10 cm $H_2O$ PEEP, and the following arterial blood gas results are obtained following this change:

pH: 7.26
$PaCO_2$: 54 mm Hg
$PaO_2$: 57 mm Hg

Based on these findings, which of the following ventilator changes should be made?

A. Increase PIP.

B. Increase $FIO_2$.

C. Increase PEEP.

D. Alter the I:E ratio to 1:2.

65. While assessing an infant at home with a tracheostomy tube in place, it is noticed that the site around the tracheostomy tube is red with swelling and tender to the touch and the infant has increased sputum production occurring over the last 3 days. These findings would indicate:

A. The need to increase humidity to the tracheostomy tube

B. The need to increase suctioning of the tracheostomy tube

C. The need to change the tracheostomy tube more often

D. The presence of an infection

66. A self-inflating resuscitation bag and mask is being used to resuscitate a child found in respiratory arrest. Over the next 2 min of resuscitation it is noticed that the oxygen saturation remains at 70% on the pulse oximeter and the heart rate correlates with the ECG. Which of the following should be done to correct this situation?

A. Increase the bagging rate.

B. Ensure that oxygen flow is entering the resuscitation bag.

C. Increase bagging volume.

D. Begin cardiac compressions.

67. A sleep apnea study has been performed on a 7-year-old. The results show that the child has cessation of airflow and continuous chest and abdominal movements. The sleep study indicates the presence of:

A. Mixed sleep apnea

B. Central sleep apnea

C. Obstructive sleep apnea

D. Apparent life threatening event

68. Which of the following maneuvers must the patient perform in order to measure the $FEF_{25-75\%}$?

A. $FEV_1$

B. FVC

C. $FEV_2$

D. Peak expiratory flowrate

69. Which of the compartments of a chest drainage unit prevents air from entering the pleural space through the chest tube?

A. Suction

B. Water seal

C. Collection

D. Accumulator

70. A 6-year-old with a 6.0 mm ID oral endotracheal tube in place is being suctioned with a 10 french suction catheter using (–) 80 mm Hg. It is noticed that with each pass of the suction catheter, it is difficult to remove secretions. The perinatal/pediatric specialist should:

A. Increase the time the suction catheter is down the endotracheal tube.

B. Increase the number of suctioning passes.

C. Increase the suction catheter size.

D. Increase the suctioning pressure.

71. A newborn infant on high-frequency oscillation has the following settings:

Rate: 12 Hz
Mean airway pressure: 10 cm $H_2O$

$FIO_2$: 0.50
Amplitude: vibration between the clavicles and umbilicus

An umbilical artery blood gas has been obtained:

pH: 7.28
$PaCO_2$: 52 mm Hg
$PaO_2$: 51 mm Hg
$HCO_3$: 20 mEq/L

Which of the following is recommended?

A. Increase rate.

B. Increase mean airway pressure.

C. Increase amplitude.

D. Increase $FIO_2$.

72. A newborn infant is presented in labor and delivery with respiratory distress. Upon examination the abdomen appears "scaphoid-shaped." Further examination reveals breath sounds are decreased in the left lung and bowel sounds are heard over the left lung. Point of maximal impulse is shifted to the right. These findings are consistent with:

A. Diaphragmatic hernia

B. Persistent pulmonary hypertension

C. Left lung hypoplasia

D. Pneumomediastinum

73. To drain air from the pleural space as a result of a pneumothorax, a chest tube is placed:

A. Between intercostal space 4 and 5, midaxillary line

B. Between intercostal space 6 and 7, midaxillary line

C. Between intercostal space 1 and 2, midclavicular line

D. Between intercostal space 2 and 3, midclavicular line

74. Which of the following would NOT indicate that endotracheal tube suctioning was successful in clearing the airways of a patient orally intubated receiving pressure-control ventilation?

A. Decreased peak inspiratory pressure

B. Increased expired tidal volume

C. Improved oxygen saturation

D. Improved breath sounds

75. Which is the most economical way of providing oxygen in the home?

A. Oxygen concentrator

B. Liquid oxygen

C. H cylinder

D. E cylinder

76. A pressure, volume, and flow scalar is present on the monitor of an 8-year-old intubated for exacerbation of his asthma condition. It is noticed that the expiratory flow waveform does not reach baseline before the next positive pressure breath is delivered. This finding is consistent with:

A. A leak around the endotracheal tube

B. Excessive flowrate delivery by the ventilator

C. Inappropriate flow waveform set on the ventilator

D. Air trapping

77. Changing the rate of blood flow through an extracorporeal membrane oxygenation circuit controls which of the following?

A. $PaO_2$

B. $PaCO_2$

C. Blood pressure

D. Body temperature

78. A patient who has been given midazolam (Versed) in preparation for intubation has been found snoring with retractions and is unresponsive. Immediate action to take at this time would be to:

A. Insert a nasopharyngeal airway.

B. Orally intubate.

C. Apply a non-rebreathing mask at 10 L/min.

D. Open the airway with a head-tilt, chin-lift maneuver.

79. A newborn has been on high-frequency oscillation with a mean airway pressure of 10 cm $H_2O$, rate 10 Hz, and the infant's chest is vibrating between the clavicles and umbilicus. While assessing the infant, the perinatal/pediatric specialist notices that chest vibrations have diminished with no change in settings. Based on this information, which of the following may be the cause of this change?

I. Improper position of the endotracheal tube

II. Pneumothorax

III. Obstructed endotracheal tube

A. I only

B. II only

C. I and II only

D. I, II, and III

80. While reading the chart of a patient, it is noticed that the patient had a significant response in $FEV_1$ before and after a bronchodilator study. This would indicate:

A. $FEV_1$ increased by 5%.

B. $FEV_1$ increased by 7 to 8%.

C. $FEV_1$ increased by 9 to 10%.

D. $FEV_1$ increased by 12 to 15%.

81. A 12-year-old patient has been on BiPAP therapy for 30 minutes with initial settings of IPAP 10 cm $H_2O$ and EPAP of 5 cm $H_2O$ with 2 L/min of oxygen running into the mask. An arterial blood gas obtained while on these settings includes: pH, 7.27; $PaCO_2$, 49 mm Hg; and $PaO_2$, 45 mm Hg. Following this blood gas the EPAP is increased to 8 cm $H_2O$. Another blood gas taken following this changes shows pH, 7.25; $PaCO_2$, 58 mm Hg; and $PaO_2$, 54 mm Hg. The perinatal/pediatric specialist should recommend to:

A. Increase the IPAP level.

B. Increase the EPAP level.

C. Increase the oxygen flowrate to 3 L/min.

D. Intubate and apply CPAP at 10 cm $H_2O$.

82. The proper instruction for parents for cleaning a nebulizer in the home is:

A. Place unassembled parts in 1 part white vinegar and 3 parts water every day.

B. Place unassembled parts in hot water and detergent every 48 h.

C. Place unassembled parts in boiling water for 30 min every 2 days.

D. Place unassembled parts in hydrogen peroxide for 30 min every 2 days.

83. A double-lumen endotracheal tube is being used for independent lung ventilation. Auscultation reveals breath sounds in the left lung only. Based on this information the perinatal/pediatric specialist should:

A. Deflate both cuffs and insert the tube until bilateral breath sounds are heard.

B. Suction the endotracheal tube.

C. Instill saline and suction the endotracheal tube.

D. Deflate both cuffs and the pull the tube back until bilateral breath sounds are heard.

84. A 10-year-old who was extubated 2 h earlier has developed laryngospasm with mild accessory muscle usage and a hoarse cough; oxygen saturation is 95% and heart rate is normal. Based on this information, which of the following should be done?

A. Administer oxygen by air-entrainment mask at 35%.

B. Administer 2.25% racemic epinephrine by small-volume nebulizer.

C. Administer ipratropium bromide by small-volume nebulizer.

D. Administer glucocorticoids by MDI.

85. A patient is intubated and receiving volume-targeted ventilation. The following volume-pressure loop has changed from loop A to loop B over the last 72 h.

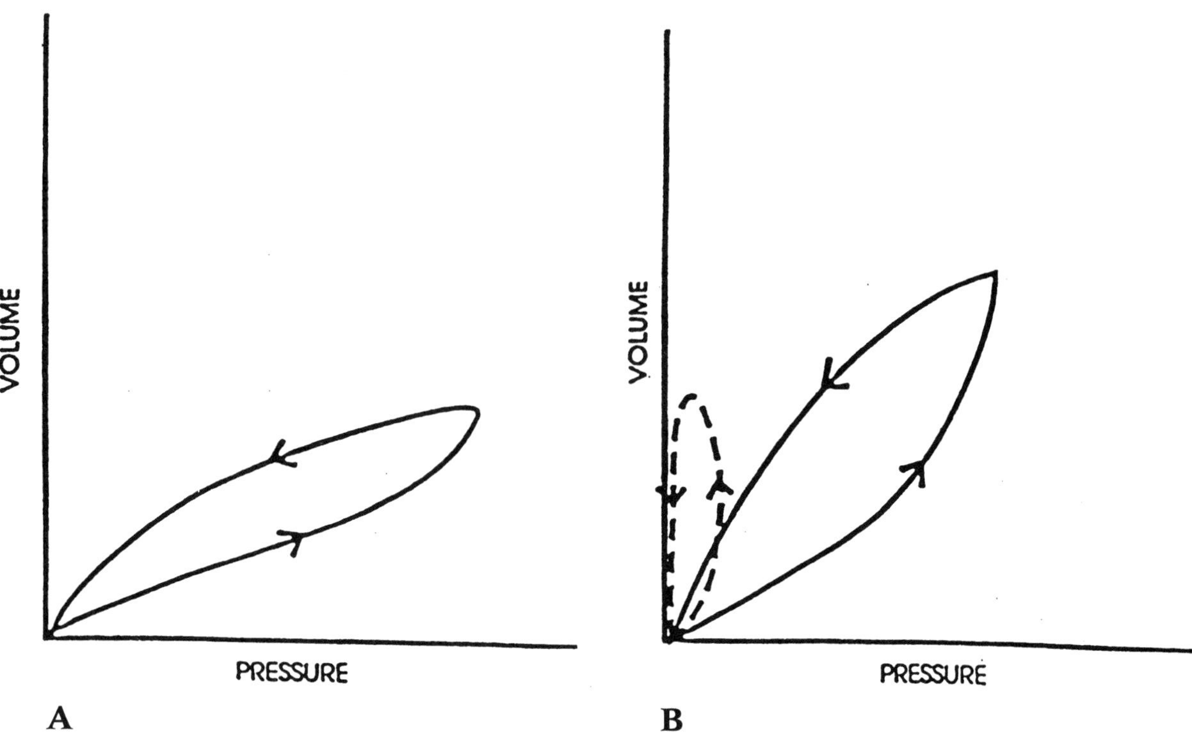


Loop B indicates:

A. Increased lung compliance

B. Insufficient sensitivity setting on the ventilator

C. Asynchrony between the patient and ventilator

D. The presence of auto-PEEP

86. A newborn infant is being suctioned through an oral endotracheal tube. Following insertion of the catheter, the heart rate decreases from 128 to 70 beats/min. The cause of this heart rate change is from:

A. Arterial hypoxemia

B. Vagal stimulation

C. Tissue hypoxia

D. Head reflex

87. A newborn infant who is being transported to another hospital is intubated and is being ventilated by pressure-limited, time-cycled ventilation. The ventilator rate is set at 30/min and I:E ratio is 1:4. What is the inspiratory time?

A. 1 s

B. 0.4 s

C. 0.8 s

D. 0.6 s

88. An 8-year-old is on mechanical ventilation with the following settings:

| | |
|---|---|
| Tidal volume: 300 mL | PEEP: 5 cm $H_2O$ |
| Mode: assist-control | $FIO_2$: 0.40 |
| Machine rate: 12 breaths/min | Total rate: 24 breaths/min |

Blood gas analysis shows:

pH: 7.51
$PaCO_2$: 30 mm Hg
$PaO_2$: 86 mm Hg

The perinatal/pediatric practitioner should:

A. Switch to SIMV mode.

B. Reduce tidal volume.

C. Decrease PEEP.

D. Reduce the machine rate to 8 breaths/min.

89. A 4-year-old has been admitted to general floor care with a diagnosis of croup. The perinatal/pediatric specialist examining the child notices that during inspiration the chest sinks in while the abdomen is pushed outward. This type of respiration is called:

A. Cheyne-Stokes

B. Apneustic

C. Paradoxical

D. Eupnea

90. Expiration is determined with pressure-limited, time-cycled ventilation by:

A. Pressure

B. Time

C. Flow

D. Volume

91. While auscultating the chest, the perinatal/pediatric specialist notices a funnel-shaped depression over the sternum. This chest configuration is:

A. Pectus excavatum

B. Kyphoscoliosis

C. Pectus carinatum

D. Pectus sternotum

92. The type of laboratory test that should be performed on pleural fluid that will determine bacterial infection is:

A. Acid-fast stain

B. Serum osmolality

C. Gram stain culture and sensitivity

D. Coombs' test

93. A patient is performing a closed-circuit helium dilution study. After 4 min of performing the test, it is noticed that the tidal volume and respiratory rate are steadily increasing. The perinatal/pediatric specialist should:

A. Reduce the helium concentration.

B. Check the carbon dioxide absorber.

C. Check for leaks in the circuit.

D. Increase the flowrate to the patient through the bellows system.

94. A resonant sound is emitted while percussing the chest of a 5-year-old. This finding is consistent with:

A. Hyperinflation

B. Pneumothorax

C. Subcutaneous emphysema

D. Normal air-filled lungs

95. A 15-year-old is receiving mechanical ventilation with the following settings:

Tidal volume: 450 mL
Mechanical rate: 12 (no assisted breaths)
Mode: Assist-control
Peak flow: 40 L/min
$FIO_2$: 0.45

Arterial blood gases are obtained:

pH: 7.31
$PaCO_2$: 50 mm Hg
$PaO_2$: 66 mm Hg

Which of the following mechanical rates will correct the $PaCO_2$ to 40 mm Hg?

A. 8 breaths/min

B. 10 breaths/min

C. 15 breaths/min

D. 18 breaths/min

96. A 3-year-old has been admitted to the general floor from the ED. Lower respiratory tract secretions need to be obtained from the patient for sputum culture and sensitivity. Which of the following would be most appropriate to obtain this sample?

A. Ultrasonic nebulizer for 30 min qid

B. Albuterol administered by small-volume nebulizer qid

C. Mucomyst administered by small-volume nebulizer every 2 h

D. Flexible bronchoscopy

97. While reviewing a patient's chart prior to administration of an aerosol, the perinatal/pediatric specialist notices that the patient has high-pitched, loud, harsh, and hollow breath sounds on inspiration and expiration. This finding would indicate that the patient has:

A. Wheezing breath sounds

B. Tracheal breath sounds

C. Bronchial breath sounds

D. Adventitious breath sounds

98. Following physical examination of a 9-year-old in the ED, the following findings have been obtained:

Inspection: dyspnea
Palpation: decreased fremitus in the right lung
Percussion: flatness in the right lung
Auscultation: absent breath sounds over the right lower lobe
Chest radiograph: blunting of the right costophrenic angle

These findings are consistent with:

A. Pleural effusion

B. Pneumothorax

C. Atelectasis

D. Bronchopneumonia

99. A medication that is administered to provide anesthesia to the upper airway prior to bronchoscopy is:

A. Lidocaine

B. Morphine sulfate

C. Atropine sulfate

D. Glycopyrrolate

100. A patient is receiving pressure-limited, time-cycled ventilation with the following settings:

PIP: 20 cm $H_2O$
Itime: 0.4 s
Flowrate: 8 L/min
$FIO_2$: 0.40

What is the estimated tidal volume?

A. 100 mL

B. 86 mL

C. 74 mL

D. 53 mL

101. A patient has a chest tube in place for drainage of air and it is connected to suction set at 15 cm $H_2O$. The wall suction is set at 15 cm $H_2O$. The physician has ordered the suction pressure to be increased to 20 cm $H_2O$. After increasing the water level in the suction control chamber to 20 cm, suction stops. The perinatal/pediatric specialist should:

I. Increase wall suction pressure to 20 cm $H_2O$.

II. Check the thoracic drainage unit for leaks.

III. Increase the water level in the suction control compartment to 25 cm $H_2O$.

A. I only

B. II only

C. III only

D. II and III only

102. Which of the following chest radiographic positions would be recommended to determine the presence of free-floating fluid?

a. Lordotic

b. Lateral decubitus

c. Oblique

d. Posterior-anterior

103. A perinatal/pediatric practitioner returns from a patient's room and charts the following information: Five-year-old female who is awake and oriented to family and place. Respiratory rate is 34 breaths/min, blood pressure is 136/88, color is pale with diaphoresis, and pulse is 128 beats/min. Patient is restless, sitting in mother's lap. This information should be placed under what part of SOAP notes?

A. Assessment

B. Plan

C. Objective

D. Subjective

104. A 7-year-old has been admitted to the general floor with symptoms of nonproductive cough, temperature of 101°F, and dyspnea. Laboratory examination returns with a finding of streptococcus infection. Which of the following laboratory tests determined this finding?

A. Acid-fast stain

B. Culture and sensitivity

C. Gram stain

D. Ziehl-Neelsen stain

105. Which of the following would NOT increase mean airway pressure?

A. Increasing PEEP

B. Changing from decelerating flow ramp to square wave flow

C. Decreasing inspiratory flowrate

D. Increasing respiratory rate

106. An infant on high-frequency oscillation requires an increase in the $PaO_2$. Which of the following adjustments is recommended?

A. Rate

B. Mean airway pressure

C. PIP

D. Amplitude

107. Which of the following is an appropriate precaution when placing a patient in strict isolation?

I. Patient should be placed in a single room.

II. Mask must be worn while in the room.

III. Gloves must be worn while in the room.

IV. Gown must be worn while in the room.

A. I and II only

B. I and III only

C. I, II, and III only

D. I, II, III, and IV

108. A physician has ordered an arterial blood gas obtained from a 3-day-old term infant to assess the pH and $PaCO_2$. After several attempts, it is determined that it is not possible to obtain the arterial blood gas. The perinatal/pediatric specialist should:

A. Insert a percutaneous arterial line.

B. Insert an umbilical artery catheter.

C. Suggest performing a cutdown at the radial artery site.

D. Obtain a capillary blood gas.

109. A parent calls the pulmonary clinic and states that her child does not feel oxygen coming from the nasal cannula that is running at 1 L/min from an oxygen concentrator. Which of the following would you instruct the parent to do to ensure that the oxygen concentrator is working properly?

I. Check the air filter.

II. Check the flow of oxygen by inserting the cannula in water.

III. Crimp the oxygen tubing and listen for an internal pop-off alarm.

A. I only

B. II only

C. III only

D. I, II, and III

110. The physician has ordered a 14-year-old with asthma to go home with a dry-powder inhaler (DPI). Orders state that the patient is to be instructed in the proper use of the inhaler. The perinatal/pediatric practitioner should instruct the patient to:

A. Exhale normally, place the DPI between the lips, and inhale slowly and deeply.

B. Exhale normally, place the DPI between the lips, inhale slowly and deeply, and breath hold for 5 seconds.

C. Exhale completely, place the DPI between the lips, inhale slowly and deeply, and breath hold for 5 seconds.

D. Exhale completely, place the DPI between the lips, and inhale slowly and deeply.

111. An arterial blood gas has been obtained from a peripheral arterial line and has been sent to the blood gas laboratory. Returning to the bedside, the perinatal/pediatric specialist notices that the arterial waveform is not present on the monitor. This would indicate:

A. The three-way stopcock is off to pressure transducer.

B. There is a leak in the fluid-filled line.

C. The fast-flush device has malfunctioned.

D. The system has not been flushed properly.

112. An intubated, premature newborn on pressure-limited, time-cycled ventilation has received the full dose of exogenous surfactant. Over the last 30 minutes the expired tidal volume has increased from 5 mL/kg to 10 mL/kg. Based on this finding the perinatal/pediatric specialist should:

A. Decrease mechanical rate.

B. Decrease PIP.

C. Decrease $FIO_2$.

D. Maintain current ventilator settings.

113. A 33-week gestational-age newborn is on nasal CPAP at 7 cm $H_2O$ and an $FIO_2$ of 0.60. Over the last 2 hours the infant has developed sternal and intercostal retractions, agitation, and periods of apnea. An umbilical artery blood gas reveals pH, 7.18; $PaCO_2$, 69 mm Hg; and $PaO_2$, 40 mm Hg. Based on these findings the perinatal/pediatric specialist should:

A. Increase CPAP to 10 cm $H_2O$.

B. Increase $FIO_2$ to 1.0.

C. Intubate and apply CPAP at 10 cm $H_2O$.

D. Intubate and mechanically ventilate.

114. A chest radiograph of a 1500-gm infant shows an umbilical artery catheter positioned at a "high" position. This would indicate the position of the umbilical artery catheter to be:

A. Between thoracic vertebrae 2 and 4

B. Between thoracic vertebrae 6 and 9

C. Below the diaphragm

D. Between lumbar vertebrae 3 and 4

115. The following data have been obtained from a pulmonary artery catheter:

Pulmonary artery pressure: 22/11
Mean pulmonary artery pressure: 14 mm Hg
Pulmonary capillary wedge pressure: 10 mm Hg
Cardiac output: 4 L/min

Based on these data, what is the pulmonary vascular resistance?

a. 40 dyn/s/$cm^{-5}$

b. 60 dyn/s/$cm^{-5}$

c. 80 dyn/s/$cm^{-5}$

d. 100 dyn/s/$cm^{-5}$

116. A patient with chronic neuromuscular disorder has been ordered to receive negative-pressure ventilation with a chest cuirass. After the device is applied, the patient complains of dizziness and parasthesis. The perinatal/pediatric specialist should:

A. Reduce the applied negative pressure.

B. Reduce the expiratory time.

C. Increase the mechanical rate.

D. Increase the $FIO_2$.

117. A child returning from heart surgery has been placed on mechanical ventilation. A pulmonary artery catheter with $SvO_2$ measuring capabilities is in place. Over the past 2 h, the $SvO_2$ has decreased from 75% to 70%. Which of the following should be done at this time?

A. Increase the $FIO_2$.

B. Decrease oxygen consumption by paralyzing the child.

C. Continue monitoring; no treatment is required.

D. Increase PEEP.

118. Which of the following is a contraindication to home mechanical ventilation?

A. Patient with a tracheostomy

B. $FIO_2$ is 0.60 while on mechanical ventilation.

C. PEEP is 5 cm $H_2O$.

D. Pressure-control ventilation is required.

119. A transcutaneous monitor measuring $PO_2$ is attached to the chest wall of a newborn infant on CPAP of 5 cm $H_2O$ and $FIO_2$ 0.30. The perinatal/pediatric specialist notices

the $PO_2$ value increasing from 52 to 76 mm Hg and is continuing to increase. There has been no change in the infant's CPAP and $FIO_2$. This finding would indicate:

A. There is an air leak between the skin and electrode.

B. The electrode needs cleaning.

C. The electrode temperature is too high.

D. There is poor perfusion under the electrode site.

120. A near-drowning victim is in cardiac arrest and is having cardiac compressions performed in the ED. An ECG strip has been obtained and shows ventricular fibrillation. Treatment for this would be:

A. A bolus of lidocaine

B. Atropine

C. Cardioversion

D. Defibrillation

# Answers and Rationales to Post-Test

1. **(A)** Increasing flowrate will prolong expiratory time, allowing more time for expiratory flow to exit the lungs.
2. **(C)** Usually seen in winter and spring, bronchiolitis, which occurs commonly in hospitalized patients under 2 years of age, is caused by respiratory syncytial virus.
3. **(D)** Successful outcome indicators for suctioning include (i) improved breath sounds, (ii) improved oxygen saturation, (iii) pulmonary secretion removal, and (iv) drop in peak inspiratory pressure with volume-targeted ventilation, or increase in tidal volume with pressure-targeted ventilation.
4. **(C)** Early decelerations are a response to uterine contractions caused from head compression. Fetal heart rate recovers to predeceleration value at the completion of the contraction.
5. **(D)** The 1-min Apgar score is 9; therefore, no treatment is necessary. Continue monitoring and repeat the Apgar score in 5 min.
6. **(A)** The radiologic appearance of pulmonary interstitial emphysema reveals a bubble appearance with cyst formation. Progression of the disease causes cysts to enlarge. The enlarged cysts are called pneumatoceles.
7. **(C)** Before beginning any resuscitation attempts with positive-pressure ventilation, the meconium should be removed from the airway. This will prevent meconium in the upper airway from being pushed down into the lungs.
8. **(B)** Coarctation of the aorta presents with a narrowed aortic lumen producing a preductal obstruction to systemic blood flow. Consequently, systemic blood pressure is reduced.
9. **(B)** An infant who remains on oxygen for more than 28 days and who has a chest radiographic finding of hyperinflation, interstitial fibrosis, and cor pulmonale has symptoms consistent with bronchopulmonary dysplasia.
10. **(C)** PEP therapy is a maneuver that provides expiratory resistance and positive expiratory pressure to keep the airways open during exhalation by altering the I/E ratio. Exhalation should be active but not forced with enough resistance to produce 10 to 20 cm $H_2O$. If the patient has difficulty exhaling, the expiratory resistance should be reduced to make the maneuver easier while still maintaining 10 to 20 cm $H_2O$.
11. **(B)** Evaporative heat loss occurs when water is converted to water vapor on the surface of the body. To conserve heat, dry the infant, cover the infant with a preheated blanket, and cover the head with a stocking cap.
12. **(A)** Signs of inspiratory effort include retractions, grunting, and nasal flaring. Tachycardia is a symptom that results from increased inspiratory effort.
13. **(A)** These instructions provide the correct maneuver for a patient using a flutter device. Following this maneuver, the patient is instructed to cough or to continue performing the flutter maneuver several more times and then cough.
14. **(C)** Assessment includes findings that indicate right main-stem intubation. Pulling the tube back until bilateral breath sounds are heard is the most correct answer.
15. **(C)** The optimal or best PEEP is at 10 cm $H_2O$. The compliance is increased; cardiac output is within normal range; the percentage of shunt is decreased; a-v$DO_2$ is within normal range; and $PaO_2$ has increased from the previous PEEP level. Going to 15 cm $H_2O$ PEEP reduces compliance, shunting, and cardiac output.

16. **(A)** According to the American Heart Association's Textbook of Neonatal Resuscitation, epinephrine should be used when the heart rate is less than 80 beats/min for at least 30 s while the patient is receiving positive-pressure ventilation and chest compressions.
17. **(B)** There is a decreased incidence of RDS when the L/S ratio is greater than 2:1. Lecithin increases in concentration over sphingomyelin at approximately 34 weeks and continues increasing in concentration thereafter.
18. **(D)** The shape of the heart is a result of contour-shaped, enlarged ventricle and an enlarged superior vena cava caused by increased pulmonary blood flow.
19. **(A)** Adjusting the pressure-relief device (closing the valve) reduces leakage of gas during the positive-pressure breath.
20. **(B)** The patient has dropped from the green zone (80% of the best PEF) to the yellow zone (50 to 80% of the best PEF). The most appropriate treatment is for the patient to take a short-acting beta$_2$-agonist and consult her physician for closer day-to-day control of her asthma.
21. **(D)** Oxygen, tolazoline, nitric oxide, and alkalotic pH by hyperventilation all reduce pulmonary artery pressure and pulmonary vascular resistance.
22. **(D)** Pain radiating to the back is associated with esophageal foreign-body enlodgement. Aphonia, hoarseness, and stridor are the result of airway obstruction.
23. **(D)** A newborn infant weighing between 1000 and 2000 gm requires a 3.0-mm-ID endotracheal tube.
24. **(D)** The oxygen saturation and heart rate remain stable during the infant's periodic breathing. During the first weeks of life, this type of breathing is normal and generally requires no treatment.
25. **(C)** The sweat chloride test is done to diagnose cystic fibrosis. Normally, sweat chloride is 45 to 60 mEq/L. Sweat chloride levels greater than 60 mEq/L are consistent with cystic fibrosis.
26. **(A)** Within the first 7 days of birth, a newborn infant can develop pneumonia. The common source of group B streptococcus is the maternal genital tract.
27. **(A)** Morphine sulfate is an analgesic that is often administered to patients on mechanical ventilation.
28. **(C)** Coarctation of the aorta is an acyanotic heart defect, but with normal pulmonary blood flow. The other defects have anomalies where pulmonary blood flow is increased.
29. **(C)** Mucus plugging in the nares can block nasal prong CPAP, resulting in desaturation. Suction each nare.
30. **(B)** Mild, persistent asthma presents with variability of peak expiratory flowrate (PEF) of 20 to 30%; nighttime symptoms more than 2 times per month; activity affected by exacerbations; and symptoms more than 2 times per week, but not more than 1 time per day.
31. **(C)** Polyhydramnios is an excessive (more than 1500 mL) amount of amniotic fluid.
32. **(C)** One method to determine pressure support ventilation level is:
    i. Determine airway resistance.
    $$\frac{\text{PIP} - \text{plateau pressure}}{\text{Peak flow (in L/s)}} = \frac{30 - 20 \text{ cm } H_2O}{40 \text{ L/min } (0.66 \text{ L/s})} = 15 \text{ cm } H_2O\text{/L/s}$$
    ii. To start, set the pressure support at 15 cm $H_2O$ and evaluate the patient's expired tidal volume.
33. **(C)** The child is instructed to stand, filling the lungs completely, and give one fast blast. The child should not bend over or do a slow expiratory maneuver. This maneuver should be done 1 to 5 times to get an average value.
34. **(B)** The thymus gland is a thin, bilobed organ located at the superior mediastinum. The sail-like appearance, or "sail sign," is the right lobe of the thymus extending into the right hemithorax.
35. **(B)** Epiglottitis causes swelling ("thumb" sign) in the supraglottic area of the upper airway. Typical clinical signs include the 4 Ds: dyspnea, distress, dysphagia, and drooling.
36. **(D)** Albuterol, methylprednisolone, and ipratropium bromide are reliever medications for the treatment of exacerbation of asthma.
37. **(D)** In spite of stimulation, the infant remains apneic and bradycardia occurs, indicating severe hypoxemia. Bag-mask resuscitation is required at this time.
38. **(A)** The PEF should be measured once in the morning and afternoon before using a bronchodilator. It will take a 2- to 3-week period of time to establish the individual's best PEF.
39. **(B)** Assessing appropriate placement would be determined by bilateral breath sounds, indicating the tube is above the carina and below the vocal cords.

40. **(D)** These findings indicate the potential presence of a pneumothorax. A transillumination can determine the presence of free air in the chest. The affected chest will "light up," as compared to the unaffected chest, which will appear darker.
41. **(B)** Birth weight is the primary predictor of infant survival.
42. **(A)** Air found in the mediastinum causes the bilobed thymus to be pushed up and away from the heart.
43. **(B)** Serum glucose levels lower than 40 mg/dL indicate hypoglycemia. Symptoms of hypoglycemia include irregular respirations, tremors, jitteriness, weak cry, convulsions, and apnea.
44. **(A)** Air bronchograms are bronchi that contain air and stand out against consolidated alveoli.
45. **(A)** To reduce intracranial pressure, minute ventilation is increased by adjusting the mechanical respiratory rate. This will reduce $PaCO_2$ and cause an alkalotic pH.
46. **(D)** When instructing parents in the use of medical equipment, immediate feedback by the parents in their own words is important.
47. **(C)** Static lung compliance is calculated by the following equation:

$$\frac{\text{Tidal volume}}{\text{Plateau pressure} - \text{PEEP}} = \frac{400 \text{ mL}}{25 - 5 \text{ cm } H_2O} = 20 \text{ mL/cm } H_2O$$

48. **(A)** The average age of onset of myasthenia gravis is 8 years of age, with females having a higher prevalence. Early presentation includes ocular weakness and generalized muscle weakness that follows a descending route. The disease can slowly progress to involving the upper airway and lungs, although it may not progress to the lungs.
49. **(C)** To drain the superior segment of the lower lobes, place the bed flat with the child lying on his or her abdomen.
50. **(A)** $OI = \text{Mean airway pressure} \times (FIO_2 \times 100) \div PaO_2$
    $OI = 20 \text{ cm } H_2O \times (1.0 \times 100) \div 40 \text{ mm Hg}$
    $OI = 2000 \div 40 = 50$
51. **(C)** There is no air movement with complete airway obstruction.
52. **(D)** All three spirometry tests are primarily used to determine the presence of obstructive disease because they all require an expiratory flow measurement.
53. **(A)** In patients breathing room air, a $PaO_2$ less than or equal to 55 mm Hg and a $SaO_2$ less than or equal to 88% are indications for home oxygen. For patients with diseases such as cor pulmonale or erythrocythemia, a $PaO_2$ 56 to 59 or a $SaO_2$ less than 89% is an indication for home oxygen.
54. **(B)** The head-tilt, chin-lift maneuver pulls the tongue (soft tissue) away from the oropharynx, reducing obstruction.
55. **(D)** The therapeutic range for oxygen is 50 to 70 mm Hg in newborn infants. Decreasing the $FIO_2$ would be appropriate at this time to decrease the incidence of oxygen toxicity or retrolental fibroplasia.
56. **(B)** Duration of flow from a liquid oxygen device is as follows:

$$\frac{\text{Pounds of oxygen in device} \times 342 \text{ (gaseous liters/lb of oxygen)}}{\text{liter flow}}$$

$$\frac{60 \text{ lb} \times 342}{2 \text{ L/min}} = 10{,}260 \text{ min} \div 60 \text{ min} = 171 \text{ h} \div 24 \text{ h} = 7.125 \text{ days}$$

57. **(D)** Each of these is an indication for placement of a chest tube to drain either air or fluid or both.
58. **(D)** The first assessment to perform when entering a patient's room and finding that patient slumped over a chair is to determine unresponsiveness.
59. **(B)** Increasing rate would be appropriate to increase minute ventilation to treat hypercarbia.
60. **(C)** The 3-mm-ID endotracheal tube is small for this size infant. An appropriate size for this infant would be 4 mm ID. More than 20% leak is inappropriate.
61. **(A)** A piston or bellows is used with high-frequency oscillation. This causes both positive-pressure and negative-pressure ventilation at the airway.
62. **(C)** An inappropriately sized oropharyngeal airway or an airway that is not inserted properly can push the tongue to the posterior oropharynx and occlude the airway. Remove the airway and ensure that it is the proper size by measuring it from the angle of the jaw to the lips.
63. **(C)** The end-tidal $CO_2$ waveform indicates an increase in the exhaled $CO_2$ as seen by the rise in the end-tidal point. Increasing minute ventilation is recommended to treat the hypercarbia.
64. **(A)** With the addition of PEEP, the driving pressure (PIP minus PEEP) was reduced. Instead of 25 cm $H_2O$ being delivered, 15 cm $H_2O$ was delivered, causing

decreased ventilation and hypercarbia. Increasing PIP to provide 35 cm $H_2O$ would establish the driving pressure the patient was receiving prior to the addition of PEEP.

65. **(D)** These observations indicate the presence of infections and require that the physician be notified.
66. **(B)** Without oxygen connected to the resuscitation bag, room air is being delivered to the infant. Check to ensure that the oxygen connecting tube is attached to the bag.
67. **(C)** The presence of chest and abdominal movement without airflow indicates obstruction to the airway.
68. **(B)** The patient performs a FVC, and the $FEF_{25-75\%}$ is measured in the middle of the expiratory flow. This flow is from the medium and small airways.
69. **(B)** The water-seal compartment has 2 to 3 cm of water in the bottom of the compartment that acts as a one-way valve, allowing air from the pleural space to escape but preventing air from entering the pleural space.
70. **(D)** Since the suction pressure is at the low end of normal, the suction pressure should be increased to see if this will remove the secretions more effectively.
71. **(C)** Amplitude is increased to decrease $PaCO_2$. Reducing the rate by 1 to 2 Hz can also improve alveolar ventilation.
72. **(A)** All clinical manifestations and the appearance of the abdomen are the result of herniation of abdominal contents into the thoracic cavity. The herniation is more common on the left than the right.
73. **(D)** Midclavicular placement between the second and third ribs is the proper placement for drainage of air from the pleural space. The chest tube is then directed anteroapically.
74. **(A)** Decreased peak inspiratory pressure would not change because the pressure is set at a constant value.
75. **(A)** An oxygen concentrator provides the most economical way of delivering oxygen but is unable to provide portable oxygen.
76. **(D)** When the expiratory flow curve does not reach baseline before the next positive-pressure breath is delivered, air trapping is present. Flow is still exiting the lungs when the positive-pressure breath is delivered. The pressure found in the lung is auto-PEEP.
77. **(A)** The rate of blood flow through an extracorporeal membrane oxygen circuit controls the $PaO_2$. Normal flow is 100 to 120 mL/kg/min.
78. **(D)** The patient has been oversedated and requires an open airway immediately to overcome the partial airway obstruction.
79. **(D)** A misplaced endotracheal tube, secretions blocking the endotracheal tube, and pneumothorax may alter chest vibrations.
80. **(D)** A significant response is an increase in $FEV_1$ of 12 to 15% before and after a bronchodilator study.
81. **(A)** The change in driving pressure between IPAP and EPAP is decreased, thus decreasing alveolar ventilation. An appropriate recommendation would be to increase the IPAP pressure to reestablish the driving pressure.
82. **(B)** Cleaning requires placing the nebulizers' unassembled parts in hot water and detergent for 30 min every 2 days. Disinfecting the nebulizer requires 1 part white vinegar and 3 parts water.
83. **(D)** Breath sounds in the left lung indicate that only the opening in the endotracheal tube to the left main-stem bronchus is patent. The opening to the right main-stem bronchus in the endotracheal tube is within the left main-stem bronchus because the endotracheal tube is too low.
84. **(B)** Because of its vasoconstrictive properties, racemic epinephrine is suggested for persistent laryngospasm. Delivery of the medication by small-volume nebulizer is appropriate.
85. **(A)** A shift of the loop from the right to the left indicates an increase in lung compliance.
86. **(B)** Vagal stimulation by the suction catheter causes a reflex bradycardia.
87. **(B)** Inspiratory time is calculated by the following:
    i. Total cycle time = 60 ÷ 30 = 2 s
    ii. I:E ratio 1:4 = 5 parts
    iii. 2 s ÷ 5 parts = 0.4 s inspiratory time
88. **(A)** The mode of ventilation should be switched to SIMV because of the hyperventilation caused by the assist-control mode. SIMV will allow the patient to receive consistent minute ventilation but allow spontaneous breaths to be taken in between the mandatory machine breaths. Decreasing the assist-control rate to 8 will not change the patient's total rate.
89. **(C)** Paradoxical respirations cause ineffective ventilation and are present with patients breathing at a high respiratory rate and indicate diaphragmatic fatigue.

90. **(B)** Pressure-limited, time-cycled ventilation meets pressure early in inspiration and remains at this pressure until inspiratory time expires. Exhalation then occurs.
91. **(A)** Pectus excavatum is a restrictive formation of the chest wall characterized by a pronounced funnel-shaped depression. This is caused by shortening of the central portion of the diaphragm, which pulls the sternum backward during inhalation.
92. **(C)** Gram stain culture and sensitivity determine bacterial infection.
93. **(B)** Changes in respiratory rate and tidal volume will occur if the carbon dioxide absorber is not in line or if the soda lime absorber has expired.
94. **(D)** When percussed, normal air-filled lungs will emit a resonant sound.
95. **(C)** Determine rate by means of the following:

$$\frac{\text{Known rate} \times \text{known PaCO}_2}{\text{Desired PaCO}_2} = \frac{12 \times 50}{40} = \frac{600}{40} = 15 \text{ beats/min}$$

96. **(D)** Flexible bronchoscopy is used to obtain lower respiratory tract secretions, cell washings, and biopsies for cytology, histology, and microbiological samples.
97. **(C)** Bronchial breath sounds are produced from air entering airways where there are collapsed alveoli. Normally these breath sounds are heard over main-stem bronchus. Abnormal findings include bronchial breath sounds heard over peripheral lung fields.
98. **(A)** Pleural effusion is an accumulation of fluid in the pleural cavity; the finding is consistent with the respiratory physical assessment and chest radiograph.
99. **(A)** Lidocaine (1%, 2%, or 4%) is used topically to anesthetize the upper airway prior to bronchoscopy.
100. **(D)**

$$\text{Estimated tidal volume} = \frac{8{,}000 \text{ mL/min}}{60 \text{ s}} = 133 \text{ mL} \times 0.4 \text{ s} = 53 \text{ mL}$$

101. **(A)** The wall suction pressure needs to be at the same water level or above the water level in the suction control compartment. Bubbling in this compartment indicates suction is occurring.
102. **(B)** A lateral decubitus position is where the patient lies on the affected side and the film plate is placed beneath the affected side. This position is used to determine the presence of pleural fluid.
103. **(C)** SOAP notes provide a plan of care. Findings obtained from the physical assessment of the patient fall under objective findings in the SOAP notes.
104. **(C)** Gram stain provides a presumptive diagnosis of bacterial pneumonia and differentiates gram-positive from gram-negative bacteria.
105. **(B)** Square wave flow pattern causes a decrease in mean airway pressure because a decelerating flow ramp causes a greater proportion of average flow in early inspiration, thus increasing mean airway pressure.
106. **(B)** Mean airway pressure improves oxygenation with high-frequency oscillation.
107. **(D)** Strict isolation requires a single room and that a mask, gloves, and gown must be worn.
108. **(D)** The pH and $PaCO_2$ of a capillary blood gas are accurate to assess the acid-base status of the newborn.
109. **(B)** Determining flow from a nasal cannula is best and quickly determined by placing the device in water and watching for bubbling.
110. **(C)** Correct instructions include exhaling completely followed by a deep and rapid inhalation (need to exceed a flow rate of 60 L/min for best deposition in the lung), followed by a breath for a few seconds. Repeat as needed to evacuate the drug capsule.
111. **(A)** If the three-way stopcock is off to the pressure transducer, arterial pressure will not be able to communicate to the pressure transducer. The stopcock should be turned so that it is off to the three-way stopcock hub where blood is obtained.
112. **(B)** Lung compliance has improved, as indicated by the increase in tidal volume. To prevent overdistention of the lungs, PIP is reduced to maintain a tidal volume of 5 mL/kg.
113. **(D)** The infant's sternum and intercostal retractions, agitation, periods of apnea, and ABG are all indications for mechanical ventilation.
114. **(B)** High-position placement of an umbilical artery catheter is between thoracic vertebra 6 to 9. Low-position placement is between lumbar vertebra 3 and 4.
115. **(C)** Pulmonary vascular resistance is calculated as follows:

$$\frac{\text{Mean PAP} - \text{PCWP}}{\text{Cardiac output}} \times 80 \quad \frac{14 - 10}{4} = \frac{4}{4} = 1 \times 80 = 80 \text{ dyn/s/cm}^{-5}$$

116. **(A)** These are signs of hyperventilation. Decrease the negative pressure to reduce alveolar ventilation.

117. **(C)** Normal $SvO_2$ is 60 to 80%. A drop in $SvO_2$ by 5% is not clinically significant and does not require intervention. A drop in $SvO_2$ by more than 10% does require intervention.
118. **(B)** $FIO_2$ greater than or equal to 0.40 is a contraindication to home mechanical ventilation. This level of $FIO_2$ is considered to be a need for a high level of care or requiring hospital personnel expertise.
119. **(A)** Room air entering between the skin of the newborn and electrode will cause the transcutaneous $PO_2$ to climb since the atmospheric $PO_2$ is greater than the infant's $PO_2$.
120. **(D)** Treatment for ventricular fibrillation is to defibrillate at 2 J/kg as soon as possible.

# Index

*A page number with an "f" indicates a figure; a page number with a "t" indicates a table.*